Trust Carol J. Buck and Elsevier
to take you through the levels
of coding success

Step 4:
Professional Resources

Step 3:
Certify

With the resources you need for every
level of coding success, Carol J. Buck
and Elsevier are with you every step
of your coding career. From beginning
to advanced, from the classroom to
the workplace, from application to
certification, the Step Series products
are your guides to greater opportunities
and successful career advancement.

Step 2:
Practice

Step 1:
Learn

Keep climbing with the most trusted name in medical coding.

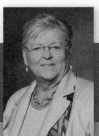

Author and Educator
Carol J. Buck, MS, CPC, CPC-H, CCS-P

B-00

Step 3: Certify

Congratulations on reaching the certification step in your career! As you know, certified coders are in top demand in today's marketplace. That's why, as a lifelong coder and educator, I have dedicated myself to providing the most up-to-date, comprehensive, and user-friendly certification review books on the market. I update these books every year so that you will have the best tools possible when studying for your certification exam. It's time to hit the books. ***You can do it! I know you can!***

— Carol J. Buck, MS, CPC, CPC-H, CCS-P

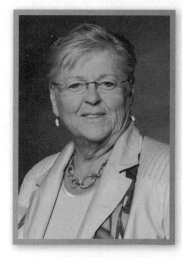

Track your progress!

See the checklist in the back of this book to learn more about your next step toward coding success!

2014

PHYSICIAN CODING EXAM REVIEW

THE CERTIFICATION STEP

with ICD-9-CM

Carol J. Buck
MS, CPC, CPC-H, CCS-P

Former Program Director
Medical Secretary Programs
Northwest Technical College
East Grand Forks, Minnesota

ELSEVIER
SAUNDERS

3251 Riverport Lane
St. Louis, Missouri 63043

PHYSICIAN CODING EXAM REVIEW 2014:
THE CERTIFICATION STEP WITH ICD-9-CM

ISBN: 978-1-4557-2287-7

Notices

Knowledge and best practice in this field are constantly changing. As new research and experience broaden our understanding, changes in research methods, professional practices, or medical treatment may become necessary.

Practitioners and researchers must always rely on their own experience and knowledge in evaluating and using any information, methods, compounds, or experiments described herein. In using such information or methods they should be mindful of their own safety and the safety of others, including parties for whom they have a professional responsibility.

With respect to any drug or pharmaceutical products identified, readers are advised to check the most current information provided (i) on procedures featured or (ii) by the manufacturer of each product to be administered, to verify the recommended dose or formula, the method and duration of administration, and contraindications. It is the responsibility of practitioners, relying on their own experience and knowledge of their patients, to make diagnoses, to determine dosages and the best treatment for each individual patient, and to take all appropriate safety precautions.

To the fullest extent of the law, neither the Publisher nor the authors, contributors, or editors assume any liability for any injury and/or damage to persons or property as a matter of products liability, negligence or otherwise, or from any use or operation of any methods, products, instructions, or ideas contained in the material herein.

Library of Congress Cataloging-in-Publication Data

Buck, Carol J., author.
  2014 physician coding exam review : the certification step with ICD-9-CM / Carol J. Buck.
    p. ; cm.
  Physician coding exam review
  Includes index.
  Preceded by: 2013 physician coding exam review / Carol J. Buck. 2013 ed. c2013.
  ISBN 978-1-4557-2287-7 (pbk. : alk. paper)
  I. Title. II. Title: Physician coding exam review.
  [DNLM: 1. International classification of diseases. 9th revision. Clinical modification.
2. Classification—Examination Questions. 3. Clinical Coding—methods—Examination Questions.
4. Terminology as Topic—Examination Questions. WB 18.2]
  RB115
  616.001′2—dc23

2013019381

Content Strategy Director: Jeanne R. Olson
Associate Content Development Specialist: Helen O'Neal
Publishing Services Manager: Pat Joiner
Senior Project Manager: Joy Moore
Senior Designer: Amy Buxton

Printed in the United States of America

Last digit is the print number: 9 8 7 6 5 4 3 2 1

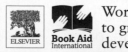

Working together to grow libraries in developing countries

www.elsevier.com • www.bookaid.org

Dedication

*To coding instructors,
who each day strive to enhance the lives
of their students and provide the next generation
of knowledgeable medical coders.*

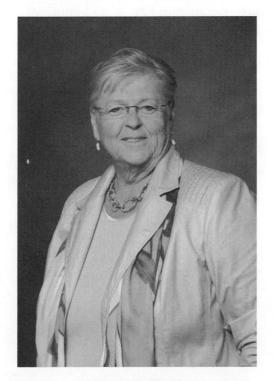

Carol J. Buck

Acknowledgments

There are so many, many people who participated in the development of this text, and only through the effort of all of the team members has it been possible to publish this text.

Sheri Poe Bernard, who has assumed responsibility for development of this text. **Jackie Grass**, who has contributed significantly to its content.

John W. Danaher, President, Education, and **Sally Schrefer,** former Executive Vice President, Nursing/Health Sciences, who possess great listening skills and the ability to ensure the publication of high-quality educational materials. **Andrew Allen,** Vice President and Publisher, Health Professions, who sees the bigger picture and shares the vision. **Jeanne R. Olson,** Content Strategy Director, who maintains an excellent sense of humor and is a valued member of the team who can always be depended upon for reasoned judgment. **Helen O'Neal,** Associate Content Development Specialist, who assumed the responsibility of shepherding this project to production with steady fortitude. **Amy Simpson,** Production Editor at Graphic World, who assumed responsibility for many projects while maintaining a high degree of professionalism. The employees of Elsevier, who have participated in the publication of this text and demonstrated exceptional professionalism and competence. **Arlene Scher,** Senior Program Coordinator at Augusta State University Division of Continuing Education, for her sharp eye and help regarding the organization of the exam questions.

Preface

Thank you for purchasing *Physician Coding Exam Review 2014: The Certification Step with ICD-9-CM,* the latest guide to the outpatient physician coding certification exam. This 2014 edition has been carefully reviewed and updated with the latest content, making it the most current guide for your review. The author and publishers have made every effort to equip you with skills and tools you will need to succeed on the exam. To this end, this review guide presents essential information about all health care coding systems, anatomy, terminology, and pathophysiology, as well as sample examinations for practice. No other review guide on the market brings together such thorough coverage of all necessary examination material in one source.

ORGANIZATION OF THIS TEXTBOOK

Following a basic outline approach, *Physician Coding Exam Review 2014: The Certification Step with ICD-9-CM* takes a practical approach to assisting you with your examination preparations. The text is divided into four units—Anatomy, Terminology, and Pathophysiology; Reimbursement Issues; Overview of CPT, ICD-9-CM, and HCPCS Coding; and Preparing for Practice Examinations—and there are several appendices for your reference. Additionally, examinations are provided on the companion Evolve website to assist you in your preparation.

Some of the CPT code descriptions for physician services include physician extender services. Physician extenders, such as nurse practitioners, physician assistants, and nurse anesthetists, etc., provide medical services typically performed by a physician. Within this educational material the term "physician" may include "and other qualified health care professionals" depending on the code. Refer to the official CPT® code descriptions and guidelines to determine codes that are appropriate to report services provided by non-physician practitioners.

Unit 1, Anatomy, Terminology, and Pathophysiology
Covers all the essential body systems and terms you'll need to get certified. Organized by body systems to follow the CPT codes, the sections also include illustrations to review each major anatomical area and quizzes to check your understanding and recall (Answers are located at the end of Unit 1).

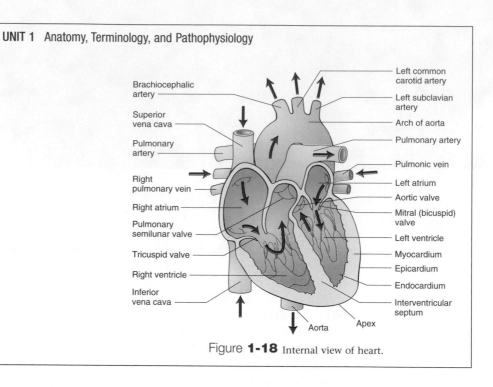

UNIT 1   Anatomy, Terminology, and Pathophysiology

Brachiocephalic artery
Superior vena cava
Pulmonary artery
Right pulmonary vein
Right atrium
Pulmonary semilunar valve
Tricuspid valve
Right ventricle
Inferior vena cava

Left common carotid artery
Left subclavian artery
Arch of aorta
Pulmonary artery
Pulmonic vein
Left atrium
Aortic valve
Mitral (bicuspid) valve
Left ventricle
Myocardium
Epicardium
Endocardium
Interventricular septum
Apex
Aorta

Figure **1-18** Internal view of heart.

Unit 2, Reimbursement Issues
Provides a review of important insurance and billing information to help you review the connections between medical coding, insurance, billing, and reimbursement.

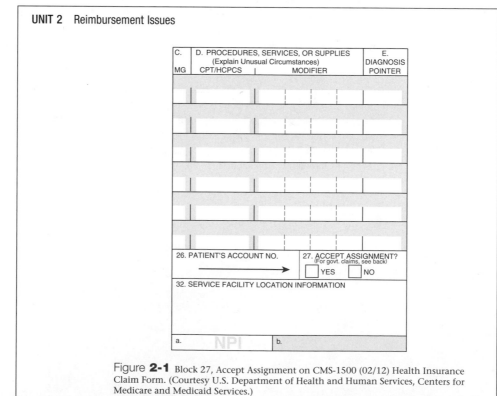

UNIT 2   Reimbursement Issues

C. MG	D. PROCEDURES, SERVICES, OR SUPPLIES (Explain Unusual Circumstances) CPT/HCPCS	MODIFIER	E. DIAGNOSIS POINTER

26. PATIENT'S ACCOUNT NO.
27. ACCEPT ASSIGNMENT? (For govt. claims, see back) ☐ YES ☐ NO
32. SERVICE FACILITY LOCATION INFORMATION
a. NPI   b.

Figure **2-1** Block 27, Accept Assignment on CMS-1500 (02/12) Health Insurance Claim Form. (Courtesy U.S. Department of Health and Human Services, Centers for Medicare and Medicaid Services.)

Unit 3, Overview of CPT, ICD-9-CM, and HCPCS Coding
Contains comprehensive coverage of the different coding systems and their applications, making other references unnecessary! Simplified text and clear examples are the highlights of this unit, and illustrations are included to clarify difficult concepts.

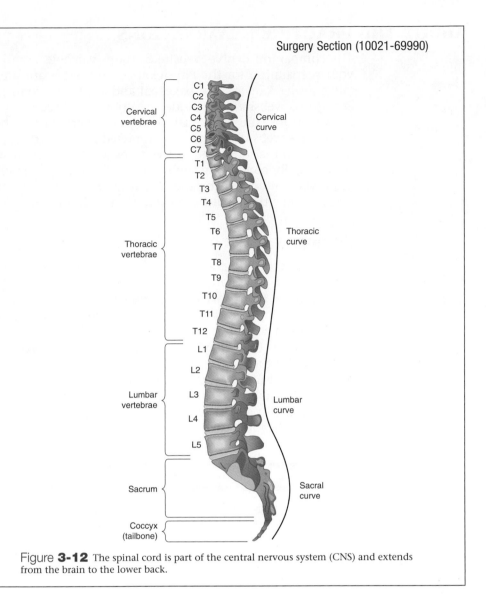

Surgery Section (10021-69990)

Figure **3-12** The spinal cord is part of the central nervous system (CNS) and extends from the brain to the lower back.

Unit 4, Preparing for Practice Examinations
Contains a Final Examination to be taken at the end of your complete program of study. To help you quantify the examination, this is meant to be taken using paper and pencil.

Final Examination

FINAL EXAMINATION

Direction: Report only the professional component unless specifically directed to do otherwise within the question.

Subject Area: Medical Terminology

1. This term means the surgical removal of the fallopian tube:
   A. ligation
   B. hysterectomy
   C. salpingostomy
   D. salpingectomy

2. This combining form means "thirst":
   A. dips/o
   B. acr/o
   C. cortic/o
   D. somat/o

ABOUT THE PRACTICE EXAMINATIONS

The companion Evolve website contains valuable resources to assist you with your preparation for the Physician coding certification examination. (See *Additional Evolve Resources* on pages xii and xiii for more information on how to access this website.) It includes two timed and scored 150-question practice examinations (the same examination is taken twice). The Pre-Examination on the Evolve website should be completed at the start of your study, and the Post-Examination, also on the Evolve website, should be taken after your study is complete. By comparing the results of these examinations, you can see your improvement after using the review guide! Once you check your scores, you are ready to take the Final Examination in Unit 4 of the text.

Summary Screen

When using the program, the Exam Sessions screen serves as home base. Here you can find information relating to your progress and performance in different subject areas. From this screen, you can choose an examination mode, submit an examination, check your progress, review your results, and access the Final Examination scoresheet and answers.

In addition to displaying your scores for completed sections and tracking the total elapsed time, this screen also shows the total, attempted, and correct questions in each subsection. You can return to the Exam Sessions screen at any point while taking or reviewing an examination, and all information related to your answers and position is saved.

Summary screen.

Taking the Examination

While taking the examination, click on the letter of your answer choice, and the circle will appear in red to the left. Click on the "Next" button at the bottom of the screen to proceed to the next question. At the top of the screen, the Quick

Jump feature is a pull-down menu that allows you jump to any question in the current section. Additionally, the Bookmark button at the bottom of the screen allows you to mark questions for later reference.

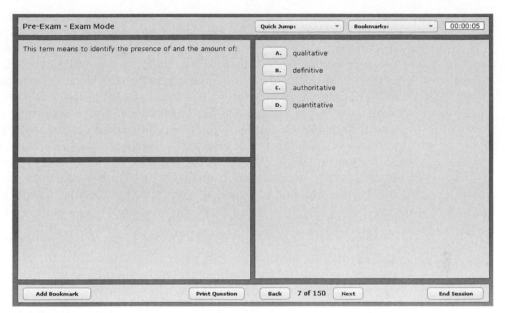

Question screen.

Reviewing Your Results

Once you have taken the Post-Examination on the companion Evolve website, you have the option to review all the Pre- and Post-Examination questions with rationales, even the ones you answered correctly, by clicking the "Review Exam" button at the bottom of the screen. The correct answer is shown for each question, and a rationale is given for each answer option. Or, if you prefer, you can review the answers and rationales using a PDF answer sheet. You can also compare your results on the Pre- and Post-Examinations by clicking on each exam on the Exam Sessions screen and viewing your results in the "Completed Exams" on the right or by printing out your results.

Once you have completed the Final Examination in Unit 4, you will access the electronic score sheet on the Evolve website and enter your answers. The software will then provide you with the answers and rationales.

SUPPLEMENTAL RESOURCES

However you decide to prepare for the certification examination, we have developed supplements designed to complement the *Physician Coding Exam Review 2014: The Certification Step with ICD-9-CM*. Each of these supplements has been developed with the needs of both students and instructors in mind.

Instructor's Electronic Resource

No matter what your level of teaching experience, this total-teaching solution, located on the companion Evolve website, will help you plan your lessons with ease, and the author has developed all the curriculum materials necessary to use the textbook in the classroom. This includes additional unit quizzes, a course calendar and syllabus, lesson plans, ready-made tests for easy assessment, and PDF files with the questions and answers for the Pre-/Post- and Final Examinations. Also included is a comprehensive PowerPoint collection for the entire text, and ExamView test banks. The PowerPoint slides can be easily customized to support your lectures or formatted as overhead transparencies or handouts for student note-taking. The ExamView test generator will help you quickly and easily prepare quizzes and exams from the ready-made test questions, and the test banks can be customized to your specific teaching methods.

Additional Evolve Resources

The companion Evolve website offers many resources that will extend your studies beyond the classroom. Related WebLinks offer you the opportunity to expand your knowledge base and stay current with this ever-changing field, and additional material is available for help and practice.

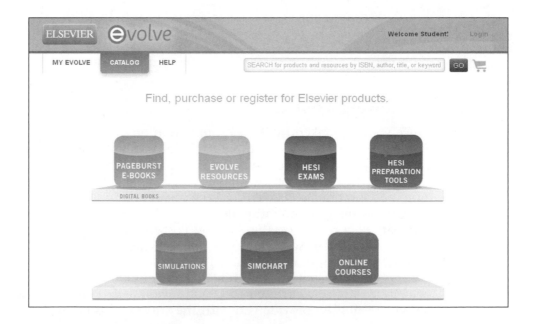

A Course Management System (CMS) is also available free to instructors who adopt this textbook. This web-based platform gives instructors yet another resource to facilitate learning and to make medical coding content accessible to students. In addition to the Evolve Resources available to both faculty and students, there is an entire suite of tools available that allows for communication between instructors and students. Students can log on through the Evolve portal to take online quizzes and practice examinations, participate in threaded discussions, post assignments to instructors, or chat with other classmates, while instructors can use the online grade book to follow class progress.

To access this comprehensive online resource, follow the instructions located on the inside front cover of this book. You will need the Course ID number provided by your instructor. If your instructor has not set up a Course Management System, you can still access the free Evolve resources at http://evolve.elsevier.com/Buck/physicianexam.

Development of This Edition

This book would not have been possible without a team of educators and professionals, including practicing coders and technical consultants. The combined efforts of the team members have made this text an incredible learning tool.

SENIOR TECHNICAL COLLABORATOR

Sheri Poe Bernard, CCS-P, CPC, CPC-H, CPC-I
Coding Education Specialist
Salt Lake City, Utah

LEAD TECHNICAL COLLABORATOR

Jacqueline Klitz Grass, MA, CPC
Coding and Reimbursement Specialist
Grand Forks, North Dakota

QUERY MANAGER

Patricia Cordy Henricksen, MS, CHCA, CPC-I, CPC, CCP-P, ASC-PCS
Auditing and Coding Educator
Soterion Medical Services
Lexington, Kentucky

SENIOR ICD-9-CM AND ICD-10-CM CODING SPECIALIST

Karla R. Lovaasen, RHIA, CCS, CCS-P
Coding and Consulting Services
Abingdon, Maryland
—Coauthor of *ICD-9-CM Coding: Theory and Practice with ICD-10, 2013/2014 Edition*, St. Louis, 2013, Saunders.

—Coauthor of *ICD-10-CM/PCS Coding: Theory and Practice, 2014 Edition*, St. Louis, 2014, Saunders.

SENIOR COLLABORATOR AND ICD-10-CM CONSULTANT

Nancy Maguire, ACS, CRT, PCS, FCS, HCS-D, APC, AFC
Physician Consultant for Auditing and Education
Winchester, Virginia

CODING SPECIALISTS

Robert H. Ekvall, PhD, CCS, CPC-H, CPC
Coder/Biller
Scripps Green Hospital
La Jolla, California

Debra Kroll, RHIT
Denial and Billing Compliance
  Supervisor
Altru Health System
Grand Forks, North Dakota

Danielle Laitres, CPC
Stuart, Florida

Sylvia Partridge, CPC, CGSC
Coding Instructor
Athens, Georgia

EDITORIAL REVIEW BOARD

Aimée Michaelis, MEd, CPC
Lead Instructor
Pima Medical Institute
Denver, Colorado

Andrea D. Potteiger, CCS, CCS-P, CPC
Senior Coder
Edaptive Systems
York, Pennsylvania

Contents

Contents

Contents

Contents

Success Strategies

This review was developed to help you as you prepare for your certification examination. First, congratulations on your initiative. Preparing for a certification examination can seem like a daunting and formidable task. You have already taken the first and hardest step: you have made a commitment. Your steely determination and organizational skills are your best tools as you prepare to complete this exciting journey successfully.

How do you prepare for a certification examination? The answers to that question are as varied as the persons preparing for it. Each person comes to the preparation with different educational, coding, and personal experiences. Therefore, each must develop a plan that meets his or her individual needs and preferences. Success Strategies will help you to develop your individual plan.

THE CERTIFICATION EXAMINATION

This text has been developed to serve as a tool in your preparation for the outpatient (physician-based) certification examination (AAPC). The CPC® certification examination consists of a total of 150 multiple choice questions covering medical terminology, anatomy, pathophysiology, CPT, ICD-9-CM, HCPCS, and coding concepts. You have 5 hours and 40 minutes to complete the examination. Exam results are reported with scores and your top three areas of weakness.

To be successful on the certification examination, you will have to know how to assign medical codes to patient services and diagnoses. This textbook focuses on providing you with that coding practice as well as anatomy, terminology, pathophysiology, reimbursement, and coding concepts in preparation for the examination.

The certification examination created specifically for the CPC® candidate is a valuable tool for candidates for the CCS-P examination, as the proficiencies for both exams are quite similar. The CCS-P exam has fewer questions, is administered for a shorter time, and has a different format. Success strategies provided are for a paper test, but the AHIMA test is administered online.

Date and Location

Although every journey begins with the first step, you have to know where you are going to make a plan to get there.

- Choose the **date and location** for taking the certification examination. The AAPC's website (www.aapc.com/certification/locate-examination.aspx) and the AHIMA website (www.ahima.org/certification/ccsp.aspx) contain detailed information about the examination sites and dates.

- The American Academy of Professional Coders has information that can be downloaded from their website at www.aapc.com or sent for by contacting:

  American Academy of Professional Coders
  2480 South 3850 West, Suite B
  Salt Lake City, UT 84120
  Telephone: 800-626-2633

- The American Health Information Management Association has information that can be downloaded from their website at www.ahima.org or sent for by contacting:

  American Health Information Management Association (AHIMA)
  233 N. Michigan Avenue, 21st Floor
  Chicago, IL 60601-5809
  Telephone: (312) 233-1100

- After you have downloaded the Candidate Guide (www.ahima.org/downloads/pdfs/certification/Candidate_Guide.pdf), read all the information carefully. Review all competencies outlined in the material to ensure that your study plan contains strategies to address each of these competencies.

- Check AHIMA examination information and examination preparation arenas on the website (www.ahima.org/certification/ccsp.aspx) for the latest information on acceptable forms of identification, coding rules to follow, and passing scores.

- After you have obtained the examination materials, read all the information carefully. Review all competencies outlined in the material to ensure that your study plan contains strategies to address each of these competencies.

- The questions within this textbook are not the same questions that are in the certification examination, but the skill and knowledge that you gain through analysis, coding, and recall will increase your ability to be successful on examination day.

MANAGING YOUR TIME

Role strain! That is what you get when you have so many different roles in your life and you cannot find time for all of them! Know that feeling? Are you a daughter/son, mother/father, wife/husband, student, friend, worker, volunteer, hobbyist—the list is endless. Each takes time from your schedule, and somehow you now need to fit into the role of successful learner. Because you have only 24 hours in your day, being a successful learner requires a time-balancing act. Maybe you will have to be satisfied with dust bunnies under your bed, dishes in your kitchen sink, or fewer visits with your friends. Whatever you have to do to juggle the time around to give yourself ample time to devote to this important task of examination preparation, you must do and make a plan for in advance; otherwise, life just takes over and you find you do not have adequate study time.

If you are planning a big event in your life—moving, a trip, and so on, think about postponing it until after the examination. Your focus right now has to be on yourself. Make your motto **"It's All About Me!"** Sounds self-centered, I know, and most likely very different from who you are, but just this once, you need to carve out the time you need to accomplish this important goal. This time is for yourself. Make it happen for yourself. Move everything you can out of the way, focus on this preparation, and give this preparation your best effort.

SCHEDULE

Each person has an individual learning style. The coding profession seems to attract those most influenced by logic and facts. The best way for a logical and factual person to learn is to problem-solve and apply the information. Hands-on practice is how you will build your skill and confidence for the examination.

- Choose a location to be your Study Central.

- Gather into Study Central the following study resources:

  - Certification packet or handbook from the certifying organization

  - CPT, current edition

  - ICD-9-CM, current edition

  - HCPCS, current edition

  - *Official Guidelines for Coding and Reporting* (Can be accessed by following the Evolve Resources link provided in Appendix A of this text)

  - Medical dictionary

  - Coding textbooks, professional journals, and magazines

  - Terminology, anatomy, or pathology text, as needed

  - See Appendix G for Further Text Resources

Make Study Central your special place where you can get away from all other responsibilities. Make it a quiet, calm getaway, even if it is a corner of your bedroom. In this quiet place have a comfortable chair, adequate lighting, supplies, and sufficient desktop surface to use all your coding books. This is your place to focus all your attention on preparation for the examination, without distractions.

- Plan your **schedule** from now until the certification examination using a calendar. Make weekly goals so that you have definite tasks to accomplish each week and you can check the tasks off—a great feeling of accomplishment comes from being able to check off a task. In this way, you can see your progress on your countdown to success.

- Choose a specific **time** each day or several times a week when you are going to study and mark them on your calendar. Make this commitment in writing. After each study session, you should check off that date on the calendar as a visual reminder that you are sticking to your plan and are one step closer to your goal.

- You should plan your study time in advance, know what you are going to be studying the next session, and **be prepared** for that upcoming study session. This will greatly increase the amount of material you are able to cover during the session. At the end of each session, decide what you are going to study next session and ensure that you have all the material and references you will need readily available. At the end of each session, you should be ready for the next study session.

- Your plan should include those areas where you know you will need improvement. For example, when is the last time you read, not referenced or reviewed, but really read, the CPT Anesthesia Guidelines? You probably do not code anesthesia services often, if ever, and as such, are not familiar with the information in these guidelines. That is an area of improvement, and your plan should include a thorough reading of all the CPT section guidelines.

- **DO THIS BEFORE YOU BEGIN YOUR STUDY: Assess** your strengths and weaknesses. By making this assessment, you will know where to concentrate your efforts and where to focus your study schedule. You know those areas where you already have strong skills and knowledge and will not need to spend as much time preparing in these areas. The **Pre-Examination,** found on the Evolve website, is an examination that you can use as a tool to assess your current skill level. This examination should be taken before you begin your study and then again immediately after you have completed your entire study schedule. Do not analyze the questions by reviewing the rationales (located on the Evolve website); rather, wait until after you have completed your studies and have taken this same examination a second time. If you review the rationales after the first time you take the examination, you will know the answers too well to provide a valid comparison between examinations. See Unit 4 of this textbook for further information.

- After you have completed your course of study, take the **Post-Examination** on the Evolve website. You should plan to cover the examination in the same amount of time as will be given for the certification examination you are going to take. Compare your scores to those from the first time you took this examination. Note the areas where you did not demonstrate sufficient skills and knowledge.

- Develop a **second plan** to improve the specific areas where you believe you need further study.

- You are now ready to take the **Final Examination** that is located in Unit 4 of this text. Take the examination in the same amount of time that will be allocated for the certification examination. It is best if you do this final in one sitting, thereby mimicking the actual examination. If your schedule does not allow for taking the examination in one sitting, plan to take it in several sessions, but always keep track of the time used to ensure that you take the examination in the same amount of time allowed for the official examination. Learning to work within the time allocated is part of the skill you are developing. Remember the certification examinations assess not only your coding knowledge but also your efficiency in completing the examination within the allocated time.

USING THIS TEXT

This text is divided into:

- Success Strategies
- Unit 1, Anatomy, Terminology, and Pathophysiology
- Unit 2, Reimbursement Issues
- Unit 3, Overview of CPT, ICD-9-CM, and HCPCS Coding
- Unit 4, Preparing for Practice Examinations
- Appendix A, Resources (Web-Based)
- Appendix B, Medical Terminology

- Appendix C, Combining Forms

- Appendix D, Prefixes

- Appendix E, Suffixes

- Appendix F, Abbreviations

- Appendix G, Further Text Resources

- Appendix H, Practice Exercises Answers and Rationales

Appendices B-F are combined lists of Medical Terminology, Combining Forms, Prefixes, Suffixes, and Abbreviations used within Unit 1, Anatomy, Terminology, and Pathophysiology.

The material in this review features the following:

- Comprehensive guide in outline format

- Photos and drawings to illustrate key points

- Pre-/Post-Examination (on the Evolve website)—150 questions

- Final Examination (in Unit 4 of this text)—150 questions

- **Unit 1** is a review of the anatomy, terminology, and pathophysiology by organ systems designed to provide you with a quick review of that organ system. In addition, there is a list of combining forms, prefixes, suffixes, and abbreviations that are often used in that organ system. At the end of each organ system, there is a quiz that will give you an opportunity to assess your knowledge.

- **Unit 2** is a review of reimbursement issues and terminology. A quiz is located at the end of the unit to assess your knowledge.

- **Unit 3** is a review of CPT, HCPCS, and ICD-9-CM. The CPT and ICD-9-CM material follows the order of the manuals. There is no quiz at the end of this unit because you will be applying this material in the practice examinations and in the Final Examination.

- **Unit 4** contains the examinations. The Pre-/Post-Examination is a 150-question examination located on the companion Evolve website. This same exam should be taken twice—once before you begin your study and the second time after you have completed your study. You should allow 5 hours and 40 minutes (340 minutes) to complete each examination. The computer software stores your scores and compares the results from the first and second time you took the examination; so you can see not only your score on each section but also the improvement from the first to the second examination. The Final Examination is also a 150-question examination, but located in the text with answers on the Evolve website.

NOTE: To enable the learner to calculate an examination score, the minimum of 70% has been identified as "passing" within this text; however, this may or may not be the percentage identified by the certifying organization as a "passing" grade. It is your responsibility to review all certification information published by the certifying organization.

There are many ways you could use this text. However you decide to prepare, you should take the examination before you begin your study to ensure that you develop a study plan that includes time and activities that will increase your knowledge in those areas where your test scores indicate areas of weakness. You could then take the units in the order they are presented, or you may want to review the anatomy, terminology, and pathophysiology for a body system and then review the CPT material for that body system. There is no one best way to approach the use of this text because each individual will have a personal learning style and preferences that will direct how the material is used. Your skills may be very strong in one or more coding or knowledge areas and you will want to delete those areas from your individual study plan.

This text is not meant to be the only study source, but only one tool of many that you will use. For example, if your terminology skills need a complete overhaul, the brief overview in this text may not meet your needs. You may want to supplement this text with a terminology text and an in-depth study of terminology.

- **Appendices** are a resource for you as you prepare your study plan.

  - **Appendix A,** Resources, is an Evolve Resources link (web-based) to the *Official Guidelines for Coding and Reporting*. This link provides the rules for use of ICD-9-CM codes and will be referenced in Unit 3 when reviewing the use of ICD-9-CM codes.

  - **Appendix B,** Medical Terminology, is a complete alphabetic list of all the medical terms listed in the Medical Terminology portion of the organ system reviews used in Unit 1.

  - **Appendix C,** Combining Forms, is a complete alphabetic list of the combining forms used in Unit 1.

  - **Appendix D,** Prefixes, is a complete alphabetic list of the prefixes used in Unit 1.

  - **Appendix E,** Suffixes, is a complete alphabetic list of the suffixes used in Unit 1.

  - **Appendix F,** Abbreviations, is a complete list of the abbreviations referenced in Unit 1.

  - **Appendix G,** Further Text Resources, is a list of texts that you may want to obtain to supplement your study plan.

  - **Appendix H,** Practice Exercise Answers and Rationales.

DAY BEFORE THE EXAMINATION

- No cramming! Your study time is now over, and cramming the day before the test is not a good idea because it just increases your anxiety level. This day is your day to prepare yourself. Do some things you enjoy this day. Take your mind off the examination. Pamper yourself: you deserve it.

- Prepare pencils (no. 2), erasers, picture identification, CPT (AMA standard or professional version only), ICD-9-CM (Vols. 1 and 2), HCPCS code manuals, and examination admission card. For a paper/pencil examination, take a ruler so that if you skip a question and want to mark that question to return to later, you can use the ruler to make certain you return to the correct question.

- You cannot have excessive writing, sticky notes, labels, etc. in your code books. Check the certifying organization's examination information to ensure that your books meet the specifications identified by the testing organization.

- Review the certification packet information one last time to ensure that you have all the required material.

- Pack quiet snacks and bottled water sufficient for 5 hours and 40 minutes.

- Listen to the weather and traffic reports. Plan your route to the examination site. If it is in a new location, drive to the location before the big day.

- Eat a light supper and get to bed early. Set the alarm in plenty of time to arrive at the site early. It is a good idea to have a friend or family member give you an early wake-up call to ensure that you do not oversleep.

DAY OF THE EXAMINATION

- Wear comfortable clothes and be prepared for any room temperature. A short-sleeved shirt with a sweater is a good plan. Dress in layers so you can ensure that you will be comfortable in any environment.

- Take a watch with you.

- Eat a good breakfast. Avoid caffeine because it initially stimulates you, but in the long run will decrease your concentration.

- Arrive early. The doors are locked to those who arrive late. This is a day to be early.

- Ensure that you have the correct room for your examination. Often there are several examinations being administered at one time, so be certain you are in the correct room for your examination.

THE CERTIFICATION EXAMINATION

You are ready for this! You have planned your work and have worked your plan. Now it is time to reap the rewards for all that hard work.

- Choose a good location in which to sit. Choose a location that will not get a lot of traffic from those leaving the room.

- Place all your supplies on the table.

- Take several deep breaths before you begin to help relax you.

- Some prefer to take the parts of the examination out of order, taking those questions they are most confident of first. Others prefer to start at the beginning and work through all questions in order. The approach that you use will depend on your individual test-taking style.

- When you come to a question for which you are unsure of the answer, you may wish to skip over and come back to all those ones you were unsure of at the end of the examination, depending on the time available. Or you may want to attempt each question and note those you are unsure of to return to when you have finished the exam section. Again, the approach you will use depends on your individual style.

- Read the directions. This may sound too simple, but many persons do not completely read the directions, only to find that the directions gave specific directions about what or what not to code on a certain case (for example, "code only this certain portion of the procedure"). Yet the choices for answers included the full coding of the case as a selection; if you did not read all the directions, you would choose the response with codes for all the items listed in the report. For example, the question may have directed you to code the service only, not the diagnosis, and yet one of the choices would be the correct service and diagnosis codes, which of course would be an incorrect answer based on the directions. So read all of the directions.

- Your speed and accuracy are being tested. You do not have time to labor over each question for a long time if you intend to complete all the questions.

Read the directions, read the question, put down your best assessment of the answer, and then move on to the next question.

- Words such as *always, every, never,* and *all* generally indicate broad terms that, with true/false questions, usually indicate a false question.

- If you do not know the answer to the question, try eliminating those that you know are incorrect first and then select that answer that seems more likely to be correct.

- Judge the time as you are moving through the examination. Keep assessing whether you are making sufficient progress or whether you can slow down or need to speed up.

- Answer all questions. Even if you have to guess quickly, at least fill in an answer. The best situation is that you answer all questions and have time left over to go back over the questions about which you are in doubt.

- Be certain to carefully complete the information sheet that accompanies the examination. This sheet will include your name, address, and other information that ensures that your test results are accurately recorded.

- Use every minute of the test time, but it is not a good idea to begin second-guessing yourself. Do not return to those questions for which you did not have serious doubts about the correct answer. Usually, your first answer is the best.

- When the time is finished, hand in your examination, and pat yourself on the back! You have done an excellent job. Now it is time to go get a good supper and a good night's sleep.

DAYS AFTER THE EXAMINATION

- You will miss the preparation! Okay, maybe not miss it exactly, but your life will be different now without that constant preparation.

- Relax and await the results in confidence. You have done your best. That is always good enough!

- Be proud of yourself; this was no small undertaking, and you did it.

My personal best wishes to you as you prepare for your certification. You can do this!

Best regards,
Carol J. Buck, MS, CPC, CPC-H, CCS-P

Our goals can only be reached through a vehicle of a plan, in which we must fervently believe, and upon which we must vigorously act. There is no other route to success.

Stephen A. Brennan

Course Syllabus and Student Calendar

The following documents are the syllabus and the course calendar that would be used in a classroom setting. It is suggested that these documents be used in development of your personal educational plan.

COURSE SYLLABUS

Course Description

The focus of this class is a review of terminology, anatomy, pathophysiology, and reimbursement as a preparation to take the coding certification examination. A review of CPT, ICD-9-CM, and HCPCS coding will be an integral part of this review course. Two practice certification review examinations will be taken under timed conditions. The course assists the learner in establishing a personal plan for continued development in preparation for a certification examination.

Texts

Physician Coding Exam Review 2014: The Certification Step with ICD-9-CM, by Carol J. Buck, Elsevier

2014 ICD-9-CM, Volumes 1 & 2, by Carol J. Buck, Elsevier

2014 HCPCS Level II, by Carol J. Buck, Elsevier

2014 CPT, American Medical Association

Medical dictionary

Performance Objectives

1. Write a personal plan for preparation for a certification examination.

2. Review the structure, function, terminology, pathophysiology, and abbreviations of the integumentary system.

3. Review the structure, function, terminology, pathophysiology, and abbreviations of the musculoskeletal system.

4. Review the structure, function, terminology, pathophysiology, and abbreviations of the respiratory system.

5. Review the structure, function, terminology, pathophysiology, and abbreviations of the cardiovascular system.

6. Review the structure, function, terminology, pathophysiology, and abbreviations of the female genital system and pregnancy.

7. Review the structure, function, terminology, pathophysiology, and abbreviations of the male genital system.

8. Review the structure, function, terminology, pathophysiology, and abbreviations of the urinary system.

9. Review the structure, function, terminology, pathophysiology, and abbreviations of the digestive system.

10. Review the structure, function, terminology, pathophysiology, and abbreviations of the mediastinum and diaphragm.

11. Review the structure, function, terminology, pathophysiology, and abbreviations of the hemic and lymphatic systems.

12. Review the structure, function, terminology, pathophysiology, and abbreviations of the endocrine system.

13. Review the structure, function, terminology, pathophysiology, and abbreviations of the nervous system.

14. Review the structure, function, terminology, pathophysiology, and abbreviations of the senses of the body.

15. Demonstrate knowledge of organ system structure, function, terminology, pathophysiology, and abbreviations.

16. Review medical reimbursement issues.

17. Demonstrate knowledge of medical reimbursement issues.

18. Review CPT E/M section.

19. Review CPT Anesthesia section.

20. Review CPT Surgery section.

21. Review CPT Radiology section.

22. Review CPT Pathology and Laboratory section.

23. Review CPT Medicine section.

24. Review HCPCS.

25. Review format and conventions of ICD-9-CM.

26. Review assignment of ICD-9-CM codes.

27. Review *ICD-9-CM Official Guidelines for Coding and Reporting.*

28. Demonstrate coding ability by assigning CPT codes.

29. Demonstrate coding ability by assigning HCPCS codes.

30. Demonstrate coding ability by assigning ICD-9-CM codes.

31. Demonstrate coding ability by completing assigned Practice Exercises.

Personal Objectives

The student will:

- Attend class sessions.

- Prepare for class sessions.

- Complete assignments in a timely manner.

- Demonstrate a high level of responsibility.

- Display respect for other members of the class.

- Participate in class discussions.

Evaluation and Grading

- Evaluation is directly related to the performance objectives.

- Performance is measured by examination, assignments, and/or quizzes.

- The letter grade is based on the percentage of the total points earned throughout the semester based on the following scale:

  - A = 93% to 100%

  - B = 85% to 92%

  - C = 79% to 84%

  - D = 70% to 78%

  - F = 69% and below

- Examinations are scheduled in advance. To qualify for the total points on the examinations, the student must take the examination at the scheduled time. Five points will be deducted from each examination if the examination is not taken at the scheduled time. This rule reinforces the need for on-time performance. Any make-up examination must be completed within 3 days of the scheduled examination or no points will be awarded for the examination.

- Assignments are scheduled in advance. To qualify for the total points on the assignment, the student must submit the completed assignment at the scheduled time. Five points are deducted from each assignment if the assignment is not submitted at the scheduled time. This rule reinforces the need for on-time performance. Any late assignment must be completed within 3 days from the date the assignment was due or no points will be awarded for the assignment.

- Quizzes are scheduled in advance. Quizzes cannot be made up, and no points are awarded for missed quizzes.

Methods of Instruction

The instructional methods used include lecture, class discussion, and assignments.

COURSE CALENDAR

Lesson 1

Reading assignment(s):	Success Strategies, pages S1-S8
Assignment(s):	Complete the Pre-Examination located on the companion Evolve website, and at **Lesson 3** class period, hand in your summary sheet with your score for 75 points. The Pre-Examination is NOT graded if each question has been attempted. 1 point will be deducted for each question not attempted.
Download certification examination information
Print one page to hand in at **Lesson 2** to demonstrate successful access to certification information from web (10 points—nongraded)

Lesson 2

Student hand in:	One printed page to demonstrate successful access to certifying organization's information from web (10 points—nongraded)
Reading assignment(s):	Unit 1, pages 1-54 (through Musculoskeletal System)
Assignment(s):	Develop a personal plan for preparation for Certification Review (20 points—graded) to be submitted at **Lesson 6** class period
Integumentary Anatomy/Terminology (10 points) and Pathophysiology Quizzes (10 points)
Musculoskeletal Anatomy/Terminology (10 points) and Pathophysiology Quizzes (10 points)

Lesson 3

Student hand in:	Integumentary System Quizzes (20 points)
Musculoskeletal Quizzes (20 points)
Pre-Examination (175 points, nongraded if each question attempted, deduct 1 point for each question not attempted)
Reading assignment(s):	Unit 1, pages 55-122 (through Female Genital System and Pregnancy)
Assignment(s):	Respiratory Anatomy/Terminology (10 points) and Pathophysiology Quizzes (10 points)
Cardiovascular Anatomy/Terminology (10 points) and Pathophysiology Quizzes (10 points)
Female Genital System and Pregnancy Anatomy/Terminology (10 points) and Pathophysiology Quizzes (10 points)

Lesson 4

Student hand in:	Respiratory Quizzes (20 points)
Cardiovascular Quizzes (20 points)

	Female Genital System and Pregnancy Quizzes (20 points)
Reading assignment(s):	Unit 1, pages 123-194 (through Mediastinum and Diaphragm)
Assignment(s):	Male Genital System Anatomy/Terminology (10 points) and Pathophysiology Quizzes (10 points) Urinary System Anatomy/Terminology (10 points) and Pathophysiology Quizzes (10 points) Digestive System Anatomy/Terminology (10 points) and Pathophysiology Quizzes (10 points) Mediastinum and Diaphragm Quiz (10 points) (There is no pathophysiology quiz for Mediastinum and Diaphragm.)

Lesson 5

Student hand in:	Male Genital System Quizzes (20 points) Urinary System Quizzes (20 points) Digestive System Quizzes (20 points) Mediastinum and Diaphragm Quiz (10 points) (There is no pathophysiology quiz for Mediastinum and Diaphragm.) Pediatrics, Neonatology, and Adolescent Medicine, Cases 5-6 (4 points)
Reading assignment(s):	Unit 1, pages 195-228 (through Endocrine System)
Assignment(s):	Hemic and Lymphatic Anatomy/Terminology (10 points) and Pathophysiology Quizzes (10 points) Endocrine Anatomy/Terminology (10 points) and Pathophysiology Quizzes (10 points) Prepare to submit Personal Plan for Preparation for Certification Examination (20 points—graded)

Lesson 6

Student hand in:	Hemic and Lymphatic Quizzes (20 points) Endocrine Quizzes (20 points) Submit Personal Plan for Preparation for Certification Examination
Reading assignment(s):	Unit 1, pages 229-276 (through end of Unit 1)
Assignment(s):	Nervous System Anatomy/Terminology (10 points) and Pathophysiology Quizzes (10 points) Senses Anatomy/Terminology (10 points) and Pathophysiology Quizzes (10 points) Prepare for Unit 1, Anatomy, Terminology, and Pathophysiology, Test 1 (50 points, 25 questions, 15 minutes)

Lesson 7

	UNIT 1: ANATOMY, TERMINOLOGY, AND PATHOPHYSIOLOGY, TEST 1 **Timed Test: 15 Minutes**
Student hand in:	Nervous System Quizzes (20 points) Senses Quizzes (20 points)

Reading assignment(s):	Unit 2, pages 277-294 (through end of Unit 2)
Assignment(s):	None

Lesson 8

Student hand in:	Reimbursement Quiz (10 points)
Reading assignment(s):	Unit 3, pages 295-301 (up to E/M section)
Assignment(s):	Prepare for Reimbursement, Test 2 (20 points, 10 questions, 10 minutes)

Lesson 9

UNIT 2: REIMBURSEMENT, TEST 2
Timed Test: 10 Minutes

Student hand in:	None
Reading assignment(s):	Unit 3, pages 302-311 (up to Contributory Factors) Read E/M Guidelines
Assignment(s):	None

Lesson 10

Student hand in:	None
Reading assignment(s):	Unit 3, pages 311-327 (up to Anesthesia section)
Assignment(s):	Complete Practice Exercises 3-1 through 3-5, pages 321-327 (10 points)

Lesson 11

Student hand in:	Practice Exercises 3-1 through 3-5, pages 321-327 (10 points) Emergency Medicine, Cases 7-10 (8 points)
Reading assignment(s):	Unit 3, pages 328-336 (up to CPT/HCPCS Level I Modifiers) Read Anesthesia Guidelines
Assignment(s):	Prepare for E/M, Test 3 (25 points, 5 Guidelines questions [10 points] and 3 cases [15 points], 15 minutes) Complete Practice Exercises 3-6 through 3-10, pages 331-336 (10 points)

Lesson 12

E/M, TEST 3
Timed Test: 15 Minutes

Student hand in:	Practice Exercises 3-6 through 3-10, pages 331-336 (10 points)
Reading assignment(s):	Unit 3, pages 337-351 (up to Surgery section)
Assignment(s):	Prepare for Anesthesia, Test 4 (20 points, 5 Guidelines questions [10 points], 2 cases [10 points], 15 minutes) Complete Practice Exercises 3-11 through 3-15, pages 344-351 (10 points)

Lesson 13

	ANESTHESIA, TEST 4 **Timed Test: 15 Minutes**
Student hand in:	Practice Exercises 3-11 through 3-15, pages 344-351 (10 points)
Reading assignment(s):	Unit 3, pages 352-353 (up to Integumentary System Subsection) Read Surgery Guidelines
Assignment(s):	None

Lesson 14

Student hand in:	None
Reading assignment(s):	Unit 3, pages 354-368 (up to Musculoskeletal System Subsection)
Assignment(s):	Complete Practice Exercises 3-16 through 3-20, pages 363-368 (10 points)

Lesson 15

Student hand in:	Practice Exercises 3-16 through 3-20, pages 363-368 (10 points)
Reading assignment(s):	Unit 3, pages 369-380 (up to Respiratory System Subsection)
Assignment(s):	Complete Practice Exercises 3-21 through 3-25, pages 375-380 (10 points)

Lesson 16

Student hand in:	Practice Exercises 3-21 through 3-25, pages 375-380 (10 points)
Reading assignment(s):	Unit 3, pages 381-385 (up to Cardiovascular System Subsection)
Assignment(s):	None

Lesson 17

Student hand in:	None
Reading assignment(s):	Unit 3, pages 385-390 (up to Venous Reconstruction)
Assignment(s):	None

Lesson 18

Student hand in:	None
Reading assignment(s):	Unit 3, pages 390-396 (up to Hemic and Lymphatic System Subsection)
Assignment(s):	Complete Practice Exercises 3-26 through 3-30, pages 398-405 (10 points)

Lesson 19

Student hand in:	Practice Exercises 3-26 through 3-30, pages 398-405 (10 points)
Reading assignment(s):	Unit 3, pages 396-418 (up to Female Genital System Subsection)
Assignment(s):	Complete Practice Exercises 3-31 through 3-35, pages 408-414 (10 points)

Lesson 20

Student hand in:	Practice Exercises 3-31 through 3-35, pages 408-414 (10 points)
Reading assignment(s):	Unit 3, pages 418-436 (through Auditory System Subsection)
Assignment(s):	Complete Practice Exercises 3-36 through 3-40, pages 425-432 (10 points)

Lesson 21

Student hand in:	Practice Exercises 3-36 through 3-40, pages 425-432 (10 points)
Reading assignment(s):	None
Assignment(s):	Complete Practice Exercises 3-41 through 3-45, pages 437-443 (10 points)

Lesson 22

Student hand in:	Practice Exercises 3-41 through 3-45, pages 437-443 (10 points)
Reading assignment(s):	Unit 3, pages 436-450 (through Nuclear Medicine Subsection)
Assignment(s):	Prepare for Surgery, Test 5 (30 points, 9 questions, 5 Guidelines questions [10 points], 4 cases [20 points], 20 minutes) Complete Practice Exercises 3-46 through 3-50, pages 451-455 (10 points)

Lesson 23

SURGERY, TEST 5
Timed Test: 20 Minutes

Student hand in:	Practice Exercises 3-46 through 3-50, pages 451-455 (10 points)
Reading assignment(s):	Unit 3, pages 456-466 (up to Medicine Section)
Assignment(s):	Prepare for Radiology, Test 6 (22 points, 5 Guidelines questions, 1 non-Guidelines question [12 points], 2 cases [10 points], 15 minutes) Complete Practice Exercises 3-51 through 3-55, pages 462-466 (10 points)

Lesson 24

RADIOLOGY, TEST 6
Timed Test: 15 Minutes

Student hand in: Practice Exercises 3-51 through 3-55,
pages 462-466 (10 points)

Reading assignment(s):   Unit 3, pages 467-471 (up to Ophthalmology)

Assignment(s):   Prepare for Pathology and Laboratory, Test 7
(47 points, 5 Guidelines questions, 1 non-Guidelines
question [12 points], 7 cases [35 points], 20 minutes)
None

Lesson 25

PATHOLOGY AND LABORATORY, TEST 7
Timed Test: 20 Minutes

Student hand in: None

Reading assignment(s):   Unit 3, pages 471-484 (up to HCPCS Coding)

Assignment(s):   Complete Practice Exercises 3-56 through 3-60,
pages 479-484 (10 points)

Lesson 26

Student hand in: Practice Exercises 3-56 through 3-60,
pages 479-484 (10 points)

Reading assignment(s):   Unit 3, pages 485-492 (up to Using the ICD-9-CM)

Assignment(s):   Prepare for Medicine/HCPCS, Test 8 (36 points, 5
Guidelines questions, 3 non-Guidelines questions
[16 points], 4 cases [20 points], 10 minutes)
None

Lesson 27

MEDICINE/HCPCS, TEST 8
Timed Test: 10 Minutes

Student hand in: None

Reading assignment(s):   Unit 3, pages 492-494 (up to Selection of Primary
Diagnosis)

Assignment(s):   None

Lesson 28

Student hand in: None

Reading assignment(s):   Unit 3, pages 494-505 (up to Chapter 8, Diseases of
Respiratory System)

Assignment(s):   Post-Examination (to hand in results at Lesson 30
class period)

Lesson 29

Student hand in: None

Reading assignment(s):   Unit 3, pages 505-512 (through end of Unit 3)

Assignment(s):   None

Lesson 30

Student hand in: Post-Examination results (75 points, nongraded if each question attempted, deduct 1 point for each question not attempted; hand in printed copy of summary of your score)

Reading assignment(s):   None

Assignment(s):   Prepare for ICD-9-CM, Test 9 (25 points, 5 cases, 20 minutes)
Bring ICD-9-CM, CPT, and HCPCS to class to begin Final Examination

Lesson 31

ICD-9-CM, TEST 9
Timed Test: 20 Minutes

Final Examination beginning

Student hand in: None

Reading assignment(s):   None

Assignment(s):   Complete Final Examination (150 points)

Lesson 32

Final grade calculation
Course evaluation

Anatomy, Terminology, and Pathophysiology

Some of the CPT code descriptions for physician services include physician extender services. Physician extenders, such as nurse practitioners, physician assistants, and nurse anesthetists, etc., provide medical services typically performed by a physician. Within this educational material the term "physician" may include "and other qualified health care professionals" depending on the code. Refer to the official CPT® code descriptions and guidelines to determine codes that are appropriate to report services provided by non-physician practitioners.

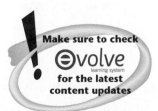

Make sure to check
evolve
learning system
for the latest
content updates

■ INTEGUMENTARY SYSTEM
INTEGUMENTARY SYSTEM—ANATOMY AND TERMINOLOGY

The skin and accessory organs (nails, hair, and glands)

Layers (Fig. 1-1)

Two layers make up skin: epidermis and dermis

Epidermis. Outermost layer; containing keratin

Stratum corneum, most superficial layer of four layers called stratum

Basal layer, deepest region of epidermis (stratum germinativum or stratum basale), is growth layer

Dermis. The second layer of skin

Two layers are papillary and reticulary and contain:

   Fibrous connective tissue or skin appendages

   Blood vessels

   Nerves

   Hair

   Nails

   Glands

Subcutaneous Tissue or Hypodermis. Not considered a layer of skin

Contains fat tissue and fibrous connective tissue

AKA: superficial fascia

Connects skin to underlying muscle

Nails

Keratin plates covering dorsal surface of each finger and toe

Lunula—semilunar or half-moon

   White area at base of nail plate is growth area

   Thickens and lengthens nail

Eponychium or cuticle: narrow band of epidermis at base and sides of nail

Paronychium: soft tissue around nail border

Glands

Sebaceous glands located in dermal layer

Secrete sebum that lubricates skin/hair

Influenced by sex hormones so they hypertrophy in adolescence and atrophy in old age

Sudoriferous glands originate in dermis. See Fig. 1-1.

AKA: sweat glands

Extend up through epidermis opening as pores

Secrete mostly water and salts to cool body

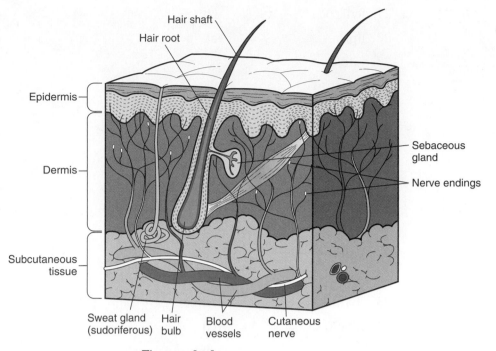

Figure **1-1** Integumentary system.

COMBINING FORMS

1.	aden/o	in relationship to a gland
2.	adip/o	fat
3.	albin/o	white
4.	aut/o	self
5.	bi/o	life
6.	caus/o	burning sensation
7.	cauter/o	burn
8.	crypt/o	hidden
9.	cutane/o	skin
10.	cyan/o	blue
11.	derm/o, dermat/o	skin
12.	diaphor/o	profuse sweating
13.	eosin/o	rosy
14.	erythem/o	red
15.	erythr/o	red
16.	heter/o	different
17.	hidr/o	sweat
18.	ichthy/o	dry/scaly
19.	jaund/o	yellow
20.	kerat/o	hard

21.	leuk/o	white
22.	lip/o	fat
23.	lute/o	yellow
24.	melan/o	black
25.	myc/o	fungus
26.	necr/o	death
27.	onych/o	nail
28.	pachy/o	thick
29.	phyt/o	plant
30.	pil/o	hair
31.	poli/o	gray matter
32.	py/o	pus
33.	rhytid/o	wrinkle
34.	rube/o	red
35.	seb/o	sebum/oil
36.	staphyl/o	clusters
37.	steat/o	fat
38.	strept/o	twisted chain
39.	steat/o	fat
40.	squam/o	flat/scalelike
41.	trich/o	hair
42.	ungu/o	nail
43.	xanth/o	yellow
44.	xer/o	dry

PREFIXES

1.	epi-	on/upon
2.	hyper-	over
3.	hypo-	under
4.	intra-	within
5.	para-	beside
6.	per-	through
7.	peri-	surrounding
8.	sub-	under

SUFFIXES

1. -coccus   spherical bacterium
2. -ectomy   removal
3. -ia   condition
4. -malacia   softening
5. -opsy   view of
6. -plasty   surgical repair
7. -rrhea   discharge
8. -tome   an instrument to cut
9. -tomy   to cut

MEDICAL ABBREVIATIONS

1. bx   biopsy
2. ca   cancer
3. derm   dermatology
4. I&D   incision and drainage
5. subcu, subq, SC, SQ   subcutaneous
6. PPD   tuberculin skin test

MEDICAL TERMS

Absence	Without
Adipose	Fatty
Albinism	Lack of color pigment
Allograft	Homograft, same species graft
Alopecia	Condition in which hair falls out
Anhidrosis	Deficiency of sweat
Autograft	From patient's own body
Avulsion	Ripping or tearing away of part either surgically or accidentally
Biopsy	Removal of a small piece of living tissue for diagnostic purposes
Causalgia	Burning pain
Collagen	Protein substance of skin
Debridement	Cleansing of or removal of dead tissue from a wound
Delayed flap	Pedicle of skin with blood supply that is separated from origin over time
Dermabrasion	Planing of skin by means of sander, brush, or sandpaper
Dermatologist	Physician who treats conditions of skin
Dermatoplasty	Surgical repair of skin
Electrocautery	Cauterization by means of heated instrument
Epidermolysis	Loosening of epidermis

Epidermomycosis	Superficial fungal infection
Epithelium	Surface covering of internal and external organs of body
Erythema	Redness of skin
Escharotomy	Surgical incision into necrotic (dead) tissue
Fissure	Cleft or groove
Free full-thickness graft	Graft of epidermis and dermis that is completely removed from donor area
Furuncle	Nodule in skin caused by *Staphylococcus* entering through hair follicle
Hematoma	A localized collection of blood, usually result of a break in a blood vessel
Hemograft	Allograft, same species graft
Ichthyosis	Skin disorder characterized by scaling
Incise	To cut into
Island pedicle flap	Contains a single artery and vein that remains attached to origin temporarily or permanently
Leukoderma	Depigmentation of skin
Leukoplakia	White patch on mucous membrane
Lipocyte	Fat cell
Lipoma	Fatty tumor
Melanin	Dark pigment of skin
Melanoma	Tumor of epidermis, malignant and black in color
Mohs surgery or Mohs micrographic surgery	Removal of skin cancer in layers by a surgeon who also acts as a pathologist during surgery
Muscle flap	Transfer of muscle from origin to recipient site
Neurovascular flap	Contains artery, vein, and nerve
Pedicle	Growth attached with a stem
Pilosebaceous	Pertains to hair follicles and sebaceous glands
Sebaceous gland	Secretes sebum
Seborrhea	Excess sebum secretion
Sebum	Oily substance
Split-thickness graft	All epidermis and some of dermis
Steatoma	Fat mass in sebaceous gland
Stratified	Layered
Stratum (strata)	Layer
Subungual	Beneath nail
Xanthoma	Tumor composed of cells containing lipid material, yellow in color
Xenograft	Different species graft
Xeroderma	Dry, discolored, scaly skin

INTEGUMENTARY SYSTEM ANATOMY AND TERMINOLOGY QUIZ
(Quiz answers are located at the end of Unit 1)

1. This is the outermost layer of skin:
   a. basal
   b. dermis
   c. epidermis
   d. subcutaneous

2. Which of the following is NOT a part of skin or accessory organs:
   a. sudoriferous glands
   b. sebaceous gland
   c. nail
   d. arterioles

3. This prefix means beside:
   a. para-
   b. intra-
   c. per-
   d. epi-

4. This combining form means hair:
   a. xanth/o
   b. trich/o
   c. ichthy/o
   d. kerat/o

5. Lunula is the:
   a. narrow band of epidermis at base of nail
   b. opening of pores
   c. outermost layer of epidermis
   d. white area at base of nail plate

6. Subcutaneous tissue is also known as:
   a. dermal
   b. adipose
   c. hypodermis
   d. stratum corneum

7. Which of the following combining forms does NOT refer to a color?
   a. cyan/o
   b. jaund/o
   c. eosin/o
   d. pachy/o

8. This medical term means surgical incision into dead tissue:
   a. onychomycosis
   b. escharotomy
   c. keratotomy
   d. curettage

9. This suffix means surgical repair:
    a. -opsy
    b. -rrhea
    c. -plasty
    d. -tome

10. Soft tissue around nail border is the:
    a. cuticle
    b. lunula
    c. paronychium
    d. corium

INTEGUMENTARY SYSTEM—PATHOPHYSIOLOGY

Lesions and Other Abnormalities (Fig. 1-2)

Macule
Flat area of color change (mostly reddened)

No elevation or depression

Example: flat moles, freckles

Papule
Solid elevation

Less than 1.0 cm in diameter

May run together and form plaques

Example: warts, lichen planus, elevated mole

Nodule
Solid elevation 1-2 cm in diameter

Extends deeper into dermis than papule

Example: lipoma, erythema nodosum, enlarged lymph nodes

Pustule
Elevated area

Filled with purulent fluid

Example: pimple, impetigo, abscess

Tumor
Solid mass

Uncontrolled, progressive growth of cells

Example: hemangioma, neoplasm, lipoma

Plaque
Flat, elevated surface

Equal or greater than 1.0 cm

Example: psoriasis, seborrheic keratosis

Wheal
Temporary localized elevation of skin

Results in transient edema in dermis

Example: insect bite, allergic reaction

Vesicle
Small blister

Less than 1 cm in diameter

Filled with serous fluid in epidermis

Example: herpes zoster (shingles), varicella (chickenpox)

Bulla
Large blister

Greater than 1.0 cm in diameter

Example: blister

MACULE
Flat area of color change; no elevation or depression

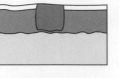

PAPULE
Solid elevation; less than 1.0 cm in diameter

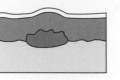

NODULE
Solid elevation 1-2 cm in diameter; extends deeper into dermis than papule

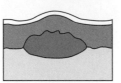

PUSTULE
Elevated, superficial lesion; similar to a vesicle but filled with purulent fluid

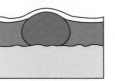

TUMOR
Solid mass; larger than 2.0 cm

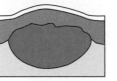

PLAQUE
Flat elevated surface found where papules, nodules, or tumors cluster

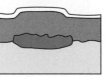

WHEAL
Temporary localized elevation of the skin; result is transient edema in dermis

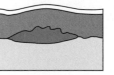

VESICLE
Small blister; fluid within or under epidermis

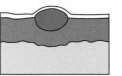

BULLA
Larger blister; greater than 1.0 cm in diameter

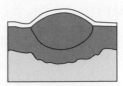

SCALES
Flakes of cornified skin layer

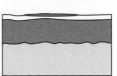

CRUST
Dried exudate on skin

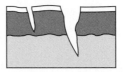

FISSURE
Cracks in skin

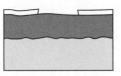

EROSION
Loss of epidermis that does not extend into dermis

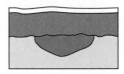

SCAR
Excess collagen production following injury

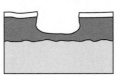

ATROPHY
Loss of some portion of the skin

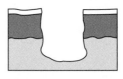

ULCER
Area of destruction of entire epidermis

Figure **1-2** Lesions of skin.

Scales
Flakes of cornified skin layer

>*Example:* dry skin

Crust
Dried exudate on skin

>*Example:* scab

Fissure
Cracks in skin

>*Example:* athlete's foot, openings in corners of mouth

Erosion
Loss of epidermis

Does not extend into dermis

>*Example:* blisters

Scar
Excess collagen production following surgery or trauma

>*Example:* healed surgical wound

Atrophy
Loss of some portion of skin and appears translucent

>*Example:* aged skin

• Not a lesion, but a physiologic response in aging process

Ulcer
Area of destruction of entire epidermis

>*Example:* missing tissue on heel, decubitus bedsore (pressure sore)

Pressure Ulcer (Decubitis Ulcer) (Fig. 1-3)
Result of pressure or force
Occludes blood flow, causing ischemia and tissue death

Develops over bony prominence

Locations
• Coccygeal (end of spine)

• Sacral (between hips)

• Heel

• Elbow

• Ischial (lower hip)

• Trochanteric (outer hip)

Staging or classification system
• Stage 1: erythema (redness) of skin

• Stage 2: partial loss of skin (epidermis or dermis)

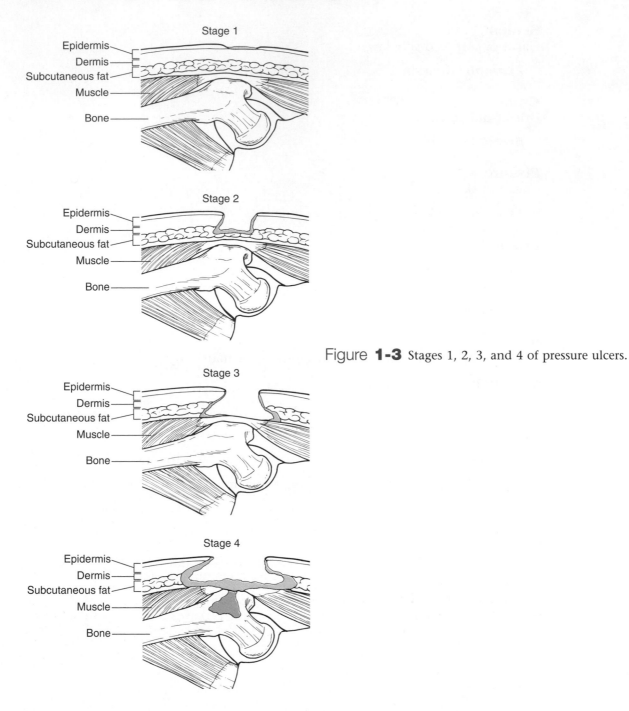

Figure **1-3** Stages 1, 2, 3, and 4 of pressure ulcers.

- Stage 3: full thickness loss of skin (up to but not through fascia)
- Stage 4: full thickness loss (extensive destruction and necrosis)

  Deep ulcers may require surgical debridement

Keloids

Sharply elevated, irregularly shaped scars that progressively enlarge

Due to excessive collagen in corneum during connective tissue repair

Result of tissue repair or trauma

Familial tendency for formation

Cicatrix
Normal scar left after wound healing

Inflammatory Disorders

Atopic Dermatitis
Unknown etiology

Exogenous (external) causes include
Irritant dermatitis

Allergic contact dermatitis

Endogenous (internal) cause includes
Seborrheic dermatitis

Results in activation of
- Mast cells
- Eosinophils
- T lymphocytes
- Monocytes

Greater in those with family history of
- Asthma
- Dry skin
- Eczema
- Allergic rhinitis

Common in
- Children
- Infants

Results in
- Chronic inflammation
- Scratching
- Erythema
- Thickened, leathery skin (lichenification)
- Secondary *Staphylococcus aureus* infection

Treatment
- Topical steroid
- Antibiotic for secondary infection
- Antihistamines

Allergic Contact Dermatitis
Most common in infants and children

Potential causes
- Hypersensitivity to allergens
  - Microorganisms
  - Drugs

- Foreign proteins
- Chemicals
- Latex
- Metals
- Plants

Manifestations
- Scaling
- Lichenification (leathery, thickened skin)
- Erythema
- Itching (pruritus)
- Vesicular lesions
- Edema

Diagnosis and treatment
- Check medical history
- Patch test
- Avoidance of irritant
- Skin lubrication and hydration
- Steroids
  - Topical
  - Systemic
- Topical tacrolimus (immunosuppressive agent)

Irritant Contact Dermatitis
Response to
- Chemical
- Exposure to irritant

Treatment
- Removal of irritant
- Topical agents

Stasis Dermatitis
Usually on the legs from venous stasis

Associated with
- Phlebitis
- Vascular trauma
- Varicosities

Progress
- Begins with erythema and pruritus
- Progresses to scaling, hyperpigmentation, petechiae (small hemorrhagic areas)
- Lesion becomes ulcerated

Treatment
- Elevate legs
- Reduce standing
- No constricting clothes
- Eliminate external compression
- Antibiotics for acute lesions
- Silver nitrate or Burow's solution dressings for chronic lesions

Seborrheic Dermatitis

Common chronic inflammation of sebaceous glands—cause unknown

Periods of remission and exacerbation

Commonly occurs on
- Scalp (cradle cap in infants)
- Ear canals
- Eyelids
- Eyebrow
- Nose
- Axillae
- Chest
- Groin

Lesions are
- Scaly (dry or greasy)
- White or yellowish
- Mildly pruritic

Treatment of mild cases
- Soap/shampoo of
  - Coal tar
  - Sulfur
  - Salicylic acid

Treatment of more severe cases
- Corticosteroid

Papulosquamous Disorders

Conditions associated with
- Scales
- Papules
- Plaque
- Erythema

Three types
- Psoriasis
- Pityriasis
- Lichen planus

Psoriasis
Chronic, relapsing, proliferating skin disorder

Usually begins by age 20

Cause unknown, suggested to be
- Exacerbated by anxiety; appears to run in families
- Immunologic
- Biochemical alterations
- Triggering agent

Commonly occurs on
- Face
- Scalp
- Forearms and elbows
- Knees and legs

Results in
- Thickened dermis and epidermis
- Well-demarcated plaque
- Cell hyperproliferation/scaly
- Inflammation (pruritus)
- Deep red lesions

Treatment
- Only palliative (treatment of symptoms)

Mild cases
- Keratolytic agents
- Corticosteroids
- Emollients

Moderate cases
- Interleukin-2 inhibitors
- Psoralens and ultraviolet A (PUVA) light therapy
- Coal tar
- Cyclosporin
- Vitamin D analogs

Severe cases
- Topical agents
- Systemic corticosteroids

- Antimetabolic
- Hospitalization

Pityriasis Rosea
Unknown cause

Self-limiting inflammatory disorder

Occurs most often in young adults

Primary lesion
- Begins with herald patch 3 to 4 cm
- Salmon-pink colored
- Circular and well-defined lesions

Secondary lesions
- 14 to 21 days

Trunk and upper extremities

- Oval lesions
- Severe pruritus

Diagnosis
May be confused with

- Secondary syphilis
- Seborrheic dermatitis
- Psoriasis

Treatment
- Antipruritics
- Antihistamines
- Corticosteroids
- Ultraviolet light
- Sunlight

Lichen Planus
Occurs on skin and mucous membranes

Unknown cause (idiopathic)

Autoimmune inflammatory disorder

Onset ages 30 to 70

Lesions
- Begin as pink lesions that turn into violet-colored pruritic papules
- Result in hyperpigmentation
- 2- to 10-mm flat lesions with central depression
- Last 12 to 18 months
- Tend to reoccur

Treatment
- Antihistamines
- Corticosteroids

  Topical

  Systemic

Acne Vulgaris

Site of lesion is sebaceous (pilosebaceous) follicles

Primarily on face and upper trunk

Occurs in 85% of the population between the ages of 12 and 25

Exact cause: unknown

Causative factor: sebum accumulation/inflammation in pores of skin

Types

Noninflammatory acne

- Whiteheads
- Blackheads

Inflammatory acne

- Follicle walls rupture
- Sebum expels into dermis
- Inflammation begins
  - Pustules, cysts, and papules result

Cause

Unknown

Treatment

Topical

- Antibiotics
- Salicylic acid
- Benzoyl peroxide
- Tretinoin

Systemic

- Antibiotic
- Hormones
- Corticosteroids
- Isotretinoin

Diaper Dermatitis

Variety of disorders

Causes

Urine

Feces

Plastic diaper cover

Allergic reaction

Secondary *Candida albicans* infection

Treatment
Clean, dry area

Expose to air

Topical antifungal medications

Topical steroids

Pruritus (Itching)
Symptom of skin disorder/dermatitis

Can be localized or generalized and is a condition not an inflammation

Results from stimulation of nerves of skin reacting to an allergen or irritation from substances in blood or foreign bodies

Causes
Primary skin disorder

Example: eczema or lice

Systemic disease

Example: chronic renal failure

Opiates

Allergic reaction

Treatment is for underlying condition
Antihistamines

Minor tranquilizers

Application of emollients (lotions)

Topical steroids

Skin Infections

■ Bacterial Impetigo
Most common in infants and children

Usually on face and begins as small vesicles

Caused primarily by *Staphylococcus*

• Sometimes by group A beta-hemolytic *Streptococcus*

It is a highly contagious pyoderma

Treatment in mild cases
Topical antibiotics

Topical antiseptics

Treatment in moderate cases
Systemic antibiotics

Local compresses

Analgesics

Cellulitis

Caused primarily by *Staphylococcus*

Often secondary to an injury

Results in
Erythema, usually of lower trunk and legs

Fever

Localized pain

Lymphangitis

Treatment
Systemic antibiotics

Burow's soaks for pain relief

Furuncles (Boils)

Infected hair follicle

Usually caused by *Staphylococcus*

Developed boil drains pus and necrotic tissue

Squeezing spreads infection

Collection of furuncles that have merged is a carbuncle

Folliculitis

Infection of hair follicles

Results in
Erythema

Pustules

Causes
Skin trauma, such as irritation or friction

Poor hygiene

Excessive skin moisture

Treatment
Cleansing of area

Topical antibiotics

Erysipelas

Infection of skin

Cause
Group A beta-hemolytic *Streptococcus*

Common occurrence: face, ears, lower legs

Prior to outbreak, presents with

- Fever
- Malaise
- Chills

Lesions appear as
Bright red and hot

- Develop raised borders

- Itching

- Burning

- Tenderness

Acute Necrotizing Fasciitis
Flesh-eating disease
Virulent strain of gram-positive, group A beta-hemolytic *Streptococcus*

Mortality rate of over 40%

Causes
Skin trauma

Skin infection

Areas secrete tissue-destroying enzyme, proteases
Extreme inflammation and pain

Rapidly increasing

Dermal gangrene develops

Systemic toxicity may develop with
Fever

Disorientation

Hypotension

Tachycardia (fast heart rate)

May lead to organ failure

Treatment
Antimicrobial therapy

Fluid replacement

Removal of areas of infection

■ Viral Herpes Simplex (Cold Sores)
Causes
Herpes simplex virus type 1 (HSV-1)

- Most common type

- Results in fever blisters or cold sores on or near lips or canker sores of the mouth

Herpes simplex virus type 2 (HSV-2)

- Genital and oral type

- Prominent sexually transmitted disease

Primary infections may show no symptoms (asymptomatic)

Virus remains in nerve tissue to later reactivate

Reactivation may be triggered by
Stress

Common cold

Exposure to sun

Presents with
Burning or tingling

Develops painful vesicles that rupture
Causes spreading

May cause secondary infection of eye

- Episode lasts several weeks

- Treatment may include antiviral medication

  • No permanent cure exists

Herpes Zoster (Shingles)
Usually older adult

Caused by varicella-zoster virus (VZV)
Virus was dormant and then reactivates

Result of varicella or chickenpox, usually in childhood

Affects
One cranial nerve or one dermatome (an area of skin supplied with afferent nerve fibers by a posterior spinal root)

Results in
Pain

Rash (unilateral)

Paresthesia (abnormal touch sensation, such as burning)

Course
Several weeks

Pain may continue even after lesion disappears

Treatment
Clears spontaneously

Antiviral medications provide symptomatic relief

Sedatives

Analgesic

Antipruritics

Warts (Verrucae)
Verruca vulgaris (common wart)

Caused by human papillomavirus (HPV)

- Numerous types of HPV

Spread by contact

Appear anywhere on body

Present with a grayish appearance

Variety of shapes and sizes

Transmitted by touch

Plantar warts (verrucae) are located on pressure points of body (such as feet; *plantar* means the bottom surface of foot)

Painful when pressure is applied

Juvenile warts occur on feet and hands of children

Venereal warts occur on genitals/anus

Treatment
Liquid nitrogen

Topical keratolytics

Laser

Electrocautery

Often persist even with treatment

Fungal (Mycoses)
Usually superficial dermatophytes (fungus)

Fungus lives off dead cells

Tinea
Superficial skin infections

Tinea capitis

- Infection of scalp

- Common in children

- Treatment with oral antifungal medication

Tinea corporis (ringworm)

- Infection of body

- Presents as a red ring

- Produces burning sensation and pruritus

- Treatment with topical antifungal medication

Tinea pedis (athlete's foot)

- Involves feet and toes

- Produces pain, inflammation, fissures, and foul odor

- Treatment with topical antifungal medication

Tinea unguium (onychomycosis)

- Nail infection

  - Usually toenails

- Nail turns white then brown, thickens and cracks

- Spreads to other nails

Candidiasis
Caused by *Candida albicans*

Normally on mucous membranes of gastrointestinal tract and vagina

Poor health and certain conditions predispose individuals to overarching infection by *Candida*

- Antibiotic therapy, which changes the balance of the normal flora in the body

Treatment is topical or oral antifungal medications

Tumors of Skin

■ Benign Tumors
Keratosis(es)
Seborrheic keratosis

Proliferation of basal cells

Dark colored lesion

Found on trunk and face

Actinic keratosis

Pigmented, scaly patch

Often caused by exposure to sun

Often in fair-skinned individuals

Premalignant lesion

May develop into squamous cell carcinoma

Treatment with cryosurgery (freezing area) or excision

Keratoacanthoma

Occurs in hair follicles

Usually in those over 60

Often on face, neck, back of hands, and other locations exposed to the sun

Resolve spontaneously or are excised

Moles (Nevi)

Located on any body part

Various shapes and sizes

May become malignant

- Especially if located in area of continual irritation

■ Malignant Tumors
Squamous Cell Carcinoma

Similar to basal cell carcinoma

Grows wherever squamous epithelium is located (skin, mouth, pharynx, esophagus, lungs, bladder)

Most often appears in areas exposed to sun (actinic keratosis—precancerous)

Scaly appearance

Rarely metastatic (spreading)

Easily treated with good prognosis

Surgical excision

Cryotherapy

Curettage

Electrodesiccation

Radiotherapy

Basal Cell Carcinoma
Common type of skin cancer

Developed in deeper skin layers (basal cells) than squamous cell carcinoma

Often occurs with sun exposure in fair-skinned individuals

Shiny appearance and slow growing

Easily treated with good prognosis

Malignant Melanoma
Originates in cells that produce pigment (melanocytes) or nevi

Increased incidence with
Sun exposure

Fair hair and skin, freckles

Genetic predisposition

Skin nevus (mole) often brown and evenly colored with irregular borders

Grow downward into tissues

• Metastasize quickly

Treatment is removal with extensive border excision

• Depending on extent, chemotherapy or radiation therapy may be used

Kaposi's Sarcoma
Rare form of vascular skin cancer

Associated with
Human immunodeficiency virus (HIV)

Acquired immunodeficiency syndrome (AIDS)

Herpes virus may be found in lesions

Cells originate from endothelium in small blood vessels

Painful lesions develop rapidly, appearing as purple papules; spread quickly to lymph nodes and internal organs

Treatment

Radiation

Chemotherapy

Merkel Cell Carcinoma
Rare form of skin cancer

Treatment is excision and chemotherapy/radiation therapy

INTEGUMENTARY SYSTEM PATHOPHYSIOLOGY QUIZ
(Quiz answers are located at the end of Unit 1)

1. A pimple is an example of a:
   a. papule
   b. vesicle
   c. pustule
   d. nodule

2. A Stage III pressure ulcer involves:
   a. erythema of skin
   b. partial loss of epidermis and dermis
   c. full thickness loss of skin up to but not through fascia
   d. full thickness loss of skin with extensive destruction and necrosis

3. This type of dermatitis may be exogenous or endogenous and is common in children and infants:
   a. atopic
   b. irritant contact
   c. stasis
   d. seborrheic

4. Psoriasis, pityriasis, and lichen planus are three types of this disorder:
   a. dermatitis
   b. inflammatory
   c. acne
   d. papulosquamous

5. This condition begins with a herald spot:
   a. psoriasis
   b. pityriasis
   c. lichen planus
   d. dermatitis

6. This skin infection is caused by group A beta-hemolytic *Streptococcus*, and the lesions appear as firm red spots with itching, burning, and tenderness:
   a. furuncles
   b. folliculitis
   c. erysipelas
   d. fasciitis

7. This type of herpes produces cold sores:
   a. herpes zoster
   b. shingles
   c. VZV
   d. herpes simplex

8. This condition is caused by human papillomavirus:
   a. mycoses
   b. verrucae
   c. shingles
   d. folliculitis

9. This type of tumor occurs in hair follicles:
   a. keratoses
   b. nevi
   c. Kaposi's sarcoma
   d. keratoacanthoma

10. This type of superficial carcinoma is rarely metastatic:
    a. squamous cell
    b. basal cell
    c. melanoma
    d. Kaposi's sarcoma

■ MUSCULOSKELETAL SYSTEM
MUSCULOSKELETAL SYSTEM—ANATOMY AND TERMINOLOGY

Skeletal System

Comprises 206 bones, cartilage, and ligaments

Provides organ protection, movement, framework, stores calcium, hematopoiesis (formation of blood cells)

Classification of Bones
Long bones (tubular)
Length exceeds width of bone

Broad at ends, such as thigh, lower leg, upper arm, and lower arm

Short bones (cuboidal)
Cubelike bones, such as carpals (wrist) and tarsals (ankle)

Flat
Thin—flattened with curved surfaces

Cover body parts, such as skull, scapula, sternum, ribs

Irregular
Varied shapes, such as zygoma of face or vertebrae

Sesamoid
Rounded

Found near joint, such as patella (kneecap)

Patella is largest sesamoid bone in body

Structure
Long Bones (Fig. 1-4)
Diaphysis: shaft

Epiphysis: both ends of long bones—bulbular shape with muscle attachments

• Articular cartilage covers epiphyses and serves as a cushion

Epiphyseal line or plate: growth plate that disappears when fully grown

Metaphysis: flared portion of bone near epiphyseal plate

Periosteum: dense, white outer covering (fibrous)

Cortical or compact bone: hard bone beneath periosteum mainly found in shaft

• Medullary cavity contains yellow marrow (fatty bone marrow)

Cancellous bones: spongy or trabecular

• Contains red bone marrow (blood cell development)

Endosteum is thin epithelial membrane lining medullary cavity of long bone

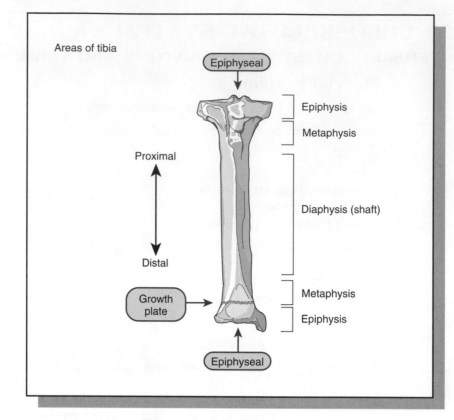

Figure **1-4** Structure of bones.

Two Skeletal Divisions
Axial (trunk)

Appendicular (appendages)

Axial Skeleton, comprised of 80 bones
Skull, hyoid bone, vertebral column, sacrum, ribs, and sternum

Skull (Fig. 1-5)
Cranial
Frontal (forehead)

Parietal (sides and top)

Temporal (lower sides)

Occipital (posterior of cranium)

Sphenoid (floor of cranium)

Ethmoid (area between orbits and nasal cavity)

Styloid process (below ear)

Zygomatic process (cheek)

Middle ear bones (Fig. 1-6)
Malleus (hammer)

Incus (anvil)

Stapes (stirrup)

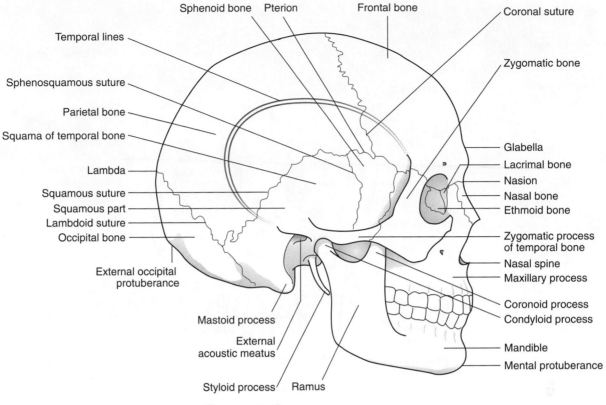

Figure **1-5** Lateral view of skull.

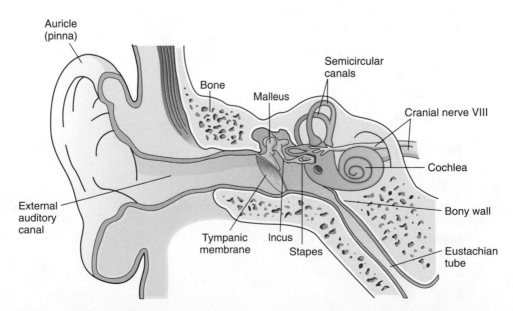

Figure **1-6** Structure of ear and three divisions of external, middle, and inner ear.

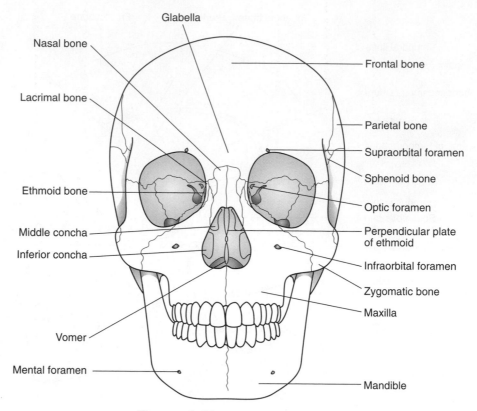

Figure **1-7** Frontal view of skull.

Face (Fig. 1-7)
Nasal (bridge of nose)

Maxilla (upper jaw)

Zygomatic (arch of cheekbone)

Mandible (lower jawbone)

Lacrimal (near orbits)

Palate (separates oral and nasal cavities)

Vomer (base, nasal septum)

Nasal conchae (turbinates)

   Interior

   Middle

   Superior

Hyoid
Supports tongue

U shaped

Attached by ligaments and muscles to larynx and skull

Spine (33 vertebrae) (Fig. 1-8)
Cervical vertebrae (7)

- C1-7

- (C1)-atlas

- (C2)-axis

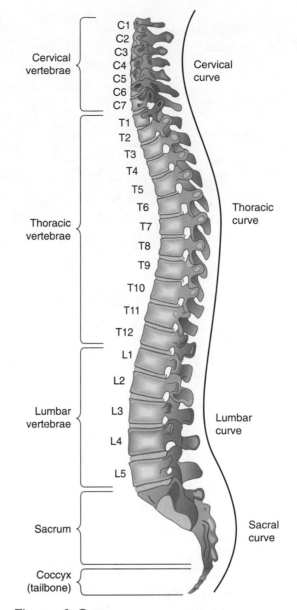

Figure **1-8** Anterior view of vertebral column.

Thoracic vertebrae (12) (T1-12)

Lumbar vertebrae (5) (L1-5)

Sacrum (5)—fused in adults

Coccyx (4)—fused in adults

Thorax (Fig. 1-9)
Ribs, 12 pairs

- True ribs, 1-7

- False ribs, 8-10

- Floating ribs, 11 and 12

Sternum

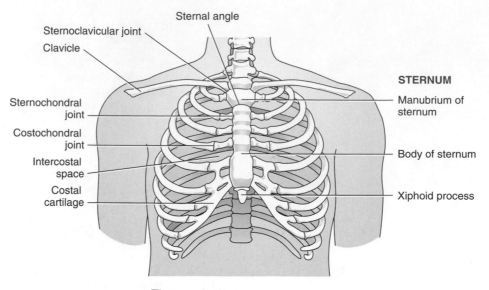

Figure **1-9** The thoracic cage.

Appendicular Skeleton, comprised of 126 bones (Fig. 1-10)

Shoulder, girdle, pelvic girdle, and extremities
Pelvis
Ilium (uppermost part) wing shaped

• Acetabulum, depression on lateral hip surface into which head of femur fits

Ischium (posterior part)

Pubis (anterior part)

Pubis symphysis (cartilage between pubic bones)

Lower extremities
Femur (thighbone)
Trochanter (processes at neck of femur)

Head fits into acetabulum

Patella (kneecap)

Tibia (shinbone)

Fibula (smaller lateral bone in lower leg)

Talus (ankle bone)

Calcaneus (heel bone)

Metatarsals (foot instep)

Phalanges (toes)

Lateral malleolus (lower part of fibula)

Medial malleolus (lower part of tibia)

Upper extremities
Clavicle (collarbone)

Scapula (shoulder blade)

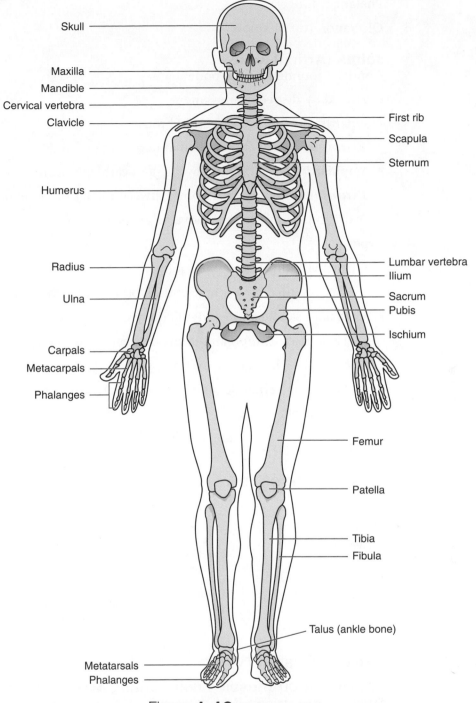

Skull

Maxilla
Mandible
Cervical vertebra
Clavicle

Humerus

Radius

Ulna

Carpals
Metacarpals

Phalanges

First rib
Scapula
Sternum

Lumbar vertebra
Ilium
Sacrum
Pubis
Ischium

Femur

Patella

Tibia
Fibula

Talus (ankle bone)

Metatarsals
Phalanges

Figure **1-10** Skeletal system.

Humerus (upper arm)

Radius (forearm, thumb side)

Ulna (forearm, little finger side)

Olecranon (projection of ulna at elbow)

Carpals (wrist)—eight bones bound by ligaments in two rows with 4 bones in each

Metacarpals (hand)—framework or palm of hand (5 bones)

Phalanges (finger)

Olecranon (tip of elbow)

Joints (Articulations)

Condyle, rounded end of bone

Classified by degree of movement

- Synarthrosis (immovable and fibrous)

  Example: joint between cranial bones

- Amphiarthrosis (slightly movable and cartilaginous)

  Example: intervertebral (joint between bodies of vertebra)

- Diarthrosis (considerably movable and synovial)

Types

- Uniaxial—hinge and pivot joints

  Example—elbow (hinge and pivot) and cervical 2 (axis) (pivot)

- Biaxial—saddle and condyloid joints

  Example—thumb and joints between radius and carpal bones

- Multiaxial—ball and socket and gliding

  Example—shoulder and hip/joints between articular surfaces of vertebrae

  Example: elbow, hip

- Bursa, sac of synovial fluid located in the tissues to prevent friction

Muscular System

Functions

Heat production

Movement

Posture

Protection

Shape

Muscle Tissue Types

Skeletal—600 muscles constituting 40% to 50% of body weight

Striated (cross stripes) (Figs. 1-11 and 1-12)

Move body

Voluntary

Attaches to bones

- Most attach to two bones with a joint in between

- Origin, point where muscle attaches to stationary bone

- Insertion, where muscle attaches to movable bone

- Body of muscle, main part of muscle

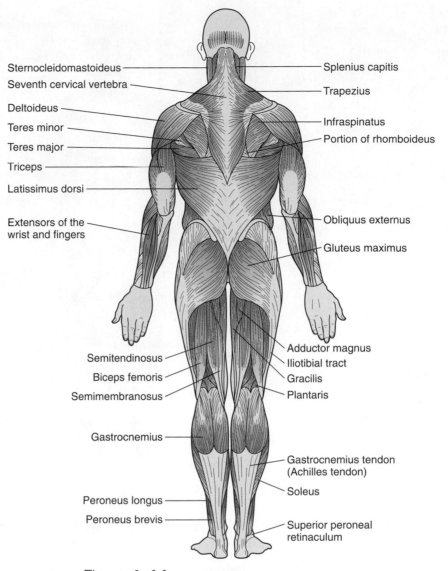

Figure **1-11** Muscular system, posterior view.

Cardiac/Heart Muscle
Striated and smooth muscle

   Specialized cells that interlock so that muscle cells contract together

Involuntary

Moves blood by means of contractions

Smooth/Visceral
Linings such as bowel, urethra, blood vessels

Nonstriated

Involuntary

Tendons Anchor Muscle to Bone

Ligaments Anchor Bones to Bones

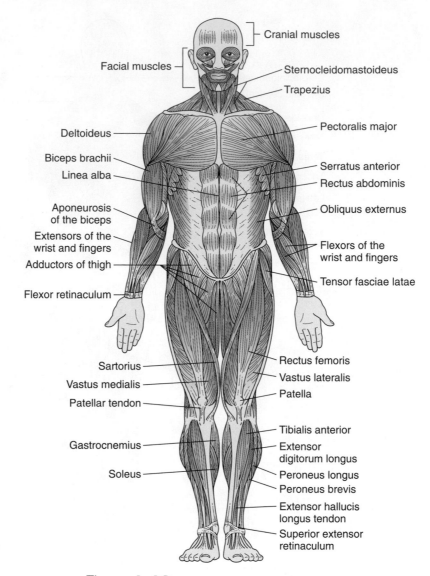

Figure **1-12** Muscular system, anterior view.

Muscle Action

Muscle Capabilities

Stretches

Contracts

Receives and responds to stimulus

Returns to original shape and length

Muscle Movement

Prime mover, responsible for movement (agonist)

Synergist, assists prime mover

Antagonist, relaxes as prime mover and synergists contract, resulting in movement

Fixator, acts as joint stabilizer

Terms of Movement—from midline of body

Flexion (bend)

Extension (straighten)

Abduction (away)

Adduction (toward)

Rotation (turn on axis)

Circumduction (circular)

Supination (turning palm upward or forward [anteriorly] or lying down with face upward)

Pronation (turning palm downward or backward or act of lying face down)

Hyperextension (overextension)

Inversion (inward)

Eversion (outward)

Names of Muscles

Head and neck
Facial expression

- Occipitofrontalis (raises eyebrows and wrinkles forehead horizontally)
- Corrugator supercilii (wrinkles forehead vertically)
- Orbicularis oris (opens mouth)
- Zygomaticus (elevates corners of mouth)
- Orbicularis oculi (opens and closes eyelid)
- Buccinator (smiling and blowing)

Mastication (chewing)

- Masseter (used to chew closing jaw)
- Temporalis (closes jaw)
- Pterygoids (grates teeth)

Muscles moving head

- Sternocleidomastoid (flexes head)
- Semispinalis capitis (complexus) (extends head)
- Splenius capitis (extends head, bends and rotates head to side where muscle is contracting)
- Longissimus capitis (trachelomastoid muscle) (extends head, bends and rotates to contracting side)
- Trapezius (extends head)

Upper extremities
Biceps brachii (flexes elbow)

Triceps brachii and anconeus (extends elbow)

Brachialis (flexes prone forearm)

Brachioradialis (flexes semi-prone/supinated forearm)

Deltoid (abducts upper arm)

Latissimus dorsi (extends upper arm)

Pectoralis major (flexes upper arm)

Trapezius (raises/lowers shoulder)

Trunk
External oblique (compresses abdomen)

Internal oblique (compresses abdomen)

Transversus abdominis (compresses abdomen)

Rectus abdominis (flexes trunk)

Quadratus lumborum (flexes vertebral column laterally)

Respiratory
Diaphragm (enlarges thorax/inspiration)

External intercostals (raise ribs)

Internal intercostal (depress ribs)

Lower extremities
Thigh

• Gluteus group, maximus, medius, minimus (abducts thigh)

• Tensor fasciae latae (abducts thigh)

• Abductor group, brevis, longus, magnus (adducts thigh)

• Gracilis (adducts thigh)

• Iliopsoas (flexes thigh)

• Rectus femoris (flexes thigh)

Hamstring group, biceps femoris, semitendinosus, semimembranosus (extends thigh)

Quadriceps group, rectus femoris, vastus lateralis, vastus medialis, vastus intermedius (extends lower leg)

Sartorius (flexes, abducts, and rotates leg)

Lower leg

Tibialis anterior (dorsiflexes foot)

Peroneus group, longus, brevis, tertius (everts foot)

Gastrocnemius (calf, with soleus extends foot, also flexes knee)

Soleus (calf, extends foot)

Extensor digitorum longus (extends toes, flexes foot)

Achilles tendon (largest tendon, extending from gastrocnemius to calcaneus)

COMBINING FORMS

1. acetabul/o   hip socket

2. ankyl/o   bent, fused

3. aponeur/o   tendon type

4. arthr/o   joint

5. articul/o   joint

6. burs/o   fluid-filled sac in a joint

7. calc/o, calci/o   calcium

8. calcane/o   calcaneus (heel)

9. carp/o   carpals (wrist bones)

10. chondr/o   cartilage

11. clavic/o, clavicul/o   clavicle (collar bone)

12. cost/o   rib

13. crani/o   cranium (skull)

14. disc/o   intervertebral disc

15. femor/o   thighbone

16. fibul/o   fibula

17. humer/o   humerus (upper arm bone)

18. ili/o   ilium (upper pelvic bone)

19. ischi/o   ischium (posterior pelvic bone)

20. kinesi/o   movement

21. kyph/o   hump

22. lamin/o   lamina

23. lord/o   curve

24. lumb/o   lower back

25. malleol/o   malleolus (process on lateral ankle)

26. mandibul/o   mandible (lower jawbone)

27. maxill/o   maxilla (upper jawbone)

28. menisc/o   meniscus

29. menisci/o   meniscus

30. metacarp/o   metacarpals (hand)

31. metatars/o   metatarsals (foot)

32. myel/o   bone marrow

33. my/o, muscul/o   muscle

34. olecran/o   olecranon (elbow)

35. orth/o   straight

36. oste/o   bone

37. patell/o   patella (kneecap)

38. pelv/i   pelvis (hip)

39. perone/o   fibula

40. petr/o	stone
41. phalang/o	phalanges (finger or toe)
42. plant/o	sole of foot
43. pub/o	pubis
44. rachi/o	spine
45. radi/o	radius (lower arm)
46. rhabdomy/o	skeletal (striated muscle)
47. rheumat/o	watery flow (collection of fluids in joints)
48. sacr/o	sacrum
49. scapul/o	scapula (shoulder)
50. scoli/o	bent
51. spondyl/o	vertebra
52. stern/o	sternum (breast bone)
53. synovi/o	synovial joint membrane
54. tars/o	tarsal (ankle/foot)
55. ten/o	tendon
56. tend/o	tendon (connective tissue)
57. tendin/o	tendon (connective tissue)
58. tibi/o	shin bone
59. uln/o	ulna (lower arm bone)
60. vertebr/o	vertebra

PREFIXES

1. inter-	between
2. supra-	above
3. sym-	together
4. syn-	together

SUFFIXES

1. -asthenia	weakness
2. -blast	embryonic
3. -clast, -clasia, -clasis	break
4. -desis	bind together
5. -listhesia	slipping
6. -malacia	softening
7. -physis	to grow
8. -porosis	passage, cavity formation
9. -schisis	split
10. -stenosis	narrowing

11. -tome   instrument that cuts

12. -tomy   incision

MEDICAL ABBREVIATIONS

1.	ACL	anterior cruciate ligament
2.	AKA	above-knee amputation
3.	BKA	below-knee amputation
4.	C1-C7	cervical vertebrae
5.	CTS	carpal tunnel syndrome
6.	fx	fracture
7.	L1-L5	lumbar vertebrae
8.	OA	osteoarthritis
9.	RA	rheumatoid arthritis
10.	T1-T12	thoracic vertebrae
11.	TMJ	temporomandibular joint

MEDICAL TERMS

Arthrocentesis	Injection and/or aspiration of joint
Arthrodesis	Surgical immobilization of a joint
Arthrography	Radiography of joint
Arthroplasty	Reshaping or reconstruction of a joint
Arthroscopy	Use of scope to view inside joint
Arthrotomy	Incision into a joint
Articular	Pertains to a joint
Aspiration	Use of a needle and a syringe to withdraw fluid
Atrophy	Wasting away
Bunion	Hallux valgus, abnormal increase in size of metatarsal head that results in displacement of great toe
Bursitis	Inflammation of bursa (joint sac)
Carpal tunnel syndrome	Compression of medial nerve
Chondral	Referring to the cartilage
Closed fracture repair	Not surgically opened with/without manipulation and with/without traction
Closed treatment	Fracture site that is not surgically opened and visualized
Colles' fracture	Fracture at lower end of radius that displaces bone posteriorly
Dislocation	Placement in a location other than original location
Endoscopy	Inspection of body organs or cavities using a lighted scope that may be inserted through an existing opening or through a small incision

Fasciectomy	Removal of band of fibrous tissue
Fissure	Groove
Fracture	Break in a bone
Ganglion	Knot or knotlike mass
Internal/External fixation	Application of pins, wires, screws, placed externally or internally to immobilize a body part
Kyphosis	Humpback
Lamina	Flat plate
Ligament	Fibrous band of tissue that connects cartilage or bone
Lordosis	Anterior curvature of the spine
Lumbodynia	Pain in lumbar area
Lysis	Releasing
Manipulation or reduction	Alignment of a fracture or joint dislocation to normal position
Open fracture repair	Surgical opening (incision) over or remote opening as access to a fracture site
Osteoarthritis	Degenerative condition of articular cartilage
Osteoclast	Absorbs or removes bone
Osteotomy	Cutting into bone
Percutaneous	Through skin
Percutaneous fracture repair	Repair of a fracture by means of pins and wires inserted through the fracture site
Percutaneous skeletal fixation	Considered neither open nor closed; fracture is not visualized, but fixation is placed across fracture site under x-ray imaging
Reduction	Replacement to normal position
Scoliosis	Lateral curvature of the spine
Skeletal traction	Application of pressure to bone by means of pins and/or wires inserted into bone
Skin traction	Application of pressure to bone by means of tape applied to the skin
Spondylitis	Inflammation of vertebrae
Subluxation	Partial dislocation
Supination	Supine position—lying on back, face upward
Synchondrosis	Union between two bones (connected by cartilage)
Tendon	Attaches a muscle to a bone
Tenodesis	Suturing of a tendon to a bone
Tenorrhaphy	Suture repair of tendon
Traction	Application of pressure to maintain normal alignment
Trocar needle	Needle with a cannula that can be removed; used to puncture and withdraw fluid from a cavity

MUSCULOSKELETAL SYSTEM ANATOMY AND TERMINOLOGY QUIZ

(Quiz answers are located at the end of Unit 1)

1. Tubular is another name for these bones:
   a. short
   b. long
   c. flat
   d. irregular

2. These bones are found near joints:
   a. irregular
   b. flat
   c. sesamoid
   d. broad

3. Zygoma is an example of this type of bone:
   a. irregular
   b. flat
   c. sesamoid
   d. broad

4. Diaphysis is this part of bone:
   a. end
   b. surface
   c. shaft
   d. marrow

5. Which is NOT a part of cranium?
   a. condyle
   b. sphenoid
   c. ethmoid
   d. parietal

6. This is NOT an ear bone:
   a. malleus
   b. stapes
   c. incus
   d. styloid

7. This term describes growth plate:
   a. endosteum
   b. epiphyseal
   c. metaphysis
   d. periosteum

8. This is a depression on lateral hip surface into which head of femur fits:
   a. ilium
   b. ischium
   c. patella
   d. acetabulum

9. Tip of elbow is the:
   a. olecranon
   b. trapezium
   c. humerus
   d. tarsal

10. This term describes an immovable joint:
   a. amphiarthrosis
   b. diarthrosis
   c. synarthrosis
   d. ischium

MUSCULOSKELETAL SYSTEM—PATHOPHYSIOLOGY

Injuries

■ Fractures

Classification of fractures

Open/closed

Open (compound): broken bone penetrates skin

Closed (simple): broken bone does not penetrate skin

Complete/incomplete

Complete: bone is broken all way through

> *Example:* oblique, linear, spiral, and transverse

Incomplete: bone is not broken all way through

> *Example:* greenstick, bowing, torus, stress, and transchondral

Treatment

Closed reduction (realignment of bone fragments by manipulation)

Reduction (the returning of the bone to normal alignment)

Immobilization (returns to normal alignment and holds in place)

Traction (application of pulling force to hold bone in alignment)

- Skeletal traction uses internal devices (pins, screws, wires, etc.) inserted into bone with ends sticking out through skin for attachment of traction device (Fig. 1-13)

- Skin traction is use of strapping, elastic wrap, or tape attached to skin to which weights are attached (Fig. 1-14)

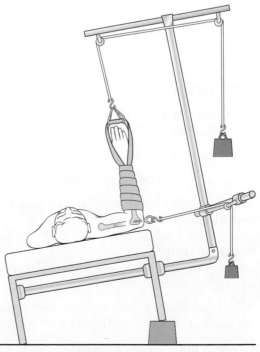

Figure **1-13** Skeletal traction uses patient's bones to secure internal devices to which traction is attached.

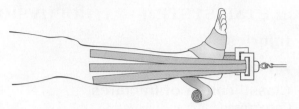

Figure **1-14** Skin traction utilizes strapping, wraps, or tape to which traction is attached.

Improper union

   Nonunion: failure of bone ends to grow together

   Malunion: incorrect alignment of bone ends

   Delayed union: delay of bone union 8 or 9 months

Dislocations

   Bone and soft tissue damage usually caused by trauma

   Any part of bone is displaced

   Can result in nerve and tissue damage

Treatment

   Reduction

   Immobilization

Sprains and strains

   Soft tissue damage usually caused by trauma to tendons and ligaments

Strain: partial tear of a tendon

Sprain results from overuse or overextension/tearing or rupture of some part of musculature

Bone Disorders

Osteomyelitis

Bone infection

Usually caused by bacteria

- Exogenous osteomyelitis is caused by bacteria that enter from outside body

- Hematogenous osteomyelitis (endogenous) is caused by a bacterial infection within body

Osteoporosis

Common disorder in postmenopausal women and elderly and most common metabolic disease

- Malabsorption of calcium and magnesium; certain trace elements and vitamins C and D contribute to bone loss

Decreased bone mass and density

- Fractures more common due to decrease in strength of bone

Treatment

Increased intake of calcium, magnesium, and vitamin D

Increased weight-bearing activity

Osteomalacia and Rickets

Osteomalacia is softened adult bones, while rickets is softened growing bones in children

Caused by vitamin D and phosphate deficiency

Osteitis Deformans (Paget's Disease)

Abnormal bone remodeling and resorption resulting in enlarged, soft bones

Unknown cause but strong genetic considerations

Treatment

Calcitonin and biophosphates

Spinal Curvatures

Lordosis: swayback

- Inward curvature of spine

Kyphosis: humpback

- Outward curvature of spine

Scoliosis

- Lateral curvature of spine

Spina Bifida

Congenital abnormality in which vertebrae do not close correctly around the spinal cord

Joint Disorders

Bursitis: inflammation of bursa (joint sac)

Arthritis: inflammation of joints

Osteoarthritis (OA)

This is degenerative or wear/tear arthritis

- DJD, degenerative joint disease

Chronic inflammation of joint

Increased pain on weightbearing or movement

Affects weight-bearing joints

- Loss of articular cartilage
- Sclerosis of bone—eburnation

    Turning bone into ivorylike mass—polished

- Osteophytes (bone spurs)

Symptoms

Pain and stiffness

Crepitation (bone on bone creates characteristic grinding sound)

Classifications

Primary (idiopathic)

- No known cause

Secondary

- Associated with joint instability, joint stress, or congenital abnormalities

Treatment

Symptomatic

Arthroplasty

Rheumatoid Arthritis (RA)

Progressive inflammatory connective tissue disease of the joints

Systemic autoimmune disease

- Can invade arteries, lungs, skin, and other organs with inflammation or nodules

Affects small joints

- Destroys synovial membrane, articular cartilage, and surrounding tissues

Leads to loss of function due to fixation and deformity

Treatment

Pharmaceuticals to modify autoimmune and inflammatory processes

Gene therapy and stem cell transplantation are being researched

Symptomatic

Arthroplasty

Infectious and Septic Arthritis

Infectious process

Usually affects single joint

Without antimicrobial intervention, permanent joint damage results

Example: Lyme disease

Treatment

Antibiotics—early intervention

Gout (Gouty Arthritis)

Inflammatory arthritis

Often affects the joint of the great toe

Caused by excessive amounts of uric acid that crystallizes in connective tissue of joints

Leads to inflammation and destruction of joint

Treatment

Pharmaceuticals—nonsteroidal antiinflammatory drugs

Ankylosing Spondylitis (AS)

Inflammatory disease that is progressive

Affects vertebral joints and insertion points of ligaments, tendons, and joint capsules

Leads to rigid spinal column and sacroiliac joints

Treatment
    Nonsteroidal anti-inflammatory drugs relieve symptoms

    Analgesics for pain

Tendon, Muscle, and Ligament Disorders

Muscular Dystrophy—Familial Disorder

Progressive degenerative muscle disorder

Multiple types of muscular dystrophy

Most often affects boys

- Genetic predisposition—Duchenne muscular dystrophy

Primary Fibromyalgia Syndrome

Symptoms
    Generalized aching and pain

    Tender points

    Fatigue

    Depression

Usually appears in
    Middle-aged women

Polymyositis

General muscle inflammation causing weakness

- With skin rash = dermatomyositis

Tumors

Bone Tumors

Origin of bone tumors
    Osteogenic (bone cells)

    Chondrogenic (cartilage cell)

    Collagenic (fibrous tissue cell)

    Myelogenic (marrow cell)

Osteoma
    Benign

    Abnormal outgrowth of bone

Chondroblastoma
    Rare

    Usually benign

Osteosarcoma
    Malignant tumor of long bones

    Usually in young adults

    Typically causes bone pain

Multiple myeloma

Malignant plasma cells in skeletal system and soft tissue

Progressive and generally fatal

Usually in those over 40

Chondrosarcoma

Malignant cartilage tumor

Usually in middle-aged and older individuals

In late stages, symptoms include local swelling and pain

• Worsens with time

Surgical excision is usually treatment of choice

If diagnosed in early stages, it is treatable with long-term survival possible

Muscle Tumors

Rare

Rhabdomyosarcoma

Aggressive, invasive carcinoma with widespread metastasis

MUSCULOSKELETAL SYSTEM PATHOPHYSIOLOGY QUIZ
(Quiz answers are located at the end of Unit 1)

1. A compound fracture is also known as:
   a. complete
   b. incomplete
   c. closed
   d. open

2. This is a common bone disorder in postmenopausal women resulting from lower levels of calcium and potassium:
   a. Paget's disease
   b. lordosis
   c. osteoporosis
   d. rheumatoid arthritis

3. This inflammatory disease is progressive and leads to a rigid spinal column:
   a. polymyositis
   b. ankylosing spondylitis
   c. primary fibromyalgia syndrome
   d. septic arthritis of spine

4. This type of tumor arises from bone cells:
   a. osteogenic
   b. chondrogenic
   c. collagenic
   d. myelogenic

5. This type of tumor is the most common type of malignant bone tumor that occurs in those over 40 and is progressive and generally fatal:
   a. rhabdomyosarcoma
   b. chondrosarcoma
   c. osteosarcoma
   d. multiple myeloma

6. A general muscle inflammation with an accompanying skin rash is:
   a. muscular dystrophy
   b. dermatologic arthritis
   c. ankylosing spondylitis
   d. dermatomyositis

7. A cartilage tumor that usually occurs in middle-aged and older individuals:
   a. chondrosarcoma
   b. osteosarcoma
   c. chondroblastoma
   d. rhabdomyosarcoma

8. Returning of bone to normal alignment is:
   a. immobilization
   b. traction
   c. reduction
   d. manipulation

9. Result of overuse or overextension of a ligament is:
   a. strain
   b. sprain
   c. fracture
   d. displacement

10. Primary osteoarthritis is also known as:
    a. secondary
    b. functional
    c. congenital
    d. idiopathic

■ RESPIRATORY SYSTEM
RESPIRATORY SYSTEM—ANATOMY AND TERMINOLOGY

Supplies oxygen to body and helps clean body of waste (carbon dioxide)

Two tracts (Fig. 1-15A)

- Upper respiratory tract (nose, pharynx, and larynx)

- Lower respiratory tract (trachea, bronchial tree, and lungs)

Lined with ciliated mucosa

- Purifies air by trapping irritants

Warms and humidifies air

Upper Respiratory Tract (URT)

Nose
Sense of smell (olfactory)

Moistens and warms air

Nasal septum divides interior

Sinuses (Paranasal or Accessory Sinuses) (4 pair)
Frontal

Ethmoid

Maxillary

Sphenoid

Turbinates (Conchae)
Bones on inside of nose

Divided into inferior, middle, and superior (Fig. 1-15B)

Warms and humidifies air

Pharynx (Throat)
Passageway for both food and air

Nasopharynx contains adenoids

Oropharynx contains tonsils

Laryngopharynx leads to larynx

Larynx (Voice Box) (opening to trachea)
Contains vocal cords

- Cartilages of larynx, thyroid, epiglottis, and arytenoid

Lower Respiratory Tract (LRT)

Trachea (Windpipe)—Air-Conducting Structure
Mucus-lined tube with C-shaped cartilage rings to hold windpipe open

Segmental Bronchi
Trachea divides into right and left main bronchus which further divide into lobar bronchii—3 on right, 2 on left

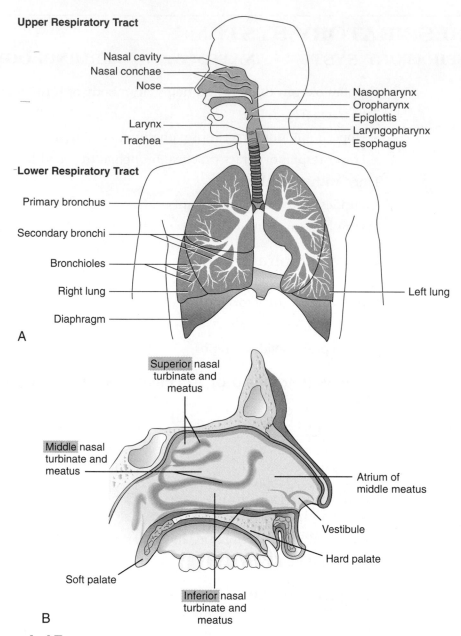

Figure **1-15 A.** Upper and lower respiratory system. **B.** Superior, inferior, and middle nasal turbinates.

Bronchioles
Branches divide into secondary bronchi, then smaller bronchioles

Alveolar Ducts (minute branches of bronchial tree)
End in alveoli (sacs) of simple squamous cells

• Primary gas-exchange units

   Surrounded by capillaries and where exchange of oxygen and carbon dioxide takes place

Lungs
Covered by pleura

Cone-shaped organs filling thoracic cavity

Base rests on diaphragm and apex (top of lungs) extends to above clavicles

Hilum is medial surface of lung where pulmonary artery, pulmonary veins, nerves, lymphatics, and bronchial tubes enter and exit

Left lung contains two lobes divided by fissures

Right lung contains three lobes

Respiration
Inspiration—oxygen moves in, downward movement of lungs enlarging thoracic cavity

Expiration—carbon dioxide moves out, upward movement of diaphragm decreasing lung space

COMBINING FORMS

1.	adenoid/o	adenoid
2.	alveol/o	alveolus
3.	atel/o	incomplete
4.	bronch/o	bronchus
5.	bronchi/o	bronchus
6.	bronchiol/o	bronchiole
7.	capn/o	carbon dioxide
8.	coni/o	dust
9.	cyan/o	blue
10.	diaphragmat/o	diaphragm
11.	epiglott/o	epiglottis
12.	laryng/o	larynx
13.	lob/o	lobe
14.	mediastin/o	mediastinum
15.	muc/o	mucus
16.	nas/o	nose
17.	orth/o	straight
18.	ox/o	oxygen
19.	oxy/o	oxygen
20.	pector/o	chest
21.	pharyng/o	pharynx
22.	phon/o	voice

23.	phren/o	diaphragm
24.	pleur/o	pleura
25.	pneum/o	lung/air
26.	pneumat/o	air
27.	pneumon/o	lung/air
28.	pulmon/o	lung
29.	py/o	pus
30.	rhin/o	nose
31.	sept/o	septum
32.	sinus/o	sinus
33.	spir/o	breath
34.	tel/o	complete
35.	thorac/o	thorax
36.	tonsill/o	tonsil
37.	trache/o	trachea

PREFIXES

1.	a-	not
2.	an-	not
3.	endo-	within
4.	eu-	good
5.	dys-	difficult
6.	pan-	all
7.	poly-	many

SUFFIXES

1.	-algia	pain
2.	-ar	pertaining to
3.	-ary	pertaining to
4.	-capnia	carbon dioxide
5.	-centesis	puncture to remove (drain)
6.	-dynia	pain
7.	-eal	pertaining to
8.	-ectasis	stretching
9.	-emia	blood
10.	-gram	record

11. -graph	recording instrument
12. -graphy	recording process
13. -itis	inflammation
14. -meter	measurement or instrument that measures
15. -metry	measurement of
16. -osmia	smell
17. -oxia	oxygen
18. -pexy	fixation
19. -phonia	sound
20. -pnea	breathing
21. -ptysis	spitting
22. -rrhage, -rrhagia	abnormal, excessive flow
23. -scopy	to examine
24. -spasm	contraction of muscle
25. -sphyxia	pulse
26. -stenosis	blockage, narrowing
27. -stomy	opening
28. -thorax	chest
29. -tomy	cutting, incision

MEDICAL ABBREVIATIONS

1. ABG	arterial blood gas
2. AFB	acid-fast bacillus
3. ARDS	adult respiratory distress syndrome
4. BiPAP	bi-level positive airway pressure
5. COPD	chronic obstructive pulmonary disease
6. CPAP	continuous positive airway pressure
7. DLCO	diffuse capacity of lungs for carbon monoxide
8. FEF	forced expiratory flow
9. FEV_1	forced expiratory volume in 1 second
10. $FEV_1:FVC$	maximum amount of forced expiratory volume in 1 second
11. FRC	functional residual capacity
12. FVC	forced vital capacity
13. HHN	hand-held nebulizer
14. IPAP	inspiratory positive airway pressure
15. IRDS	infant respiratory distress syndrome

16. MDI	metered-dose inhaler
17. MVV	maximum voluntary ventilation
18. PAWP	pulmonary artery wedge pressure
19. PCWP	pulmonary capillary wedge pressure
20. PEAP	positive end-airway pressure
21. PEEP	positive end-expiratory pressure
22. PFT	pulmonary function test
23. PND	paroxysmal nocturnal dyspnea
24. RDS	respiratory distress syndrome
25. RSV	respiratory syncytial virus
26. RV	respiratory volume
27. RV:TLC	ratio of respiratory volume to total lung capacity
28. TLC	total lung capacity
29. TLV	total lung volume
30. URI	upper respiratory infection
31. V/Q	ventilation/perfusion scan

MEDICAL TERMS

Ablation	Removal or destruction by cutting, chemicals, or electrocautery
Adenoidectomy	Removal of adenoids
Apnea	Cessation of breathing
Asphyxia	Lack of oxygen
Asthma	Shortage of breath caused by contraction of bronchi
Atelectasis	Incomplete expansion of lung, collapse
Auscultation	Listening to sounds, such as to lung sounds
Bacilli	Plural of bacillus, a rod-shaped bacteria
Bilobectomy	Surgical removal of two lobes of a lung
Bronchiole	Smaller division of bronchial tree
Bronchoplasty	Surgical repair of bronchi
Bronchoscopy	Inspection of bronchial tree using a bronchoscope
Catheter	Tube placed into body to put fluid in or take fluid out
Cauterization	Destruction of tissue by use of cautery
Cordectomy	Surgical removal of vocal cord(s)
Crackle	Abnormal sound when breathing (heard on auscultation)
Croup	Acute viral infection (obstruction of larynx), stridor
Cyanosis	Bluish discoloration

Drainage	Free flow or withdrawal of fluids from a wound or cavity
Dysphonia	Speech impairment
Dyspnea	Shortage of breath, difficult breathing
Emphysema	Air accumulated in organ or tissue
Epiglottidectomy	Excision of covering of larynx
Epistaxis	Nose bleed
Glottis	True vocal cords
Hemoptysis	Bloody sputum
Intramural	Within organ wall
Intubation	Insertion of a tube
Laryngeal web	Congenital abnormality of connective tissue between vocal cords
Laryngectomy	Surgical removal of larynx
Laryngoplasty	Surgical repair of larynx
Laryngoscope	Fiberoptic scope used to view inside of larynx
Laryngoscopy	Direct visualization and examination of interior of larynx with a laryngoscope
Laryngotomy	Incision into larynx
Lavage	Washing out
Lobectomy	Surgical excision of a lobe of lung
Nasal button	Synthetic circular disc used to cover a hole in the nasal septum
Orthopnea	Difficulty in breathing, relieved by assuming upright position
Percussion	Tapping with sharp blows as a diagnostic technique
Pertussis	Whooping cough—highly contagious bacterial infection of pharynx, larynx, and trachea
Pharyngolaryngectomy	Surgical removal of pharynx and larynx
Pleura	Covers lungs and lines thoracic cavity
Pleurectomy	Surgical excision of pleura
Pleuritis	Inflammation of pleura
Pneumocentesis/ pneumonocentesis	Surgical puncturing of a lung to withdraw fluid
Pneumonia	Inflammation of lungs with consolidation
Pneumonolysis/ pneumolysis	Surgical separation of lung from chest wall to allow lung to collapse
Pneumonotomy/ pneumotomy	Incision of lung
Pulmonary edema	Accumulation of fluid in pulmonary tissues and air spaces
Pulmonary embolism	Thrombus or other foreign material lodged in pulmonary artery or one of its branches
Rales	An abnormal respiratory sound heard in auscultation, indicating some pathologic condition

Rhinoplasty	Surgical repair of nose
Rhinorrhea	Free discharge of a thin nasal mucus
Sarcoidosis	Chronic inflammatory disease with nodules developing in lungs, lymph nodes, other organs
Segmentectomy	Surgical removal of the smaller subdivisions (segment) of lobes of a lung
Septoplasty	Surgical repair of nasal septum
Sinusotomy	Surgical incision into a sinus
Spirometry	Measuring breathing capacity
Tachypnea	Quick, shallow breathing
Thoracentesis/ thoracocentesis (pleuracentesis/ pleurocentesis)	Surgical puncture of thoracic cavity, usually using a needle, to remove fluids
Thoracoplasty	Surgical procedure that removes rib(s) and thereby allows collapse of a lung
Thoracoscopy	Use of a lighted endoscope to view pleural spaces and thoracic cavity or to perform surgical procedures
Thoracostomy	Surgical incision into chest wall and insertion of a chest tube
Thoracotomy	Surgical incision into chest wall
Total pneumonectomy	Surgical removal of an entire lung
Tracheostomy	Creation of an opening into trachea
Tracheotomy	Incision into trachea
Transtracheal	Across trachea
Tuberculosis	Infection of the lungs caused by bacteria (tubercle bacillus)

RESPIRATORY SYSTEM ANATOMY AND TERMINOLOGY QUIZ
(Quiz answers are located at the end of Unit 1)

1. This is NOT a part of lower respiratory tract:
   a. trachea
   b. larynx
   c. bronchi
   d. lungs

2. Another name for voice box is:
   a. oropharynx
   b. pharynx
   c. laryngopharynx
   d. larynx

3. This is the windpipe:
   a. pharynx
   b. larynx
   c. trachea
   d. sphenoid

4. Interior of nose is divided by the:
   a. septum
   b. sphenoid
   c. oropharynx
   d. apical

5. This combining form means "incomplete":
   a. atel/o
   b. alveol/o
   c. ox/i
   d. pneumat/o

6. This combining form means "breath":
   a. py/o
   b. lob/o
   c. spir/o
   d. pleur/o

7. This prefix means "all":
   a. a-
   b. an-
   c. pan-
   d. poly-

8. This abbreviation refers to a syndrome that involves difficulty in breathing:
   a. ABG
   b. ARDS
   c. BiPAP
   d. FEF

9. This abbreviation refers to amount of air patient can expel from the lungs in 1 second:
   a. PFT
   b. PND
   c. RDS
   d. FEV_1

10. This suffix means "breathing":
    a. -stenosis
    b. -spasm
    c. -pexy
    d. -pnea

RESPIRATORY SYSTEM—PATHOPHYSIOLOGY

Signs and Symptoms of Pulmonary Disorders

Dyspnea
Difficult breathing (sense of air hunger)

Increased respiratory effort

Hypoventilation
Decreased alveolar ventilation

Hyperventilation
Increased alveolar ventilation

Hemoptysis
Bloody sputum

Hypoxia
Reduced oxygenation of tissue cells

Cough
Caused by irritant

Protective reflex

Acute cough is up to 3 weeks

Chronic cough is over 3 weeks

Tachypnea
Rapid breathing

Apnea
Lack of breathing

Orthopnea
Requiring sitting upright to facilitate breathing

Pulmonary Diseases and Disorders

Hypercapnia
Increased carbon dioxide in arterial blood

Caused by inadequate ventilation of alveoli

Can result in respiratory acidosis

Hypoxemia
Reduced oxygenation of arterial blood

Acute Respiratory Failure
Inadequate gas exchange

Hypoxemia

Can result from trauma or disease

Adult Respiratory Distress Syndrome (ARDS)
Acute injury to alveolocapillary membrane

Results in edema and atelectasis

In infants, infant respiratory distress syndrome (IRDS)

Pulmonary Edema
Accumulation of fluid in lung tissue

Most common cause is left ventricular failure

Aspiration
Passage of fluid and solid particles into lung

Can cause severe pneumonitis

- Localized inflammation of lung

Atelectasis
Collapse of lung

Three most common types are:

- Adhesive
- Compression
- Obstruction

May be chronic or acute

- Acute, such as compression as a result of an automobile accident
- Chronic from structural defect

Absorption Atelectasis
Results from absence of air in alveoli

Caused by

Foreign body

Tumor

Abnormal external pressure

Bronchiectasis
Chronic, irreversible dilation of bronchi

Common types that describe severity of condition
- Cylindrical
- Varicose
- Sacular or cystic

Respiratory Acidosis
Decreased level of pH

Due to excess retention of carbon dioxide

Bronchiolitis
Inflammation and obstruction of bronchioles

Usually in children younger than 2 years old—preceded by URI

Viral infection (respiratory syncytial virus, or RSV)

Common types
- Constrictive
- Proliferative
- Obliterative

Pneumothorax
Air collected in pleural cavity

Leads to lung collapse

Communicating pneumothorax is barometric air pressure in pleural space

Spontaneous pneumothorax is spontaneous rupture of visceral pleura

Secondary pneumothorax is a result of trauma to chest

Pneumoconiosis
Dust particles or other particulate matter in lung

Common types
- Coal
- Asbestos
- Fiberglass

Pleural Effusion-Fluid in Pleural Space
Common types
- Hemothorax—hemorrhage into pleural cavity
- Empyema—Infectious materials in pleural space
- Exudate—Fluid remaining after infection, inflammation, malignancy

Empyema
Infectious pleural effusion
Pus in pleural space

Complication of respiratory infection

Commonly follows pneumonia and is treated like pneumonia

Pulmonary Embolism
Air, tissue, or clot occlusion

Lodges in pulmonary artery or branch of artery

Risk with congestive heart failure

Most clots originate in leg veins

Cor Pulmonale
Hypertrophy or failure of right ventricle

Result of lung, pulmonary vessels, or chest wall disorders

Acute is secondary to pulmonary embolus

Chronic is secondary to obstructive lung disease

Pleurisy (Pleuritis)
Inflammation of pleura

Often preceded by an upper respiratory infection

Infectious Disease
Upper respiratory infection (URI)
Acute inflammatory process of mucous membranes in trachea and above

Common types
- Common cold
- Croup
- Sinusitis
- Laryngitis

Lower Respiratory Infection (LRI)

Pneumonia
Inflammation of lungs with consolidation

Categorized according to causative organism

Can be caused by

    Aspiration

    Bacteria

    Protozoa

    Fungi

    Chlamydia

    Virus

Common types

    Aspiration pneumonia

    Bacterial

    Chlamydial

    Drug resistant

    Eosinophil

    Fungal

    Hospital acquired (nosocomial)

    Legionnaires' disease

    Mycoplasma

    Pneumococcal

    Viral

Tuberculosis
Communicable lung disease—airborne droplet

Caused by *Mycobacterium tuberculosis* (bacilli)

Chronic Obstructive Pulmonary Disease (COPD)
Irreversible airway obstruction that decreases expiration

Includes

Chronic bronchitis

- Bronchial spasms
- Dyspnea
- Wheezing
- Productive cough
- Cyanosis
- Chronic hypoventilation
- Polycythemia
- Cor pulmonale
- Prolonged expiration

Emphysema

- Loss of elasticity and enlargement of alveoli
- Mimics symptoms of chronic bronchitis but more exaggerated

RESPIRATORY SYSTEM PATHOPHYSIOLOGY QUIZ
(Quiz answers are located at the end of Unit 1)

1. Acute injury to alveolocapillary membrane that results in edema and atelectasis:
   a. hypoxemia
   b. adult respiratory distress syndrome
   c. bronchiolitis
   d. pneumoconiosis

2. Condition in which pus is in pleural space and is often a complication of pneumonia:
   a. empyema
   b. cor pulmonale
   c. pneumothorax
   d. atelectasis

3. Which of the following is NOT one of the most common types of atelectasis?
   a. adhesive
   b. compression
   c. obstruction
   d. expansion

4. This condition is a result of accumulation of dust particles in lung:
   a. pleurisy
   b. tuberculosis
   c. chronic obstructive pulmonary disease
   d. pneumoconiosis

5. An irreversible airway obstructive disease in which symptoms are bronchial spasm, dyspnea, and wheezing:
   a. pleurisy
   b. empyema
   c. bronchiolitis
   d. COPD

6. Cylindrical, varicose, and secular/cystic are examples of:
   a. bronchiectasis
   b. cor pulmonale
   c. pneumothorax
   d. atelectasis

7. Condition in which there is a loss of elasticity and enlargement of alveoli:
   a. chronic bronchitis
   b. asthma
   c. emphysema
   d. empyema

8. Definition of a chronic cough is one that lasts for more than this number of weeks:
   a. 2
   b. 3
   c. 4
   d. 5

9. A condition marked by an increase in carbon dioxide in arterial blood and decreased ability to breathe that can result in respiratory acidosis:
   a. hypercapnia
   b. hypoxemia
   c. acute respiratory failure
   d. pulmonary edema

10. This condition often follows a viral infection and occurs in children under 2 years of age. Examples of various types of this condition are constrictive, proliferating, and obliterative.
    a. pneumoconiosis
    b. pulmonary edema
    c. bronchiolitis
    d. bronchiectasis

■ CARDIOVASCULAR SYSTEM
CARDIOVASCULAR SYSTEM—ANATOMY AND TERMINOLOGY

Consists of blood, blood vessels, and heart

Blood (function is to maintain a constant environment)

Composed of cells suspended in plasma (clear, straw-colored liquid)

Carries
Oxygen and nutrients to cells

Waste and carbon dioxide to kidneys, liver, and lungs

Hormones from endocrine system

Regulates
Temperature by circulating blood

Protection
White cells (leukocytes) produce antibodies

Composed of Two Parts
Liquid part (extracellular) is plasma
  Water 91%

  Protein 1%, albumin, globulins, fibrinogen, ferritin, transferrin

  2% ions, nutrients, waste products, gases, regulating substances

Cellular structures
Leukocytes (WBCs)—granular and agranular—fight infections
- Neutrophils
- Lymphocytes
- Monocytes
- Eosinophils
- Basophils

Erythrocytes (red blood cells)—hemoglobin carries oxygen

Thrombocytes (platelets)—important for hemostasis

Blood types: A, B, AB, and O are genetically endowed
- Blood type O negative is known as universal donor (no Rh and no red cell antigens present)

Vessels—Circulatory System

Function

To carry blood delivering nutrients and oxygen (arterial system) and carry away cell waste and carbon dioxide (venous system)

Types
Arteries (Fig. 1-16) carrying oxygenated blood
Inner layer, endothelium

Lead away from heart

Branches are arterioles

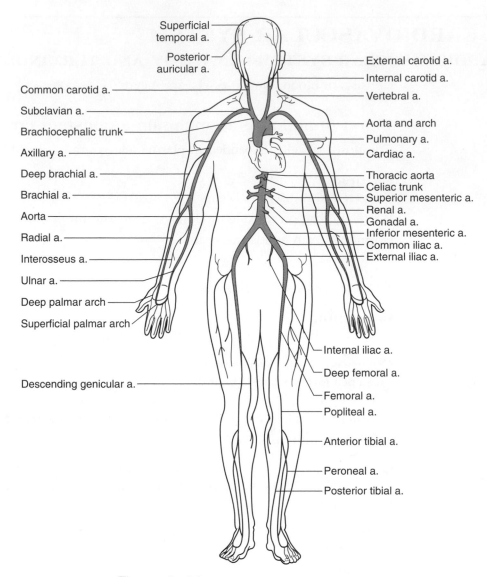

Figure **1-16** Arteries of circulatory system.

Capillaries

Connection between arterioles and venules

Exchange structure (oxygen and carbon dioxide, nutrients, and waste)

Veins (Fig. 1-17) carrying deoxygenated blood

Carry blood to heart

Venules are small branches

Heart

Circulates blood

Four Chambers (Fig. 1-18)

Two upper

Right and left atria (singular: atrium) receive blood

Two lower

Right and left ventricles discharge blood (pump)

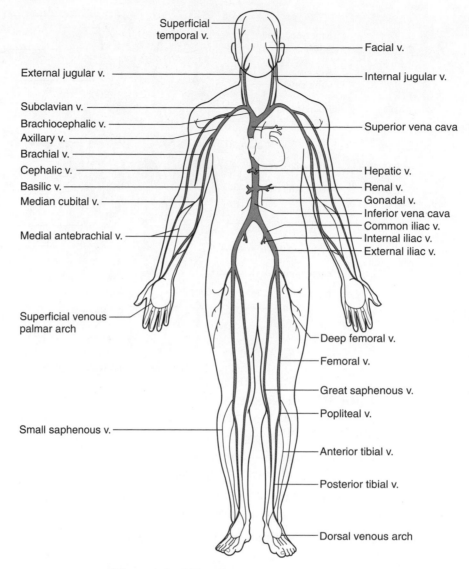

Figure **1-17** Veins of circulatory system.

Chamber Walls
Composed of three layers

- Endocardium: smooth inner layer

- Myocardium: middle muscular layer

- Epicardium: outer layer

Septa (singular: septum)
Divide chambers

- Interatrial septum

   Separates two upper chambers

- Interventricular septum

   Separates two lower chambers

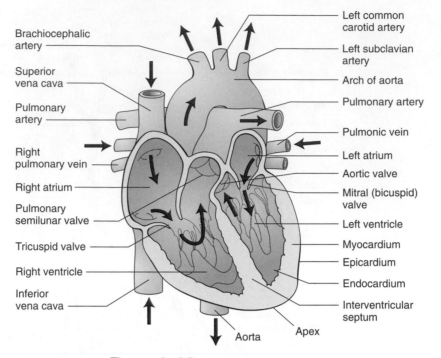

Figure **1-18** Internal view of heart.

Major Blood Vessels

Inferior vena cava—carries deoxygenated blood from lower extremities, pelvic and abdominal viscera to right atrium

Superior vena cava—drains deoxygenated blood from head, neck, upper extremities, and chest to right atrium

Pulmonary artery bifurcates and becomes right and left pulmonary artery—carries deoxygenated blood from right ventricle to lungs

Right and left pulmonary veins (4)—carry oxygenated blood from lungs to left atrium

Aorta—carries oxygenated blood from left side of heart to body

Pericardium

Sac comprised of two layers that cover heart

• Parietal pericardium: outermost covering

• Visceral pericardium: innermost (epicardium)

• Pericardial cavity: contains about 30 cc of fluid

Valves (4 in heart)

Tricuspid: between right atrium and right ventricle

Pulmonary: at entrance of pulmonary artery leading from right ventricle

Aortic: at entrance of aorta leading from left ventricle

Bicuspid (mitral): between left atrium and left ventricle

Conduction System (Fig. 1-19)

Sinoatrial node: SAN, nature's pacemaker, sends impulses to atrioventricular node

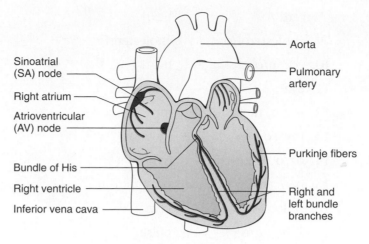

Figure **1-19** Electrical system of heart.

Atrioventricular node (AVN): located on interatrial septum and sends impulses to bundle of His

Bundle of His: divides into right bundle branch (RBB) and left bundle branch (LBB) in septum

Purkinje fibers: merge from bundle branches into specialized cells of myocardium, located in ventricular endocardium

Heartbeat

Two Phases—Correspond to Blood Pressure Readouts

Systole: contraction—top number reading

Diastole: relaxation—lower number reading

Trace a drop of blood from trunk of body (deoxygenated) to trunk of body (oxygenated)

Inferior vena cava to right atrium

Through tricuspid valve to right ventricle

From right ventricle to pulmonary artery to lung capillaries

From lung capillaries to pulmonary veins

To left atrium through mitral (bicuspid) valve to left ventricle

Though aortic valve to aorta

COMBINING FORMS

1.	angi/o	vessel
2.	aort/o	aorta
3.	ather/o	yellow plaque (fat)
4.	arter/o	artery
5.	arteri/o	artery
6.	atri/o	atrium
7.	brachi/o	arm

8.	cardi/o	heart
9.	cholesterol/o	cholesterol
10.	coron/o	heart
11.	cyan/o	blue
12.	my/o, muscul/o	muscle
13.	myx/o	mucous
14.	ox/o	oxygen
15.	pericardi/o	pericardium
16.	phleb/o	vein
17.	sphygm/o	pulse
18.	steth/o	chest
19.	thromb/o	clot
20.	valv/o	valve
21.	valvul/o	valve
22.	vascul/o	vessel
23.	vas/o	vessel
24.	ven/o	vein
25.	ventricul/o	ventricle

PREFIXES

1.	a-	not
2.	an-	not
3.	bi-	two
4.	brady-	slow
5.	de-	lack of
6.	dys-	bad, difficult, painful
7.	endo-	in
8.	hyper-	over
9.	hypo-	under
10.	inter-	between
11.	intra-	within
12.	meta-	change, after
13.	peri-	surrounding
14.	tachy-	fast
15.	tetra-	four
16.	tri-	three

SUFFIXES

1. -dilation   widening, expanding
2. -emia   blood
3. -graphy   recording process
4. -lysis   separation
5. -megaly   enlargement
6. -oma   tumor
7. -osis   condition
8. -plasty   repair
9. -sclerosis   hardening
10. -stenosis   blockage, narrowing
11. -tomy   cutting, incision

MEDICAL ABBREVIATIONS

1. ASCVD   arteriosclerotic cardiovascular disease
2. ASD   atrial septal defect
3. ASHD   arteriosclerotic heart disease
4. AV   atrioventricular
5. CABG   coronary artery bypass graft
6. CHF   congestive heart failure
7. CK   creatine kinase
8. CPK   creatine phosphokinase
9. CVI   cerebrovascular insufficiency
10. DSE   dobutamine stress echocardiography
11. HCVD   hypertensive cardiovascular disease
12. LBBB   left bundle branch block
13. LVH   left ventricular hypertrophy
14. MAT   multifocal atrial tachycardia
15. MI   myocardial infarction
16. NSR   normal sinus rhythm
17. PAC   premature atrial contraction
18. PAT   paroxysmal atrial tachycardia
19. PST/PSVT   paroxysmal supraventricular tachycardia
20. PTCA   percutaneous transluminal coronary angioplasty
21. PVC   premature ventricular contraction
22. RBBB   right bundle branch block
23. RSR   regular sinus rhythm

24.	RVH	right ventricular hypertrophy
25.	SVT	supraventricular tachycardia
26.	TEE	transesophageal echocardiography
27.	TST	treadmill stress test

MEDICAL TERMS

Acute coronary syndrome (ACS)	An umbrella term used to cover clinical symptoms compatible with acute myocardial ischemia
Anastomosis	Surgical connection of two tubular structures, such as two pieces of the intestine
Aneurysm	Abnormal dilation of vessels, usually an artery
Angina	Spasmotic, choking, or suffocative pain
Angiography	Radiography of blood vessels
Angioplasty	Procedure in a vessel to dilate vessel opening
Atherectomy	Removal of plaque from an artery (can be done by a percutaneous or open procedure)
Auscultation	Listening for sounds within body
Bundle of His	Muscular cardiac fibers that provide heart rhythm to ventricles
Bypass	To go around
Cardiopulmonary	Refers to heart and lungs
Cardiopulmonary bypass	Blood bypasses heart through a heart-lung machine
Cardioverter-defibrillator	Surgically placed or wearable device that directs an electric shock to the heart to restore rhythm
Circumflex	A coronary artery that circles heart
Cutdown	Incision into a vessel for placement of a catheter
Edema	Swelling due to abnormal fluid collection in tissue spaces
Electrode	Lead attached to a generator that carries electric current from the generator to atria or ventricles
Electrophysiology	Study of electrical system of heart, including study of arrhythmias
Embolectomy	Removal of blockage (embolism) from vessel
Endarterectomy	Incision into an artery to remove inner lining
Epicardial	Over heart
False aneurysm	Sac of clotted blood that has completely destroyed vessel and is being contained by tissue that surrounds vessel
Fistula	Abnormal opening from one area to another area or to outside of the body
Hematoma	Mass of blood that forms outside vessel
Hemolysis	Breakdown of red blood cells
Hypoxemia	Low level of oxygen in blood

Hypoxia	Low level of oxygen in tissue
Intracardiac	Inside heart
Invasive	Entering body, breaking skin
Noninvasive	Not entering body, not breaking skin
Nuclear cardiology	Diagnostic specialty that uses radiologic procedures to aid in diagnosis of cardiologic conditions
Order	Shows subordination of one thing to another; family or class
Pericardiocentesis	Procedure in which a surgeon withdraws fluid from pericardial space by means of a needle inserted percutaneously
Pericardium	Membranous sac enclosing heart and ends of great vessels
Swan-Ganz catheter	A catheter that measures pressure in right side of heart and in pulmonary artery
Thoracostomy	Incision into chest wall and insertion of a chest tube
Thromboendarterectomy	Removal of thrombus and atherosclerotic lining from an artery (percutaneous or open procedure)
Transvenous	Through a vein

CARDIOVASCULAR SYSTEM ANATOMY AND TERMINOLOGY QUIZ
(Quiz answers are located at the end of Unit 1)

1. These carry blood to the heart:
   a. capillaries
   b. arteries
   c. arterioles
   d. veins

2. Relaxation phase of heartbeat:
   a. diastole
   b. systole

3. Nature's pacemaker is this node:
   a. atrioventricular
   b. Bundle of His
   c. sinoatrial
   d. mitral

4. Node located on interatrial septum:
   a. atrioventricular
   b. Bundle of His
   c. sinoatrial
   d. Purkinje

5. Which of the following is NOT one of the three layers of chamber walls of the heart?
   a. endocardium
   b. myocardium
   c. epicardium
   d. parietal

6. Septum that divides upper two chambers of heart:
   a. intraventricular
   b. interatrial
   c. tricuspid
   d. myocardium

7. Valve between right atrium and right ventricle:
   a. pulmonary
   b. aortic
   c. bicuspid
   d. tricuspid

8. Outer two-layer covering of heart:
   a. pericardium
   b. mitral
   c. myocardium
   d. epicardium

9. These are chambers that receive blood:
   a. right and left ventricle
   b. left ventricle and right atrium
   c. right atrium and right ventricle
   d. right and left atria

10. This combining form means "plaque":
    a. atri/o
    b. brachi/o
    c. cyan/o
    d. ather/o

CARDIOVASCULAR SYSTEM—PATHOPHYSIOLOGY

Vascular Disorders

Coronary Artery Disease (CAD)/Ischemic Heart Disease (IHD)

Thickening and hardening of arterial intima (innermost layer) with lipid and fibrous plaque (atherosclerosis)

- Produces narrowing and stiffening of vessel

Location of lesions leads to various vascular diseases

- Femoral and popliteal arteries = peripheral vascular disease
- Carotid arteries = stroke
- Aorta = aneurysms (dilation/weakening of vessel walls)
- Coronary arteries = ischemic heart disease or myocardial infarction

Resulting in decreased oxygen supply

Risk factors increased by:

- Age
- Family history of CAD
- Hyperlipidemia
- Low HDL-C (good cholesterol)
- Hypertension
- Cigarette smoking
- Diabetes mellitus
- Obesity, particularly abdominal

Ischemia

Deficiency of oxygenated blood

- Often due to constriction or obstruction of blood vessel

Localized myocardial ischemia—most common cause: atherosclerosis of vessels
Oxygen demand of tissues greater than supply

Presenting symptoms

- Chest pain (angina pectoris)
- Hypotension
- Changes in ECG

Transient ischemia
Heart muscle begins to perform at a low level due to lack of oxygen (reversible ischemia)

Irreversible ischemia—is cause of an MI (myocardial infarction)
Heart muscle dies—necrosis (myocardial infarction)

- Prolonged ischemia of 30 minutes or more
- Reestablishment of blood flow reduces residual necrosis
  - Thrombolytic agents to dissolve or split up thrombus
  - Primary percutaneous transluminal coronary angioplasty (PTCA)

Cardiac enzymes are released from damaged cells

- Blood test reveals elevation of enzymes, confirming myocardial infarction

Hypertension (HTN)

Normal is less than 120/80 for adults

- Figure 1-20 illustrates new hypertension classifications

Leading cause of death in United States due to damage to brain, heart, kidneys, eyes, and arteries of the lower extremities

Cause is unknown in 95% of cases

- Known as
  - Primary hypertension
  - Essential hypertension

5% of cases are secondary to underlying disease

Increased resistance damages heart and blood vessels

- Retinal vascular changes are monitored to assess therapy and disease progression

Chronic hypertension often leads to end-stage renal disease

- Result of progressive sclerosis of renal vessels

Treatment

Medications

- ACE (angiotensin-converting enzyme) inhibitor
- Alpha-adrenergic or beta-adrenergic receptor blocker
- Diuretic
- Calcium channel blocker

Lifestyle changes

Classification of blood pressure for
adults aged 18 years or older[1]

Category	Systolic (mm Hg)	Diastolic (mm Hg)
Normal	<120	<80
Prehypertension (stays between)	120–139	80–89
Hypertension[2]		
Stage 1 (mild)	140–159	90–99
Stage 2 (moderate)	160–179	100–109
Stage 3 (severe)	≥180	≥110

[1] Not taking antihypertensive drugs and not acutely ill. When systolic and diastolic pressures fall into different categories, the higher category should be selected.

[2] Based on the average of two or more readings taken at each of two or more visits after an initial screening.

Figure **1-20** Classification of blood pressure.

Hypotension

Abnormally low blood pressure

Types

Orthostatic (postural) hypotension

- Fall in both systolic and diastolic arterial blood pressure on standing

- Associated with

  - Dizziness

  - Blurred vision

  - Fainting (syncope)

- Caused by insufficient oxygenated blood flow through brain

- Can be acute (temporary) or chronic

Chronic orthostatic hypotension—types

- Primary of unknown cause

- Secondary to certain disease processes

- Such as:

  - Endocrine

  - Metabolic

  - Central nervous system disorders

- Treatment for secondary hypotension is correction of underlying disease

Aneurysm

Dilation of an arterial blood vessel wall or cardiac chamber

- Danger is rupture of aneurysm

Atherosclerosis is common cause

Arteriosclerosis and hypertension also common in persons with aneurysms

True aneurysm

Involves all three layers of arterial wall

Causes weakening and ballooning of arterial wall

False or pseudoaneurysm

Usually result of trauma

Also known as saccular

Separation of arterial wall layers (dissecting) in artery wall (crisis situation—a medical emergency)

Bleeds into dissected space and is contained by arterial connective tissue wall

Thrombus

Blood clot that remains attached to vessel wall and occludes vessel

Dislodged thrombus is a thromboembolus

Causes

Trauma

Interior wall lining irritation/roughening

Infection

Inflammation

Low blood pressure/blood stagnation

Obstruction

Atherosclerosis

Risks related to thrombus

Dislodges and moves to lungs, brain, heart

Grows to occlude blood flow

Treatment

Pharmacologic, anticoagulants

Heparin

Warfarin derivatives

Noninvasive intervention

Balloon-tipped catheter to remove or compress thrombus

Thrombophlebitis Caused by Inflammation (Phlebitis)

Causes

Trauma

Infection

Immobility

Commonly associated with

Endocarditis

Rheumatic heart disease

Embolism

Mass that is present and circulating in blood

Common types

Air bubble

Fat

Bacterial mass

Cancer cells

Foreign substances

Dislodged thrombus

Amniotic fluid

Obstructs vessel

Pulmonary emboli travel through venous side or right side of the heart to the pulmonary artery

Systemic or arterial emboli originate in left side of the heart

Associated with

- Myocardial infarction

- Left-sided heart failure

- Endocarditis
- Valvular conditions
- Dysrhythmias

Peripheral Arterial Disease

Thromboangiitis obliterans (Buerger's disease)
Occurs most often in young men who are heavy smokers

Inflammatory disease of peripheral arteries creating thombi and vasospasms

Involves small or medium arteries of feet and often hands

- May necessitate amputation

Raynaud's disease
Vasospasms and constriction of small arterioles of fingers and toes

Affects young women as a secondary condition

Triggered by cold temperatures, emotional stress, cigarette smoking

Fingertips thicken and nails become brittle

Raynaud's phenomenon is secondary to primary disease, such as

- Scleroderma
- Pulmonary hypertension

Treatment of underlying condition
No known origin or treatment

Varicose Veins
Blood pools in veins, distending them

Tends to be progressive/vein valve failure

Occurs most commonly in saphenous veins

Hemorrhoids are varicose veins of anus

Leads to
Swelling and discomfort

Fatigue when in legs

Possible ulcerations

Heart Disorders

Congestive Heart Failure (CHF)—heart cannot pump required amounts of blood
Can be left-sided or right-sided heart failure

Left-sided heart failure (systolic); cannot generate adequate output, causing pulmonary edema

Common causes:

Myocardial infarction

Myocarditis

Cardiomyopathies leading to ischemia

Symptoms of left-sided congestive heart failure include:

Shortness of breath

Fatigue

Exercise intolerance

Right-sided heart failure (diastolic) results in right ventricle stasis, inadequate pulmonary circulation, and peripheral edema/hepatosplenomegaly

Abnormal Heart Rhythms (Conduction Irregularities)

Bradycardia and heart block (atrioventricular block)

Inadequate conduction impulses from SA node though AV node to AV bundle

Treatment

Cardiac pacemaker to maintain proper heart rate

Flutter—rapid regular contractions (most commonly of atria)

Symptoms—palpitations

Treatment

Cardioversion (electronic shock to heart)

Ablation (radiofrequency catheter destroying tissue causing arrhythmia)

Fibrillation—rapid, erratic, inefficient contractions of atria and ventricles

Atrial fibrillation—most common (electrical impulses move randomly in atria)

Symptoms—palpitation, risk of stroke due to clot formations from poor atrial outputs

Treatment

Cardioversion

Ablation

Ventricular fibrillation—life-threatening, random electrical impulses throughout ventricles

Symptoms—cardiac death or arrest without immediate treatment

Treatment

Cardioversion

Digoxin—drug used to slow heart rate

Implantable cardioverter-defibrillator (ICD)

Emergency treatment—automatic external defibrillators (AEDs)

Radiofrequency catheter ablation (RFA) is a minimally invasive technique used to treat cardiac arrhythmias

Infective Endocarditis

Inflammation of interior-most lining of heart

Leads to destruction and permanent damage to heart valves

Caused by

    Bacteria (most common: streptococci and staphylococci)

    Virus

    Fungi

    Parasites

Patients with heart defects or damage usually take antibiotics prior to invasive procedures

Pericarditis
Inflammation of pericardium of heart

Common types

- Acute

- Pericardial effusion

- Constrictive

Rheumatic Fever/Rheumatic Heart Disease
Results in formation of scar tissue of the endocardium and heart valves

In 10% of cases leads to rheumatic heart disease

Family tendency to develop

Begins as carditis (inflammation of all layers of heart wall)

Long-term effects:

Mitral and/or aortic valve disease

    Stenosis

    Regurgitation

    Insufficiency

Tricuspid valve

    Affected in about 10% of cases

Pulmonary valve

    Rarely affected

Valvular Heart Disease

Valves are extensions of endocardial tissue

Endocardial damage can be congenital or acquired

Damage leads to stenosis and/or incompetent valve

Includes

- Valvular stenosis is narrowing, stiffness, thickening, fusion, or blockage of valve, creating resistance, resulting in increased pressure in cardiac chamber behind valve

- Valvular regurgitation is failure of valve leaflet to close tightly, allowing backflow of blood

  - Result of lesions causing valve leaflets to shrink

  - Functional valvular regurgitation results in increased chamber size (cardiomegaly)

Stenosis

Aortic valve stenosis

Caused by

Congenital malformation

Degeneration

Infection

Results in slowing blood circulatory rate

Symptoms

Bradycardia

Faint pulse

May lead to heart murmur and hypertrophy

Mitral valve stenosis

Impaired flow from left atrium to left ventricle

Caused by

Rheumatic fever

Bacterial infections

Symptom

Decreased cardiac output

May lead to

- Pulmonary hypertension

- Right ventricular heart failure

- And/or edema

Valvular Regurgitation

Flow in opposite direction from normal

Mitral regurgitation (MR)

Backflow of blood from left ventricle into left atrium

Aortic regurgitation (AR)

Backflow of blood from aorta into left ventricle

Pulmonic regurgitation (PR)

Backflow of blood from pulmonary artery into right ventricle

Tricuspid regurgitation (TR)

Backflow of blood from right ventricle into right atrium

Heart Wall Disorders

Acute Pericarditis

Roughening and inflammation of pericardium (sac around heart)

Treatment

Anti-inflammatory drugs and pain medication

Constrictive Pericarditis (Restrictive Pericarditis)
Forms fibrous lesions that encase heart

Compresses heart—thickened pericardial sac prevents heart from expanding when blood enters it

> Tamponade occurs when fluid builds up in pericardial space

> Pressure stops heart from beating—pericardial effusion or bleeding after heart surgery

Reduces output

Pericardial Effusion
Accumulation of fluid in pericardial cavity

Results in pressure on heart

- Sudden development of pressure on heart is tamponade

Cardiomyopathies

Myocardium: muscular wall (middle layer) of heart musculature

Group of diseases that affect myocardium

Cause

> Idiopathic (most common)

> Underlying condition

Types of Cardiomyopathy
Dilated cardiomyopathy (congestive cardiomyopathy)

- Ventricular distention and impaired systolic function

Hypertrophic cardiomyopathy

- Cause is often hypertensive or valvular heart disease
- Results in thickened interventricular septum (septum between the ventricle chambers)

Restrictive cardiomyopathy

- Myocardium becomes stiffened
- Heart enlarges (cardiomegaly)
- Dysrhythmias common
- Caused by infiltrative diseases such as amyloidosis

Congenital Heart Defects

Coarctation of aorta (CoA)—narrowing of the aorta

- Treatment

> Surgical removal of narrow segment/end-to-end anastomosis

Patent ductus arteriosus (PDA)—opening between aorta and pulmonary artery

- Treatment

> Drugs to close/embolize or plug ductus or tying off surgically

Tetralogy of Fallot—malformation of heart includes four defects

1. Pulmonary artery stenosis
   - Narrowing/obstruction
2. Ventricular septal defect
   - Hole between two bottom chambers (ventricles) of heart
3. Overriding aorta
   - Shift of aorta to right—aorta overrides the interventricular septum
4. Hypertrophy of right ventricle
   - Myocardium enlarges to pump blood through narrowed pulmonary artery

Treatment

- Open-heart technique with heart-lung machine support to relieve right ventricular outflow tract stenosis and repair of ventriculoseptal defect

CARDIOVASCULAR SYSTEM PATHOPHYSIOLOGY QUIZ
(Quiz answers are located at the end of Unit 1)

1. Lesion of carotid artery may lead to:
   a. heart attack
   b. stroke
   c. peripheral vascular disease
   d. ischemic heart disease

2. This blood pressure is hypertension:
   a. 120/80
   b. 130/70
   c. 140/90
   d. 110/70

3. Infective endocarditis is inflammation of the interior of the lining of the heart, and when caused by streptococci or staphylococci, the infection is:
   a. viral
   b. fungal
   c. bacterial
   d. parasitic

4. Angina pectoris is:
   a. heart block
   b. heart murmur
   c. chest pain
   d. barrel chest

5. In this type of regurgitation, there is a backflow of blood from left ventricle into left atrium:
   a. aortic
   b. pulmonic
   c. tricuspid
   d. mitral

6. In this type of heart wall disorder, fibrous lesions form and encase the heart:
   a. constrictive pericarditis
   b. acute pericarditis
   c. pericardial effusion
   d. cardiomyopathy

7. Which of the following terms means "of unknown cause"?
   a. etiology
   b. manifestation
   c. idiopathic
   d. late effect

8. This condition is also known as congestive cardiomyopathy:
   a. hypertrophic
   b. valvular
   c. dilated
   d. restrictive

9. This peripheral arterial disease most often occurs in young men who are heavy smokers:
   a. Buerger's
   b. Pick's
   c. Addison's
   d. Glasser's

10. This cardiomyopathy results in a thickened interventricular septum:
    a. restrictive
    b. congestive
    c. dilated
    d. hypertrophic

■ FEMALE GENITAL SYSTEM AND PREGNANCY

FEMALE GENITAL SYSTEM AND PREGNANCY—ANATOMY AND TERMINOLOGY

Terminology

Ovaries (Pair)

Produce ova (single female gamete) and hormones; ova: plural; ovum: singular (Fig. 1-21). Each ovum/gamete contains 23 chromosomes.

Fallopian Tubes (Uterine Tubes or Oviducts)

Ducts from ovary to uterus

Uterus (Womb)

Muscular organ that holds embryo

Three layers

- Endometrium: inner mucosa
- Myometrium: middle layer/muscle
- Perimetrium/Uterine serosa: outer layer
  - Cervix: lower narrow portion of uterus
  - Fundus: the upper rounded part of the uterus

Vagina

Tube from uterus to outside of body

Vulva

External genitalia

- Clitoris: erectile tissue
- Labia majora: outer lips of vagina
- Labia minora: inner lips of vagina
- Urinary meatus: opening to urethra
- Bartholin's gland: glands on either side of vagina
- Hymen: membrane partially or wholly occludes entrance to vagina

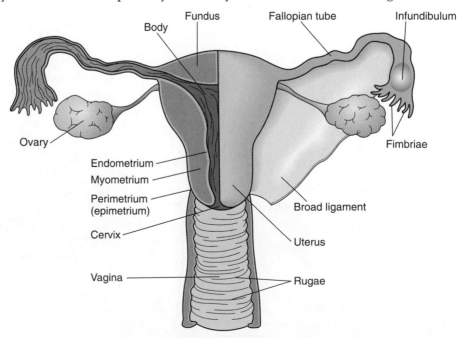

Figure **1-21** Female reproductive system.

Perineum

Area between anus and vaginal orifice

Accessory Organs (Fig. 1-22)

Breasts

Mammary glands

Composed of glandular tissue containing milk glands/lactiferous ducts

In response to hormones from pituitary gland, milk is produced in acini (also known as alveolua) (lactation)

Lactiferous ducts transfer milk to nipple

Nipple, surrounded by areola

Menstruation and Pregnancy

Proliferation Phase

Menstruation (Days 1-5): discharge of blood fluid containing endometrial cells, blood cells, and glandular secretions from endometrium

Endometrium repair (Days 6-12): maturing follicle in ovary produces estrogen (hormone) which causes endometrium to thicken and ovum (egg) to mature in graafian follicle

Secretory Phase

Ovulation (Days 13-14): occurs when graafian follicle ruptures and ovum travels down fallopian tube

Usually only one graafian follicle develops each month

Premenstruation (Days 15-28): a period of time in which graafian follicle converts to corpus luteum secreting progesterone to stimulate build-up of uterine lining. If after 5 days no fertilization occurs, cycle repeats.

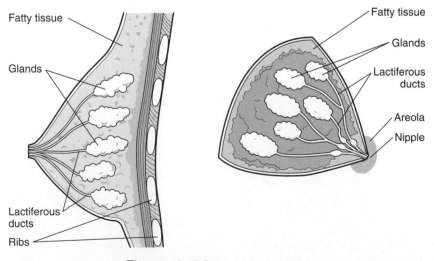

Figure **1-22** Breast structure.

Pregnancy

Prenatal stage of development from fertilization to birth (39 weeks)

Fertilized ovum or zygote develops in a double cavity: yolk sac (produces blood cells) and amniotic cavity (contains amniotic fluid)

Embryo, stage of development from 4th to 8th week

Fetus, unborn offspring, 9 weeks until birth

Placenta Forms Within Uterine Wall and Produces Hormone—Human Chorionic Gonadotropin (HCG)

HCG is hormone tested in urine pregnancy tests

HCG stimulates corpus luteum to produce estrogen and progesterone until the third month of pregnancy

Placenta then produces hormones

Expelled after delivery (afterbirth)

Gestation, Approximately 266 Days

280 days used when calculating estimated date of delivery (EDD) or time from last menstrual period (LMP)

Three trimesters

- First   LMP-12 weeks
- Second   13-27 weeks
- Third   28 weeks-EDD

COMBINING FORMS

1. amni/o	amnion
2. arche/o	first
3. cephal/o	head
4. cervic/o	cervix
5. chori/o	chorion
6. colp/o	vagina
7. crypt/o	hidden
8. culd/o	cul-de-sac
9. episi/o	vulva
10. fet/o	fetus
11. galact/o	milk
12. gynec/o	female
13. gyn/o	female
14. hymen/o	hymen
15. hyster/o	uterus
16. lact/o	milk

17.	lapar/o	abdominal wall
18.	mamm/o	breast
19.	mast/o	breast
20.	men/o	menstruation, month
21.	metr/o	uterus, measure
22.	metr/i	uterus
23.	my/o, muscul/o	muscle
24.	nat/a	birth
25.	nat/i	birth
26.	obstetr/o	pregnancy/childbirth
27.	olig/o	few
28.	oo/o	egg
29.	oophor/o	ovary
30.	ov/o	egg
31.	ovari/o	ovary
32.	ovul/o	ovulation
33.	perine/o	perineum
34.	peritone/o	peritoneum
35.	phor/o	to bear
36.	salping/o	uterine tube, fallopian tube
37.	top/o	place
38.	uter/o	uterus
39.	vagin/o	vagina
40.	vulv/o	vulva

PREFIXES

1.	ante-	before
2.	dys-	painful
3.	ecto-	outside
4.	endo-	in
5.	extra-	outside
6.	in-	into
7.	intra-	within
8.	multi-	many
9.	neo-	new
10.	nulli-	none
11.	nulli-	none

12. post-   after
13. primi-   first
14. pseudo-   false
15. retro-   backwards
16. uni-   one

SUFFIXES

1. -arche   beginning
2. -cyesis   pregnancy
3. -gravida   pregnancy
4. -rrhexis   rupture
5. -para   woman who has given birth
6. -parous   to bear
7. -rrhea   discharge
8. -salpinx   uterine tube
9. -tocia   labor
10. -version   turning

MEDICAL ABBREVIATIONS

1. AFI   amniotic fluid index
2. AGA   appropriate for gestational age
3. ARM   artificial rupture of membrane
4. BPD   biparietal diameter
5. BPP   biophysical profile
6. BV   bacterial vaginosis
7. CHL   crown-to-heel length
8. CNM   certified nurse midwife
9. CPD   cephalopelvic disproportion
10. CPP   chronic pelvic pain
11. D&C   dilation and curettage
12. D&E   dilation and evacuation
13. DUB   dysfunctional uterine bleeding
14. ECC   endocervical curettage
15. EDC   estimated date of confinement
16. EDD   estimated date of delivery
17. EFM   electronic fetal monitoring
18. EFW   estimated fetal weight

19.	EGA	estimated gestational age
20.	EMC	endometrial curettage
21.	ERT	estrogen replacement therapy
22.	FAS	fetal alcohol syndrome
23.	FHR	fetal heart rate
24.	FSH	follicle-stimulating hormone
25.	HPV	human papillomavirus
26.	HSG	hysterosalpingogram
27.	HSV	herpes simplex virus
28.	IVF	in vitro fertilization
29.	LEEP	loop electrosurgical excision procedure
30.	LGA	large for gestational age
31.	PID	pelvic inflammatory disease
32.	PROM	premature rupture of membranes
33.	SHG	sonohysterogram
34.	SROM	spontaneous rupture of membranes
35.	SUI	stress urinary incontinence
36.	TAH	total abdominal hysterectomy
37.	VBAC	vaginal birth after cesarean

MEDICAL TERMS

Abortion	Termination of pregnancy
Amniocentesis	Percutaneous aspiration of amniotic fluid
Amniotic sac	Sac containing fetus and amniotic fluid
Antepartum	Before childbirth
Cesarean	Surgical opening through abdominal wall for delivery
Chorionic villus sampling	CVS, biopsy of outermost part of placenta
Cordocentesis	Procedure to obtain a fetal blood sample; also called a percutaneous umbilical blood sampling
Curettage	Scraping of a cavity using a spoon-shaped instrument
Cystocele	Herniation of bladder into vagina
Delivery	Childbirth
Dilation	Expansion (of cervix)
Ectopic	Pregnancy outside uterus (i.e., in fallopian tube)
Hysterectomy	Surgical removal of uterus
Hysterorrhaphy	Suturing of uterus
Hysteroscopy	Visualization of canal and cavity of uterus using a scope placed through vagina

Introitus	Opening or entrance to vagina
Ligation	Binding or tying off, as in constricting blood flow of a vessel or binding fallopian tubes for sterilization
Multipara	More than one pregnancy
Oophorectomy	Surgical removal of ovary(ies)
Perineum	Area between vulva and anus; also known as pelvic floor
Placenta	A structure that connects fetus and mother during pregnancy
Postpartum	After childbirth
Primigravida	First pregnancy
Primipara	First delivered infant/given birth to only one child
Salpingectomy	Surgical removal of uterine tube
Salpingostomy	Creation of a fistula into uterine tube
Tocolysis	Repression of uterine contractions
Vesicovaginal fistula	Abnormal opening/channel between vagina and bladder

**FEMALE GENITAL SYSTEM AND PREGNANCY ANATOMY
AND TERMINOLOGY QUIZ**
(Quiz answers are located at the end of Unit 1)

1. This is NOT one of the three layers of uterus:
   a. perimetrium
   b. endometrium
   c. myometrium
   d. barametrium

2. Located at the lower end of uterus is the:
   a. cervix
   b. vagina
   c. perineum
   d. labia majora

3. Approximate gestation of a human fetus is:
   a. 266 days
   b. 276 days
   c. 290 days
   d. 292 days

4. LMP is the:
   a. later maternity phase
   b. last menstrual period
   c. low metabolic pregnancy
   d. late menstruation phase

5. Name of stage that describes development of fetus from fertilization to birth is:
   a. postpartum
   b. antepartum
   c. prenatal
   d. natal

6. Which of the following correctly identifies three trimesters of gestation?
   a. LMP-12 weeks, 13-27 weeks, 28 weeks-EDD
   b. LMP-14 weeks, 15-27 weeks, 28 weeks-EDD
   c. LMP-14 weeks, 15-28 weeks, 29 weeks-EDD
   d. LMP-11 weeks, 12-26 weeks, 27 weeks-EDD

7. Combining form meaning "few":
   a. oopho/o
   b. olig/o
   c. nati/i
   d. top/o

8. Combining form meaning "hidden":
   a. amni/o
   b. crypt/o
   c. chori/o
   d. fet/o

9. Suffix meaning "beginning":
   a. -cyesis
   b. -rrhea
   c. -arche
   d. -orrhexis

10. Prefix meaning "within":
   a. ante-
   b. dys-
   c. ecto-
   d. endo-

FEMALE GENITAL SYSTEM AND PREGNANCY—PATHOPHYSIOLOGY

Menstrual and Hormonal Disorders

Dysmenorrhea

Painful menstruation

Common types
- Primary and secondary

Primary dysmenorrhea

No underlying condition but begins with commencement of ovulation

Cramping is caused by excess of prostaglandin

- Causes contractions and uterine ischemia
- Develops 24 to 48 hours prior to menstruation

Treatment
- Nonsteroidal antiinflammatory agents
- Progesterone

Secondary dysmenorrhea

Caused by an underlying disorder, such as

- Polyps
- Tumors
- Endometriosis
- Pelvic inflammatory disease

Treatment

Directed at underlying disorder

Amenorrhea

Amenorrhea is absence of menstruation

Common types
- Primary and secondary

Primary amenorrhea

Menstruation has never occurred

May be genetic disorder

- Turner's syndrome (ovaries do not function)

Secondary amenorrhea

Cessation of menstruation for 3 cycles or 6 months

- Individual has previously menstruated

Various causes of annovulation/amenorrhea

> ***Examples:***
> - Tumors
> - Stress
> - Eating disorders
> - Competitive sports participation

Dysfunctional Uterine Bleeding (DUB)
Abnormal bleeding patterns

Occurs when no organic cause can be identified

Abnormal Menstruation Types
Oligomenorrhea: in excess of 6 weeks between periods

Polymenorrhea: less than 3 weeks between periods

Metrorrhagia: bleeding between cycles

Menorrhagia: increase in amount and duration of flow

Hypomenorrhea: light or spotty flow

Menometrorrhagia: irregular cycle with varying amounts and duration of flow

Menorrhea: lengthy menstrual flow

Dysmenorrhea: painful menstruation

Premenstrual Syndrome (PMS)
Also known as premenstrual tension (PMT)

Occurs before onset of menses (luteal phase) and ends at onset of menses

Cluster of common symptoms
Weight gain

Breast tenderness

Sleep disturbances

Headache

Irritability

Cause is unknown

Treatment
- Varies depending on individual symptoms

Endometriosis
Endometrial tissue (uterine lining) develops outside the uterus (on ovaries, fallopian tubes, small intestine, etc.)

Responses to hormone cycle
Ectopic (out of place) endometrial tissue degenerates, sheds, and bleeds

Causes
- Irritation

- Inflammation

- Pain

Continued cycles produce fibrous tissue

- Adhesions and obstructions can then form

- Interferes with normal bodily function

- For example, fallopian tube endometriosis may lead to obstructed tubes

Primary symptom is dysmenorrhea

- May also cause painful intercourse (dyspareunia)

Risks
Increased risk for cancers

- Breast

- Ovaries

- Non-Hodgkin lymphoma

Treatment Includes
Hormonal suppression

Surgical removal of endometrial tissue

- May require hysterectomy and BSO (bilateral salpingo-oophorectomy)

Infection, Inflammation, and Sexually Transmitted Diseases

Pelvic Inflammatory Disease (PID)

Infection and inflammation of reproductive tract

- Primarily ovaries and fallopian tubes

- Usually originates in cervix or vagina

  - Migrates up through reproductive tract

Types
Acute

Chronic

Commonly forms adhesions and strictures

- May lead to infertility

Candidiasis

Yeast infection

- *Candida albicans (Monilia)*

Not sexually transmitted

Opportunistic infection may follow

- Infection treated with antibiotics

- Period of reduced resistance

- Increased glucose or glycogen levels (often associated with diabetes mellitus)

Affects mucous membranes

Produces a white, thick, curdlike discharge

Result may be dyspareunia and dysuria

Treatment
Antifungal substances such as nystatin

Identification and treatment of underlying condition

Chlamydia

Most common sexually transmitted disease (STD)

Cause
　Bacteria, *Chlamydia trachomatis*

Symptoms
　Asymptomatic or mild discharge and dysuria

Treatment
　Antimicrobial

Genital Herpes
Cause
　Virus, herpes simplex 2 (HSV-2)

Symptoms
　Ulcers and vesicles

Treatment
　Antiviral, manage outbreaks

There is no cure for genital herpes

Genital Warts
Cause
　Virus, human papillomavirus

Symptoms
　Polyps or grey lesions

Treatment
　Excision

Prevention
　Vaccine

There is no cure for genital warts

Gonorrhea
Cause
　Bacteria, *Neisseria gonorrhoeae*

Symptoms
　Dysuria

　Discharge

Treatment
　Antibacterial drugs

Some strains are drug-resistant

Syphilis
Cause
　Bacteria, *Treponema pallidum*

Symptoms
　Primary syphilis

　　• Ulcer or chancre at site of entry

Secondary syphilis

- Headache

- Fever

- Rash

- Tertiary

  - Affects cardiovascular and nervous systems

Treatment
Penicillin

Trichomoniasis

Cause
Protozoan, *Trichomonas vaginalis*

Symptoms
Usually asymptomatic

Treatment
Antimicrobial drugs

Benign Lesions

Leiomyomas—Uterine Fibroids
Well-defined, solid uterine tumor

Also known as

- Uterine fibroids

- Fibromyoma

- Fibroma

- Myoma

- Fibroid

Classification is based on location of tumor within uterine wall

Submucous: beneath endometrium

Subserous: beneath serosa

Intramural: in muscle wall

Symptoms
May be asymptomatic

Abnormal uterine bleeding

Pressure on nearby structures, such as bladder and rectum

Constipation

Pain

Sensation of heaviness

Treatment
Surgical excision of lesions

Hysterectomy may be necessary

Adenomyosis
Within uterine myometrium

Symptoms
> Usually asymptomatic
>
> Abnormal menstrual bleeding
>
> Enlarged uterus

Commonly develops in late reproductive years

Common in those taking Tamoxifen

Treatment
> Symptomatic in mild cases
>
> Surgical in severe cases
>
> - Excision of adenomyosis or hysterectomy

Malignant Lesions

Carcinoma of Breast
Accessory of reproductive system

Most often develops in upper outer quadrant

- Due to location, often spreads to lymph nodes
- May metastasize to lungs, brain, bone, liver, etc.

Majority arise from epithelial cells of ducts and lobules

Second most common cancer of women

Most are adenocarcinoma

- Invasive ductal carcinoma most common type
- Invasive lobular carcinoma second most common type
- Lymph node spread is determined by sentinel node biopsy (SNB)
- Small primary tumors are excised in a lumpectomy (tumor and immediate surrounding tissue only)
- Mastectomy is alternative surgical procedure removing entire breast
- Chemotherapy and radiation may be indicated to prevent reoccurrence

If neoplasm is responsive to hormone, hormone-blocking agents are administered

Increased risks
> - Heredity
>   - Especially history of mother or sister who developed breast cancer
>   - Mutated breast cancer gene (BRCA-1)
>   - Familial breast cancer syndrome associated with BRCA-2
> - Lower socioeconomic status
> - Radiation exposure

Carcinoma of Uterus (Endometrial Cancer)

Most frequent pelvic cancer

Usually postmenopausal

Associated with higher levels of estrogen

Increases risk

Obesity (estrogen produced by fat tissue)

Early menarche

Delayed menopause

Hypertension

Diabetes mellitus

Nulliparity (no viable births)

Some types of colorectal cancer

Oral contraceptives (estrogen)

Estrogen-producing tumors

Symptoms

Abnormal, excessive uterine bleeding

Postmenopausal bleeding

No simple screening test available

• Uterine cells may be aspirated for evaluation

Staging of endometrial, cervical, and ovarian malignancies

I—Confined to corpus

II—Involves corpus and cervix

III—Extends outside uterus but not outside true pelvis

IV—Extends outside true pelvis or involves rectum or bladder

Treatment

Pharmaceutical

Surgical

Irradiation

Chemotherapy

Combination of above

Carcinoma of Cervix

Routinely found on Papanicolaou (Pap) smear

Dysplasia is an early change in cervical epithelium

Increases risks

Herpes simplex virus type 2 (HSV-2)

Human papillomavirus (HPV)

Young age of sexual activity

Smoking

Lower socioeconomic status

Stages of cervical cancer

Stage 1—Carcinoma of cervix

Stage 2—Carcinoma spread from cervix to upper vagina

Stage 3—Carcinoma spread to lower portion of vagina/pelvic wall

Stage 4—Most invasive stage spreading to other body parts

Symptoms

Early stages asymptomatic

Later stages

- Bleeding

- Discharge

Biopsy is used to confirm

Treatment

Pharmaceutical

Surgical

Irradiation

Chemotherapy

Combination of above

Carcinoma of Ovary

Cause is unknown—considered silent killer

Increased risks

Genetic factors (BRCA-1)

Endocrine

- Nulliparous

- Early menarche

- Late menopause

- Non–breast feeding

- Late first pregnancy

- Postmenopausal estrogen replacement therapy (ERT)

Tumor categories

Germ cell tumors

Arise from primitive germ cells, usually the testis and ovum

Types

- Germinoma

- Yolk sac

- Endodermal sinus tumor
- Teratoma
- Embryonal carcinoma
- Polyembryoma
- Gonadoblastoma
- Some types of choriocarcinoma

Categories

- Dermoid cysts (benign)
- Malignant tumors
- Primitive malignant
  - Embryonic
  - Extraembryonic cells

Epithelial tumors
Most common gynecologic cancer

Gonadal stromal tumors
Symptoms
  Pelvic heaviness

  Dysuria

  Increased urinary frequency

  Sometimes vaginal bleeding

Treatment
  Excision

    Hysterectomy, including bilateral salpingo-oophorectomy with omentectomy (fold of peritoneum)

  Chemotherapy

  Radiation therapy

  Combination of above

Carcinoma of Fallopian Tubes
Primary fallopian tube tumors
Rare

Must be located within tube to be considered primary

- Adenocarcinoma most common primary tumor

Most tumors are secondary

Symptoms
  Often asymptomatic

  Bleeding or discharge

  Irregular menstruation

  Pain

Treatment

> Hysterectomy, including bilateral salpingo-oophorectomy with any necessary omentectomy (fold of peritoneum)
>
> Chemotherapy
>
> Radiation therapy
>
> Combination of above

Carcinoma of Vulva

Usually squamous cell carcinoma (90%)

Increased risk with STDs

Symptoms

> Can be asymptomatic
>
> Pruritic vulvular lesion

Treatment

> Radical vulvectomy with node dissection
>
> Wide local excision

Carcinoma of Vagina

Usually squamous cell carcinoma

Increased risk

> Human papillomavirus (HPV)
>
> Postmenopausal hysterectomy
>
> History of abnormal Pap
>
> History of other carcinomas

Symptoms

> Often asymptomatic
>
> Vaginal pain, discharge, or bleeding

Treatment

> Squamous cell—radiation
>
> Early tumors may be excised
>
> Vaginectomy
>
> Hysterectomy
>
> Lymph node dissection

Pregnancy

Placenta Previa

Opening of cervix is obstructed by displaced placenta

Types (Fig. 1-23)

> Marginal
>
> Partial
>
> Total

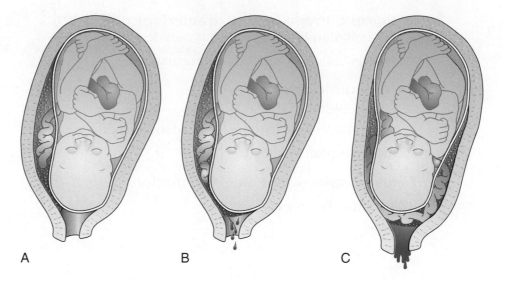

Figure **1-23** **A.** Marginal placenta previa. **B.** Partial placenta previa. **C.** Total placenta previa.

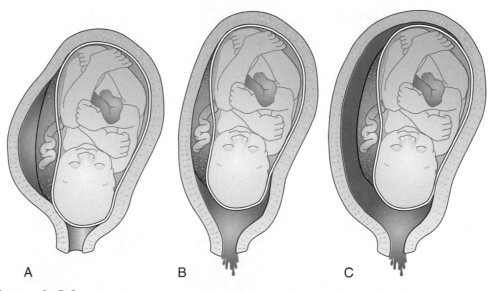

Figure **1-24** Abruptio placentae is classified according to the grade of separation of the placenta from uterine wall. **A.** Mild separation in which hemorrhage is internal. **B.** Moderate separation in which there is external hemorrhage. **C.** Severe separation in which there is external hemorrhage and extreme separation.

Abruptio Placentae (Fig. 1-24)
Premature separation of placenta from uterine wall

Eclampsia
Serious condition of pregnancy characterized by

- Hypertension
- Edema
- Proteinuria

Ectopic Pregnancy (Extrauterine) (Fig. 1-25)
Implantation of fertilized ovum outside uterus

- Often fallopian tubes (tubal pregnancy)

Hydatidiform Mole
Benign tumor of placenta

Secretes hormone (chorionic gonadotropic hormone, CGH)

Indicates positive pregnancy test

Malpositions and Malpresentations (Fig. 1-26)
Vaginal Delivery

Breech

Vertex

Face

Brow

Shoulder

Abortion
Types

Spontaneous

- Miscarriage
- Happens naturally
- Uterus completely empties

Incomplete

- Uterus does not completely empty
- Requires intervention to remove remaining fetal material

Missed

- Fetus dies naturally
- Requires intervention to remove fetal material

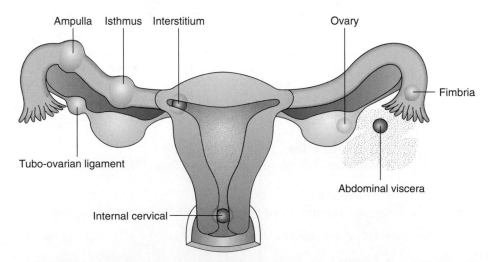

Figure **1-25** Ectopic pregnancy most often occurs in fallopian tube. Pregnancy outside the uterus may end in life-threatening rupture.

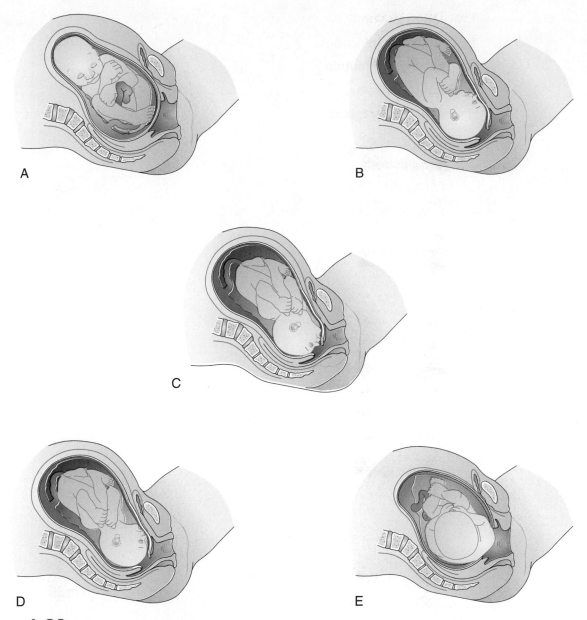

Figure **1-26** Five types of malposition and malpresentation of fetus: **A.** Breech. **B.** Vertex. **C.** Face. **D.** Brow. **E.** Shoulder.

Septic

- Similar to missed

- Has added complication of infection

- Requires intervention to remove fetal material

- Vigorous treatment of infection

Methods
    D&C

- Dilation and curettage (scraping)

Evacuation (suction)

Intra-amniotic injections

- Saline (salt) solution

Vaginal suppositories

- Such as prostaglandin

FEMALE GENITAL SYSTEM AND PREGNANCY PATHOPHYSIOLOGY QUIZ
(Quiz answers are located at the end of Unit 1)

1. Most common solution used for intra-amniotic injections is:
   a. prostaglandin
   b. saline
   c. estrogen
   d. chorionic gonadotropic hormone

2. This type of dysmenorrhea is treated with nonsteroidal antiinflammatory agents and progesterone:
   a. secondary
   b. constrictive
   c. periodic
   d. primary

3. In this type of amenorrhea there is a cessation of menstruation:
   a. secondary
   b. constrictive
   c. periodic
   d. primary

Match the abnormal menstruation type with correct definition.

4. oligomenorrhea _____   a. increased amount and duration of flow

5. metrorrhagia _____   b. bleeding between cycles

6. menorrhagia _____   c. in excess of 6 weeks

7. Increased risks of breast cancer, ovarian cancer, and non-Hodgkin lymphoma exist with this condition:
   a. endometriosis
   b. pelvic inflammatory disease
   c. sexually transmitted disease
   d. dysfunctional uterine bleeding

8. This benign lesion is also known as uterine fibroids:
   a. adenomyosis
   b. squamous cell
   c. leiomyoma
   d. extraembryonic cell primitive

9. Marginal, partial, and total are types of this condition:
   a. abruptio placentae
   b. placenta previa
   c. ectopic pregnancy
   d. hydatidiform mole

10. Which of the following is NOT a malposition of fetus?
    a. breech
    b. shoulder
    c. back
    d. brow

■ MALE GENITAL SYSTEM
MALE GENITAL SYSTEM—ANATOMY AND TERMINOLOGY

Function, reproduction

Structure, essential organs, and accessory organs (Fig. 1-27)

Essential Organs

Testes (Gonads)
Produce sperm (male gamete with 23 chromosomes) in seminiferous tubules

Covered by tunica albuginea, located in scrotum

Produce testosterone in Leydig cells

Vas Deferens
Is a tube

End of epididymis

Accessory Organs

Ducts (carry sperm from testes to exterior), sex glands (produce solutions that mix with sperm), and external genitalia

Seminal vesicles produce most seminal fluid

Prostate gland produces some seminal fluid and activates sperm

Bulbourethral gland (Cowper's gland) secretes a very small amount of seminal fluid

External genitalia: penis and scrotum

- Penis contains three columns of erectile tissue: two corpora cavernosa and one spongiosum

- Urethra passes through corpora spongiosum

- Scrotum encloses testes

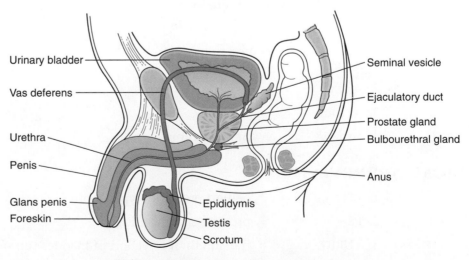

Figure **1-27** Male reproductive system.

Passage of sperm from production to exterior

Sperm are produced in seminiferous tubules (testes) and pass into

Epididymis then to vas deferens (within seminal vesicles) to

Ejaculatory duct then through urethra (prostate gland and Cowper's [bulbourethral] gland)

Pass though penis to outside of body

COMBINING FORMS

1.	andr/o	male
2.	balan/o	glans penis
3.	cry/o	cold
4.	crypt/o	hidden
5.	epididym/o	epididymis
6.	gon/o	seed
7.	hydr/o	water, fluid
8.	orch/i	testicle
9.	orch/o	testicle
10.	orchi/o	testicle
11.	orchid/o	testicle
12.	prostat/o	prostate gland
13.	semin/i	semen
14.	sperm/o	sperm
15.	spermat/o	sperm
16.	test/o	testicle
17.	varic/o	varicose veins
18.	vas/o	vessel, vas deferens
19.	vesicul/o	seminal vesicles

SUFFIXES

1.	-one	hormone
2.	-pexy	fixation
3.	-ectomy	removal
4.	-stomy	new opening

MEDICAL ABBREVIATIONS

1.	BPH	benign prostatic hypertrophy
2.	PSA	prostate-specific antigen
3.	TURBT	transurethral resection of bladder tumor
4.	TURP	transurethral resection of prostate

MEDICAL TERMS

Cavernosa	Connection between cavity of penis and a vein
Cavernosography	Radiographic recording of a cavity, e.g., pulmonary cavity or main part of penis
Cavernosometry	Measurement of pressure in a cavity, e.g., penis
Chordee	Condition resulting in penis being bent downward
Corpora cavernosa	The two cavities of penis
Epididymectomy	Surgical removal of epididymis
Epididymis	Tube located at the top of testes that stores sperm
Epididymovasostomy	Creation of a new connection between vas deferens and epididymis
Meatotomy	Surgical enlargement of opening of urinary meatus
Orchiectomy	Castration, removal of testes
Orchiopexy	Surgical procedure to release undescended testis and fixate within scrotum
Penoscrotal	Referring to penis and scrotum
Plethysmography	Determining changes in volume of an organ part or body
Priapism	Painful condition in which penis is constantly erect
Prostatotomy	Incision into prostate
Transurethral resection, prostate	Procedure performed through urethra by means of a cystoscopy to remove part or all of prostate
Tumescence	State of being swollen
Tunica vaginalis	Covering of testes
Varicocele	Swelling of a scrotal vein
Vas deferens	Tube that carries sperm from epididymis to ejaculatory duct and seminal vesicles
Vasectomy	Removal of segment of vas deferens
Vasogram	Recording of the flow in vas deferens
Vasotomy	Incision in vas deferens
Vasorrhaphy	Suturing of vas deferens
Vasovasostomy	Reversal of a vasectomy
Vesiculectomy	Excision of seminal vesicle
Vesiculotomy	Incision into seminal vesicle

MALE GENITAL SYSTEM ANATOMY AND TERMINOLOGY QUIZ
(Quiz answers are located at the end of Unit 1)

1. This gland activates sperm and produces some seminal fluid:
   a. seminal vesicle
   b. bulbourethral gland
   c. prostate gland
   d. scrotum

2. Carries sperm from testes to ejaculatory duct:
   a. vas deferens
   b. sex gland
   c. tunica
   d. seminal

3. Penis contains these erectile tissues:
   a. one corpora cavernosa and two spongiosa
   b. two corpora cavernosa and two spongiosa
   c. one corpora cavernosa and one spongiosum
   d. two corpora cavernosa and one spongiosum

4. Also known as Cowper's gland:
   a. seminal vesicles
   b. bulbourethral gland
   c. prostate gland
   d. scrotum

5. Which of the following is NOT an accessory organ?
   a. gonads
   b. seminal vesicles
   c. prostate
   d. penis

6. Combining form meaning "male":
   a. andr/o
   b. balan/o
   c. orchi/o
   d. test/o

7. Combining form meaning "glans penis":
   a. balan/o
   b. vas/o
   c. vesicul/o
   d. orch/o

8. Testes are covered by the:
   a. seminal vesicles
   b. androgen
   c. chancre
   d. tunica albuginea

9. This abbreviation describes a surgical resection of prostate that is accomplished by means of an endoscope inserted into the urethra:
   a. TURBT
   b. BPH
   c. UPJ
   d. TURP

10. This abbreviation describes a condition of prostate in which there is an enlargement that is benign:
   a. TURBT
   b. BPH
   c. UPJ
   d. TURP

MALE GENITAL SYSTEM—PATHOPHYSIOLOGY

Male Genital System Disorders

Disorders of Scrotum, Testes, and Epididymis

Cryptorchidism

Undescended testes—condition at birth

- Unilateral or bilateral

- Primarily result from obstruction

- Risk neoplastic processes

- May descend spontaneously

Treatment

- Administration of hormone to stimulate testosterone production

- Surgical intervention (orchiopexy) near age 1 to avoid risk of infertility

Orchitis

Inflammation of testes

Most common cause is virus

- Such as mumps orchitis

- Atrophy with irreversible loss of sperm production at risk

May be associated with

- Mumps or epidemic parotitis

- Gonorrhea

- Syphilis

- Tuberculosis

Symptoms

- Mild to severe pain in testes

- Mild to severe edema

- Feeling of weight in testicular area

Treatment

- Depends upon presence of underlying condition

Epididymitis

Inflammation of epididymis

Inflammatory response to trauma or infection

Abscess may form

Types

Sexually transmitted epididymitis

- Gonorrhea

- *T. pallidum*

- *T. vaginalis*

Nonspecific bacterial epididymitis

- *E. coli*
- Streptococci
- Staphylococci
- Associated with underlying urological disorder

Symptoms

Scrotal pain

Swelling

Erythema

Perhaps hydrocele formation

Treatment

Antibiotic

Bed rest

Ice packs

Scrotal support

Analgesics

Hydrocele (Fig. 1-28)

Collection of fluid in membranes of tunica vaginalis

May be congenital or acquired (response to infection or tumors)

Congenital hydrocele may reabsorb due to a communication between the scrotal sac and peritoneal cavity and require no intervention

Symptoms

Scrotal enlargement

Usually painless

- Unless infection is present

Varicocele

Abnormal dilation of plexus of veins

Decreases sperm production and motility

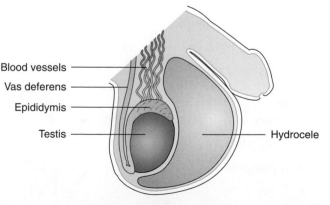

Figure **1-28** Hydrocele.

Symptoms
Usually painless

In elderly, may signal renal tumor

Treatment
Surgical intervention

Torsion of testes (Fig. 1-29)
Twisting of testes

Congenital abnormal development of tunica vaginalis and spermatic cord

Trauma may precipitate

Symptoms
Sudden onset of severe pain

Nausea

Vomiting

Scrotal edema and tenderness

Fever

Treatment
Immediate surgical intervention

Cancer of testes
Rare form of cancer

Cure rate high (95%)

Cause unknown

Usually occurs in younger men

Two main groups

• Germ cell tumors (GCT)—90% of testicular tumors

• Sex cord-stromal tumors

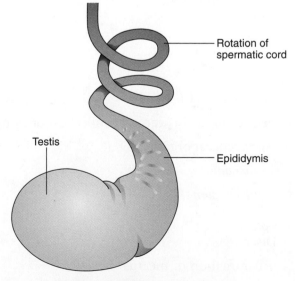

Figure **1-29** Torsion of testis.

Cancer of scrotum
Rare form of cancer

- Squamous cell carcinoma

Symptoms
Asymptomatic in early stages

Ulcerations in later stages

Treatment
Wide local excision

Mohs micrographic surgery

- Precise removal of tumor

- Layers are removed until no further microscopic evidence of abnormal cells is seen

Laser therapy

Lymph nodes are examined for metastasis

Disorders of Urethra
Epispadias
Congenital anomaly

Urethral meatus is located on dorsal side of penis

Usually occurs in conjunction with other abnormalities

Treatment
Surgical reconstruction

Hypospadias
Most common abnormality of penis

Urethral opening on ventral side of penis

Results in curvature of penis

- Due to chordee

Treatment
Surgical reconstruction

Urethritis
Inflammation of urethra

Infectious urethritis can be gonococcal or nongonococcal

Nongonococcal organisms

- *C. trachomatis*

- *U. urealyticum*

Symptoms
Discharge

Inflammation of meatus

Burning

Itching

Urgent and frequent urination

In nongonococcal, symptoms are fewer

Treatment
Antibiotics based on organism

Disorders of Penis
Balanitis
Inflammation of glans

Causes
Syphilis

Trichomoniasis

Gonorrhea

Candida albicans

Tinea

Underlying disease—diabetes mellitus and candidiasis

No circumcision

Symptoms
Irritation

Tenderness

Discharge

Edema

Ulceration

Swelling of lymph nodes

Treatment
Culture of discharge

Saline irrigation

Antibiotics

Phimosis and paraphimosis
Phimosis
Condition in which prepuce (foreskin) is constricted

• Prepuce cannot be retracted over glans penis

Can occur at any age

Associated with poor hygiene and chronic infection in uncircumcised males

Symptoms
Erythema

Edema

Tenderness

Purulent discharge

Treatment
Surgical circumcision

Paraphimosis
Condition in which prepuce (foreskin) is constricted

Prepuce is retracted over glans penis and cannot be moved forward

Symptom
Edema

Treatment
Surgical

Peyronie's disease
Also known as bent nail syndrome

Fibrotic condition

• Results in lateral curvature of penis during erection

Occurs most often in middle-aged men

Cause is unknown but associated with

• Diabetes

• Keloid development

• Dupuytren's contracture (flexion deformity of toes and fingers)

Treatment
Sometimes spontaneous remission

Pharmacologic oxygenation increasing therapies

Surgical resection of fibrous bands

Cancer of penis
Rare form of cancer

Occurs most often in men over age 60

Squamous cell carcinoma

Increased risks

• More common in uncircumcised men

• Sexual partner with cervical carcinoma

• Human papillomavirus

Usually begins with small lesion beneath prepuce

Intraepithelial neoplasia is also known as

• Bowen's disease

• Erythroplasia of Queyrat

• Begins as noninvasive

Progresses to invasive if untreated

Metastasis to lymph nodes

Treatment

Excision

Mohs micrographic surgery

Radiation therapy

Laser therapy

Cryosurgery

Advanced tumors are treated with partial or total penectomy and chemotherapy

Disorders of Prostate Gland

Benign prostatic hyperplasia/hypertrophy (BPH)
Multiple fibroadenomatous nodules; usually located on outside of gland, so easily palpable on digital exam

- Related to aging; common in men over 60 years of age

- Enlarging prostate obstructs bladder neck and urethra

- Decreases urine flow

It is thought that increased levels of estrogen/androgen cause BPH

Symptoms
Increased frequency and urgency of urination

Nocturia

Incontinence

Hesitancy

Diminished force

Postvoiding dribble

Screening
Prostate-specific antigen (PSA)

Digital rectal examination (DRE)

Treatment
Partial prostatectomy

Transurethral resection of prostate (TURP)

Excision of nodules

Hormone therapy

Placement of urethral stents

Pharmaceuticals—those that inhibit production of testosterone and those that relax smooth muscle of gland and neck of bladder

Prostatitis
Inflammation of prostate

- Acute or chronic bacterial prostatitis

Bacterial Causes
Escherichia coli

Enterococci

Staphylococci

Streptococci

Chlamydia trachomatis

Ureaplasma urealyticum

Neisseria gonorrhea

Nonbacterial Causes
Spontaneous

Prostatodynia

Symptoms
 Acute prostatitis
Fever and chills

Lower back pain

Perineal pain

Dysuria

Tenderness, suprapubic

Urinary tract infection

 Chronic prostatitis
Recurring

Same as acute only with no infection in urinary tract

Treatment
 Acute
Antibiotic based on culture

 Chronic
No treatment available

Cancer of prostate
Most common diagnosed malignancy in men, occurring in men over age 60

Indications are that the cause is related to androgens

Predominately adenocarcinoma (95%)

No relationship between BPH and cancer of prostate

Symptoms
Asymptomatic in early stages

Later symptoms include

- Dysuria

- Back pain

- Hematuria

- Frequent urination

- Urinary retention

- Increased incidence of uremia

Stages
Two systems used to stage prostate cancer

- Whitmore-Jewett stages as indicated in Fig. 1-30

- Tumor-node-metastasis (TNM) as indicated in Fig. 1-31

Treatment
Dependent upon stage

WHITMORE-JEWETT STAGES:

Stage A is clinically undetectable tumor confined to the gland and is an incidental finding at prostate surgery.
A1: well-differentiated with focal involvement
A2: moderately or poorly differentiated or involves multiple foci in the gland
Stage B is tumor confined to the prostate gland.
B0: nonpalpable, PSA-detected
B1: single nodule in one lobe of the prostate
B2: more extensive involvement of one lobe or involvement of both lobes
Stage C is a tumor clinically localized to the periprostatic area but extending through the prostatic capsule; seminal vesicles may be involved.
C1: clinical extracapsular extension
C2: extracapsular tumor producing bladder outlet or ureteral obstruction
Stage D is metastatic disease.
D0: clinically localized disease (prostate only)
but persistently elevated enzymatic serum acid phosphatase
D1: regional lymph nodes only
D2: distant lymph nodes, metastases to bone or visceral organs
D3: D2 prostate cancer patients who relapse after adequate endocrine therapy

Figure **1-30** Whitmore-Jewett stages.

TNM STAGES:

Primary Tumor (T)

TX: Primary tumor cannot be assessed

T0: No evidence of primary tumor

T1: Clinically inapparent tumor not palpable or visible by imaging

   T1a: Tumor incidental histologic finding in 5% or less of tissue resected

   T1b: Tumor incidental histologic finding in more than 5% of tissue resected

   T1c: Tumor identified by needle biopsy (e.g., because of elevated PSA)

T2: Tumor confined within the prostate

   T2a: Tumor involves half a lobe or less

   T2b: Tumor involves more than half of a lobe, but not both lobes

   T2c: Tumor involves both lobes; extends through the prostatic capsule

T3a: Unilateral extracapsular extension

T3b: Bilateral extracapsular extension

T3c: Tumor invades the seminal vesicle(s)

T4: Tumor is fixed or invades adjacent structures other than the seminal vesicle(s)

   T4a: Tumor invades any of bladder neck, external sphincter, or rectum

   T4b: Tumor invades levator muscles and/or is fixed to the pelvic wall

Regional lymph nodes (N)

NX: Regional lymph nodes cannot be assessed

N0: No regional lymph node metastasis

N1: Metastasis in a single lymph node, 2 cm or less in greatest dimension

N2: Metastasis in a single lymph node, more than 2 cm but not more than 5 cm in greatest dimension; or multiple lymph node metastases, none more than 5 cm in greatest dimension

N3: Metastasis in a single lymph node more than 5 cm in greatest dimension

Distant metastases (M)

MX: Presence of distant metastasis cannot be assessed

M0: No distant metastasis

M1: Distant metastasis

   M1a: Nonregional lymph node(s)

   M1b: Bone(s)

   M1c: Other site(s)

Figure **1-31** TNM stages.

MALE GENITAL SYSTEM PATHOPHYSIOLOGY QUIZ
(Quiz answers are located at the end of Unit 1)

1. What is the condition in which testes do not descend?
   a. cryptorchidism
   b. Bowen's disease
   c. torsion
   d. hypospadias

2. Orchitis is most often caused by a:
   a. bacteria
   b. virus
   c. parasite
   d. fungus

3. A condition that can be either congenital or acquired through trauma and that involves twisting of testes is:
   a. hydrocele
   b. hypospadias
   c. cryptorchidism
   d. torsion

4. Cancer of the _____ is divided into two main groups of germ cell tumors and sex stromal cord tumors.
   a. testes
   b. penis
   c. scrotum
   d. prostate

5. This type of surgical technique involves excision of a lesion in layers until no further evidence of abnormality is seen:
   a. Bowen's
   b. Addison's
   c. Mohs
   d. laser

6. Epispadias is a disorder of urethra in which urethral meatus is located on the _____ side of penis:
   a. ventral
   b. dorsal
   c. lateral
   d. medial

7. Inflammation of glans is:
   a. phimosis
   b. paraphimosis
   c. urethritis
   d. balanitis

8. This disease is also known as bent nail syndrome:
   a. Bowen's
   b. Peyronie's
   c. Addison's
   d. Whitmore-Jewett

9. Condition in which multiple fibroadenomatous nodules form and lead to decreased urine flow. Condition is thought to be related to increased levels of estrogen/androgen.
   a. BPH
   b. DRE
   c. GCT
   d. TNM

10. Cancer of prostate is predominately this type of cancer:
    a. sex cord
    b. adenocarcinoma
    c. squamous cell
    d. seminoma

■ URINARY SYSTEM

URINARY SYSTEM—ANATOMY AND TERMINOLOGY

Removes metabolic waste materials (nitrogenous waste: urea, creatinine, and uric acid)

Conserves nutrients and water

Balances: electrolytes (acids/bases balance)

Electrolytes are electrically charged molecules required for nerve and muscle function

Assists liver in detoxification

Organs (Fig. 1-32)

Kidneys

Ureters

Urinary bladder

Urethra

Kidneys (Fig. 1-33)

Electrolytes and fluid balance

Control pH balance (acid/base)

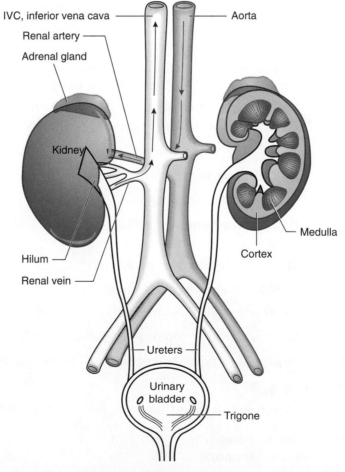

Figure **1-32** Urinary system.

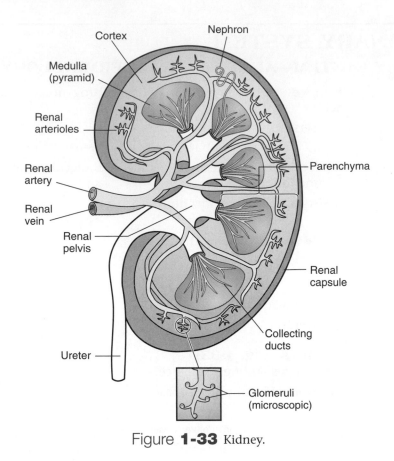

Figure **1-33** Kidney.

Secrete renin (which affects blood pressure) and erythropoietin (which stimulates red blood cell production in bone marrow)

Secrete active vitamin D required for calcium absorption from intestines

Two organs located behind peritoneum (retroperitoneal space)

Kidney Structure

Cortex (outer layer)

Medulla (inner portion)

Hilum (depression on medial border through which blood vessels and nerves pass)

Pyramids (divisions of medulla)

Papilla (inner part of pyramids)

Pelvis (receptacle for urine within kidney)

Calyces surround top of renal pelvis

Nephrons (3 types) are operational units of kidney

Ureters
Narrow tubes transporting urine from kidneys to bladder

Urinary Bladder
Reservoir for urine

Shaped like an upside-down pear with three surfaces

- Posterior (base)

- Anterior (neck)

- Superior (peritoneum)

Trigone

- Smooth triangular area inside bladder—size never changes

- Formed by openings of ureters and urethra

Urethra

Canal from bladder to exterior of body

Urinary meatus, outside opening of urethra

COMBINING FORMS

1.	albumin/o	albumin
2.	azot/o	urea
3.	bacteri/o	bacteria
4.	cali/o	calyx
5.	cyst/o	urinary
6.	dips/o	thirst
7.	glomerul/o	glomerulus
8.	glyc/o	sugar
9.	glycos/o	sugar
10.	hydr/o	water
11.	ket/o	ketone bodies/ketoacidosis
12.	lith/o	stone
13.	meat/o	meatus
14.	nephr/o	kidney
15.	noct/i	night
16.	olig/o	scant, few
17.	pyel/o	renal pelvis
18.	ren/o	kidney
19.	son/o	sound
20.	tripsy	to crush
21.	tryg/o	trigone region/kidney
22.	ur/o	urine
23.	ureter/o	ureter
24.	urethr/o	urethra
25.	uria	urination/urinary condition
26.	urin/o	urine
27.	vesic/o	bladder

PREFIXES

1.	dys-	painful
2.	peri-	surrounding
3.	poly-	many
4.	retro-	behind

SUFFIXES

1.	-eal	pertaining to
2.	-lithiasis	condition of stones
3.	-lysis	separation
4.	-plasty	repair
5.	-rrhaphy	suture
6.	-tripsy	crush

MEDICAL ABBREVIATIONS

1.	ARF	acute renal failure
2.	BUN	blood urea nitrogen
3.	ESRD	end-stage renal disease
4.	HD	hemodialysis
5.	IVP	intravenous pyelogram
6.	KUB	kidney, ureter, bladder
7.	pH	symbol for acid/base level
8.	PKU	phenylketonuria
9.	sp gr	specific gravity
10.	UA	urinalysis
11.	UPJ	ureteropelvic junction
12.	UTI	urinary tract infection

MEDICAL TERMS

Bulbocavernosus	Muscle that constricts vagina in a female and urethra in a male
Bulbourethral	Gland with duct leading to urethra
Calculus	Concretion of mineral salts, also called a stone
Calycoplasty	Surgical reconstruction of recess of renal pelvis
Calyx	Recess of renal pelvis
Cystolithectomy	Removal of a calculus (stone) from urinary bladder
Cystometrogram	CMG, measurement of pressures and capacity of urinary bladder
Cystoplasty	Surgical reconstruction of bladder
Cystorrhaphy	Suture of bladder

Cystoscopy	Use of a scope to view bladder
Cystostomy	Surgical creation of an opening into bladder
Cystotomy	Incision into bladder
Cystourethroplasty	Surgical reconstruction of bladder and urethra
Cystourethroscopy	Use of a scope to view bladder and urethra
Dilation	Stretching or expansion
Dysuria	Painful urination
Endopyelotomy	Procedure involving bladder and ureters, including insertion of a stent into renal pelvis
Extracorporeal	Occurring outside of body
Fundoplasty	Repair of the bottom of bladder
Hydrocele	Sac of fluid
Kock pouch	Surgical creation of a urinary bladder from a segment of the ileum
Nephrocutaneous fistula	An abnormal channel from kidney to skin
Nephrolithotomy	Removal of a kidney stone through an incision made into the kidney
Nephrorrhaphy	Suturing of kidney
Nephrostomy	Creation of a channel into renal pelvis of kidney
Transureteroureterostomy	Surgical connection of one ureter to other ureter
Transvesical ureterolithotomy	Removal of a ureter stone (calculus) through bladder
Ureterectomy	Surgical removal of a ureter, either totally or partially
Ureterocutaneous fistula	Channel from ureter to exterior skin
Ureteroenterostomy	Creation of a connection between intestine and ureter
Ureterolithotomy	Removal of a stone from ureter
Ureterolysis	Freeing of adhesions of ureter
Ureteroneocystostomy	Surgical connection of ureter to a new site on bladder
Ureteropyelography	Ureter and renal pelvis radiography
Ureterotomy	Incision into ureter
Urethrocystography	Radiography of bladder and urethra
Urethromeatoplasty	Surgical repair of urethra and meatus
Urethropexy	Fixation of urethra by means of surgery
Urethroplasty	Surgical repair of urethra
Urethrorrhaphy	Suturing of urethra
Urethroscopy	Use of a scope to view urethra
Vesicostomy	Surgical creation of a connection of viscera of bladder to skin

URINARY SYSTEM ANATOMY AND TERMINOLOGY QUIZ
(Quiz answers are located at the end of Unit 1)

1. The outer covering of kidney:
   a. medulla
   b. pyramids
   c. cortex
   d. papilla

2. Which is not a division of kidneys?
   a. pelvis
   b. pyramids
   c. cortex
   d. trigone

3. The inner portion of kidneys:
   a. medulla
   b. pyramids
   c. cortex
   d. papilla

4. The smooth area inside bladder:
   a. pyramids
   b. calyces
   c. trigone
   d. cystocele

5. The narrow tube connecting kidney and bladder:
   a. urethra
   b. ureter
   c. meatus
   d. trigone

6. Which of the following is NOT a surface of urinary bladder?
   a. posterior
   b. anterior
   c. superior
   d. inferior

7. Combining form that means "stone":
   a. azot/o
   b. cyst/o
   c. lith/o
   d. olig/o

8. Term meaning "painful urination":
   a. pyuria
   b. dysuria
   c. diuresis
   d. hyperemia

9. Combining form meaning "scant":
   a. glyc/o
   b. hydr/o
   c. meat/o
   d. olig/o

10. Term that describes renal failure that is acute:
    a. ARF
    b. ESRD
    c. HD
    d. BPH

URINARY SYSTEM—PATHOPHYSIOLOGY

Renal Failure

Acute Renal Failure
Sudden onset of renal failure

Causes
Extreme hypotension

Trauma

Infection

Inflammation

Toxicity

Obstructed vascular supply

Symptoms
Uremia

Oliguria (decreased output) or anuria (no output)

Hyperkalemia (high potassium in blood)

Pulmonary edema

Types
Prerenal

- Associated with poor systemic perfusion
- Decreased renal blood flow
  - Such as with congestive heart failure

Intrarenal

- Associated with renal parenchyma disease (functional tissue of kidney)
  - Such as acute interstitial nephritis, glomerulopathies, and malignant hypertension

Postrenal

- Resulting from urine flow obstruction outside kidney (ureters or bladder neck)

Treatment
Underlying condition

Dialysis

Monitoring of fluid and electrolyte balance

Chronic Renal Failure
Gradual loss of function

- Progressively more severe renal insufficiency until end stage of
  - Renal disease
  - Irreversible kidney failure

Stages—based on level of creatinine clearance
Stage 1: Blood flow through kidney increases, kidney enlarges

Stage 2 (mild): Small amounts of blood protein (albumin) leak into urine (microalbuminuria)

Stage 3 (moderate): Albumin and other protein losses increase; patient may develop high blood pressure and kidney loses ability to filter waste

Stage 4 (severe): Large amounts of urine pass through kidney; blood pressure increases

Stage 5: End-stage renal failure. Ability to filter waste nearly stops; dialysis or transplant only option

Causes
Long-term exposure to nephrotoxins

Diabetes

Hypertension

Symptoms
No symptoms until well advanced

Polyuria

Nausea or anorexia

Dehydration

Neurologic manifestations

Stages of nephron loss
Decreased reserve

- 60% loss

Renal insufficiency

- 75% loss

End-stage renal failure

- 90% loss

Treatment
No cure

Dialysis

Kidney transplant

Urinary Tract Infections (UTI)

Cystitis—Bacterial
Cause
Bacteria, usually *E. coli*

Symptoms
Lower abdominal pain

Dysuria

Lower back pain

Urinary frequency and urgency

Cloudy, foul-smelling urine

Systemic signs
Fever

Malaise

· Nausea

Treatment
Antibiotics

Increased fluid intake

Cystitis—Noninfectious, Nonbacterial
Cause
Radiation, chemotherapy, autoimmune disorder, etc.

May later produce bacterial infection

Symptoms
Urinary frequency and urgency

Dysuria

Negative urine culture

Treatment
No known treatment

Acute Pyelonephritis (Fig. 1-34)
Bacterial infection with multiple abcesses of renal pelvis and medullary tissue

• May involve one or both kidneys

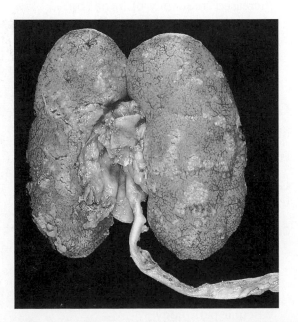

Figure **1-34** Acute pyelonephritis. Cortical surface exhibits grayish white areas of inflammation and abscess formation.

Causes
E. coli

Proteus

Pseudomonas

Obstruction and reflux of urine from bladder

Symptoms
Fever

Chills

Groin or flank pain

Dysuria

Pyuria

Nocturia

Treatment
Antibiotics

Surgical correction of obstruction

Chronic Pyelonephritis

Recurrent infection that causes scarring of kidney

Cause is difficult to determine

- Repeated infections
- Obstructive conditions

Symptoms
Hypertension

Dysuria

Flank pain

Increased frequency of urination

Treatment
Antibiotics for extended periods when reoccurring

Surgical reduction of obstruction

Glomerular Disorders

May be acute or chronic

Function of glomerulus is blood filtration

Glomerulonephritis

Inflammation of glomerulus

Causes
Drugs or toxins

Systemic disorder affecting many organs or idiopathic

May follow acute infections—most commonly streptococcal infections

Vascular pathology

Immune disorders

Treatment
Follows cause

Nephrotic Syndrome (Nephrosis)

Disease of kidneys that includes damage to membrane of the glomerulus causing excessive protein loss to urine

Accompanied by

- Hypoalbuminemia
- Hypercholesterolemia
- Hypercoagulability (excessive clotting)
- Prone to infections
- Edema
- Protein loss of >3.5 g

Damage to glomerulus results from

- Infection
- Immune response
  - Most predominant cause of dysfunction is exposure to toxins

May be a manifestation of an underlying condition, such as diabetes

Symptoms
Edema

Weight gain

Pallor

Proteinuria

Lipiduria

Treatment
Glucocorticoids, such as prednisone

- Reduces inflammation

Sodium- and fat-reduced diet

Protein supplements

Careful monitoring for continued inflammation

Acute Poststreptococcal Glomerulonephritis (APSGN)

Cause
Streptococcus infection

- With certain types of group A beta-hemolytic *Streptococcus*

Creates an antigen-antibody complex

- Infiltrates glomerular capillaries
- Results in inflammation in kidneys
- Inflammation interferes with normal kidney function
- Fluid and waste build-up
- Can lead to acute renal failure and scarring

Usually occurs in children 3 to 7 years of age

- Most often in boys

Symptoms

Back and flank pain

Cloudy, dark urine

Oliguria (decreased output)

Edema

Elevated blood pressure

Fatigue

Malaise

Headache

Nausea

Treatment

Sodium reduction

Antibiotics

Careful monitoring for continued inflammation

Urinary Tract Obstructions

Interference with urine flow

Causes urine backup behind obstruction of urinary system

Damage occurs to structures behind blockages

Increased urinary tract infection

Obstruction can be

- Functional

- Anatomic

  - Also known as obstructive uropathy

Kidney Stones (nephrolithiasis—renal calculi)

Formed of mineral salts (uric and calcuim)

Develop anywhere in urinary tract

Tend to form in presence of excess salt and decreased fluid intake

- Most stones are formed of calcium salts

- Staghorn calculus forms in renal pelvis

Symptoms

Asymptomatic until obstruction occurs

Obstruction results in renal colic

- Extremely intense pain in flank

- Nausea

- Vomiting

- Cold, clammy skin

- Increased pulse rate

Treatment

Stone usually passes spontaneously

May use extracorporeal ultrasound or laser lithotripsy to break up stone (also known as extracorporeal shock wave lithotripsy, or ESWL)

Drugs may be used to dissolve stone

Preventative treatment to adjust pH level

- Increased fluid intake

Bladder Carcinoma

Malignant tumor

Most common site of malignancy in urinary system

Tumors originate in transitional epithelial lining

Tends to recur

Often metastatic to liver and bone

Tumor staging for renal cancer

Stage I—Tumor of kidney capsule only

Stage II—Tumor invading renal capsule/vein but within fascia

Stage III—Tumor extending to regional lymph nodes/vena cava

Stage IV—Other organ metastasis

Symptoms

Often asymptomatic in early stage

Hematuria

Dysuria

Frequent urination

Infections common

Increased Risks

Cigarette smoking

Males age 50+

Working with industrial chemicals

Analgesics used in large amounts

Recurrent bladder infections

Treatment

Immunotherapy (Bacillus Calmette-Guérin [BCG] vaccine)

Excision

Chemotherapy

Radiation therapy

Hydronephrosis

Distention of kidney with urine

- Due to an obstruction

- Usually as a result of a kidney stone

- May also be due to scarring, tumor, edema from infection, or other obstruction

Symptoms
Usually asymptomatic

Mild flank pain

Infection may develop

May lead to chronic renal failure

Treatment
Treat underlying condition, such as removal of stone or antibiotics for infection

Dilation of stricture

Vascular Disorders

Nephrosclerosis
Excessive hardening and thickening of vascular structure of kidney

- Reduces blood supply

  - Increases blood pressure

  - Results in atrophy and ischemia of structures

  - May lead to chronic renal failure

Symptoms
Asymptomatic in early stages

Treatment
Diuretics

ACE (angiotensin-converting enzyme) inhibitors

Beta blockers that block release of resin

Antihypertensive drugs

Sodium intake reduction

Congenital Disorders

Polycystic Kidney (PKD)
Numerous kidney cysts

Genetic disease

Symptoms
Asymptomatic until 40s

Cysts progressive in development (both kidneys)

Nephromegaly, hematuria, URT, hypertension, uremia

Develops chronic renal failure

Cysts may spread to other organs, such as liver

Treatment
As for chronic renal failure

Wilms' Tumor—Nephroblastoma
Usually unilateral kidney tumors

Most common tumor in children

Usually advanced at time of diagnosis

- Metastasis to lungs at time of diagnosis is common

Symptoms
Asymptomatic until abdominal mass becomes apparent at age 1 to 5

Treatment
Excision

Radiation therapy

Chemotherapy

Usually a combination of above

URINARY SYSTEM PATHOPHYSIOLOGY QUIZ
(Quiz answers are located at the end of Unit 1)

1. Which of the following is NOT a type of acute renal failure?
   a. prerenal
   b. intrarenal
   c. interrenal
   d. postrenal

2. The loss of nephron function in end-stage renal disease is:
   a. 60%
   b. 70%
   c. 80%
   d. 90%

3. The cause of bacterial cystitis is usually:
   a. *Proteus*
   b. *Pseudomonas*
   c. Staphylococcus
   d. *E. coli*

4. The primary treatment for acute pyelonephritis would be:
   a. prednisone
   b. sodium reduction
   c. antibiotics
   d. BCG

5. APSGN stands for:
   a. advanced poststaphylococcal glomerulonephritis
   b. acute poststreptococcal glomerulonephritis
   c. acute poststaphylococcal glomerulonephritis
   d. advanced poststreptococcal glomerulonephritis

6. Obstructive uropathy is also known as:
   a. pyelonephritis
   b. renal failure
   c. urinary tract obstruction
   d. nephrotic syndrome

7. A treatment for kidney stone may be:
   a. ESWL
   b. prednisone
   c. open surgical procedure
   d. diuretics

8. The treatment for hydronephrosis involves:
   a. an open surgical procedure
   b. use of diuretics
   c. treatment of the underlying condition
   d. BCG

9. This is a congential condition in which numerous cysts form in the kidney:
   a. Wilms' tumor
   b. polycystic kidney
   c. nephrosclerosis
   d. nephrotic syndrome

10. The treatment of Wilms' tumor would NOT include which of the following?
    a. excision
    b. chemotherapy
    c. diuretic
    d. radiation therapy

■ DIGESTIVE SYSTEM

DIGESTIVE SYSTEM—ANATOMY AND TERMINOLOGY

Function: digestion, absorption, and elimination

Includes gastrointestinal tract (alimentary canal) and accessory organs

Mouth (Fig. 1-35)

Roof: hard palate, soft palate, uvula (projection at back of mouth)

Floor: contains tongue (Fig. 1-36), muscles, taste buds, and lingual frenulum, which anchors tongue to floor of mouth

Teeth

Thirty-two teeth (permanent)

Names of teeth: incisor, cuspid, bicuspid, and tricuspid

Tooth has crown (outer portion), neck (narrow part below gum line), root (end section), and pulp cavity (core)

Salivary Glands (Fig. 1-37)

Surround mouth and produce saliva—1.5 liters daily

Parotid

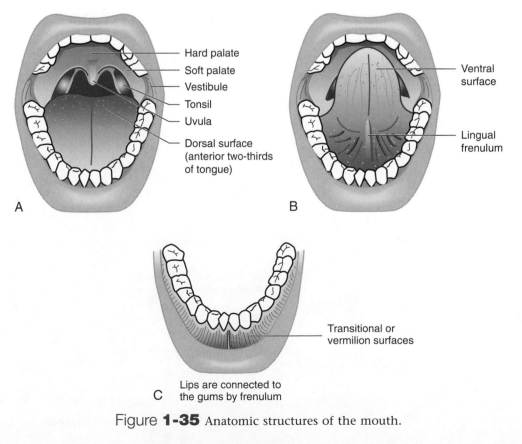

Figure **1-35** Anatomic structures of the mouth.

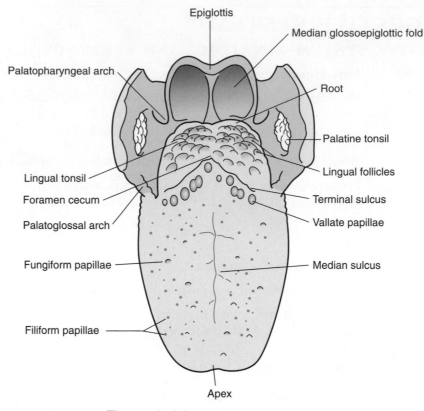

Epiglottis

Median glossoepiglottic fold

Palatopharyngeal arch

Root

Palatine tonsil

Lingual tonsil

Lingual follicles

Foramen cecum

Terminal sulcus

Palatoglossal arch

Vallate papillae

Fungiform papillae

Median sulcus

Filiform papillae

Apex

Figure **1-36** Dorsum of the tongue.

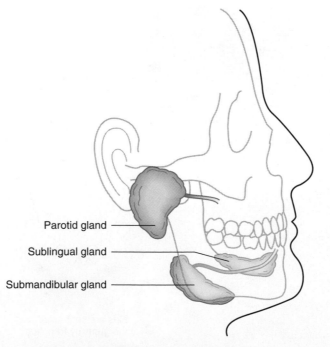

Parotid gland

Sublingual gland

Submandibular gland

Figure **1-37** Major salivary glands.

Submandibular

Sublingual

Pharynx or Throat (Fig. 1-38)

Muscular tube (5 inches long) lined with mucous membrane through which air and food/water travel

Epiglottis covers larynx/esophagus when swallowing

Esophagus

Muscular tube (9-10 inches long) that carries food from pharynx to stomach by means of peristalsis (rhythmic contractions)

Stomach

Sphincter (ring of muscles) at entry into stomach (gastroesophageal or cardiac)

Three parts of stomach:

    Fundus (upper part)

    Body (middle part)

    Antrum/pylorus (lower part)

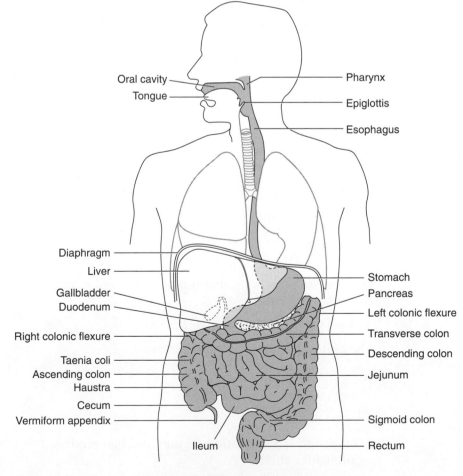

Figure **1-38** Digestive system.

Lined with rugae (folds of mucosal membrane)

Pyloric sphincter opens to allow chyme (thick liquid) to leave stomach and enter small intestine

Small Intestine

Duodenum (2 inches long): first portion beyond stomach—bile and pancreatic juice delivered here

Jejunum (96 inches long): connects duodenum to ileum

Ileum (132 inches long): attaches to large intestine

Large Intestine

Extends from ileum to anus

Cecum, from which appendix extends, connects ileum and colon

Colon (60 inches long), divided into:

    Ascending

    Transverse

    Descending

    Sigmoid

Sigmoid colon connected to rectum, which terminates at anus

Accessory Organs

Liver produces bile, sent to gallbladder via hepatic duct and cystic duct

Gallbladder stores bile, sent to duodenum from cystic duct into common bile duct

Bile emulsifies fat (breaks up large globules)

Pancreas produces enzymes sent through pancreatic duct to hepatopancreatic ampulla (ampulla of Vater) then to duodenum

Pancreatic cells—islets of Langerhans produce insulin and glucagon

Peritoneum

Serous membrane lines abdominal cavity and maintains organs in correct anatomic position

Food passes through digestive tract via:

    Mouth—including salivary glands

    Pharynx

    Esophagus

    Stomach

    Duodenum—pancreatic enzymes and bile produced in liver and stored in gallbladder enter

    Jejunum

Ileum

Cecum

Ascending colon

Transverse colon

Descending colon

Sigmoid colon

Rectum

Anus

COMBINING FORMS

1.	abdomin/o	abdomen
2.	an/o	anus
3.	appendic/o	appendix
4.	bil/i	bile
5.	bilirubin/o	bile pigment
6.	bucc/o	cheek
7.	cec/o	cecum
8.	celi/o	abdomen
9.	cheil/o	lip
10.	chol/e	gall/bile
11.	cholangio/o	bile duct
12.	cholecyst/o	gallbladder
13.	choledoch/o	common bile duct
14.	col/o	colon
15.	dent/i	tooth
16.	diverticul/o	diverticulum
17.	duoden/o	duodenum
18.	enter/o	small intestine
19.	esophag/o	esophagus
20.	faci/o	face
21.	gastr/o	stomach
22.	gingiv/o	gum
23.	gloss/o	tongue
24.	hepat/o	liver
25.	herni/o	hernia
26.	ile/o	ileum
27.	jejun/o	jejunum

28. labi/o	lip
29. lapar/o	abdomen
30. lingu/o	tongue
31. lip/o	fat
32. lith/o	stone
33. or/o	mouth
34. ordont/o	tooth
35. palat/o	palate
36. pancreat/o	pancreas
37. peritone/o	peritoneum
38. pharyng/o	throat
39. polyp/o	polyp
40. proct/o	rectum
41. pylor/o	pylorus
42. rect/o	rectum
43. sial/o	saliva
44. sialaden/o	salivary gland
45. sigmoid/o	sigmoid colon
46. steat/o	fat
47. stomat/o	mouth
48. uvul/o	uvula

SUFFIXES

1. -ase	enzyme
2. -cele	hernia
3. -chezia	defecation
4. -iasis	abnormal condition
5. -phagia	eating
6. -prandial	meal

MEDICAL ABBREVIATIONS

1. EGD	esophagogastroduodenoscopy
2. EGJ	esophagogastric junction
3. ERCP	endoscopic retrograde cholangiopancreatography
4. GERD	gastroesophageal reflux disease
5. GI	gastrointestinal
6. HJR	hepatojugular reflux

7.	LLQ	left lower quadrant
8.	LUQ	left upper quadrant
9.	PEG	percutaneous endoscopic gastrostomy
10.	RLQ	right lower quadrant
11.	RUQ	right upper quadrant

MEDICAL TERMS

Anastomosis	Surgical connection of two tubular structures, such as two pieces of intestine
Biliary	Refers to gallbladder, bile, or bile duct
Cholangiography	Radiographic recording of bile ducts
Cholecystectomy	Surgical removal of gallbladder
Cholecystoenterostomy	Creation of a connection between gallbladder and intestine
Colonoscopy	Fiberscopic examination of entire colon that may include part of terminal ileum
Colostomy	Artificial opening between colon and abdominal wall
Diverticulum	Protrusion in wall of an organ
Dysphagia	Difficulty swallowing
Enterolysis	Releasing of adhesions of intestine
Eventration	Protrusion of bowel through an opening in abdomen
Evisceration	Pulling viscera outside of the body through an incision
Exstrophy	Condition in which an organ is turned inside out
Fulguration	Use of electric current to destroy tissue
Gastrointestinal	Pertaining to stomach and intestine
Gastroplasty	Operation on stomach for repair or reconfiguration
Gastrostomy	Artificial opening between stomach and abdominal wall
Hernia	Organ or tissue protruding through wall or cavity that usually contains it
Ileostomy	Artificial opening between ileum and abdominal wall
Imbrication	Overlapping
Incarcerated	Regarding hernias, a constricted, irreducible hernia that may cause obstruction of an intestine
Intussusception	Slipping of one part of intestine into another part
Jejunostomy	Artificial opening between jejunum and abdominal wall
Laparoscopy	Exploration of the abdomen and pelvic cavities using a scope placed through a small incision in abdominal wall
Lithotomy	Incision into an organ or a duct for the purpose of removing a stone
Lithotripsy	Crushing of a stone by sound wave or force

Paraesophageal or hiatal hernia	Protrusion of any structure through esophageal hiatus of diaphragm
Proctosigmoidoscopy	Fiberscopic examination of sigmoid colon and rectum
Sialolithotomy	Surgical removal of a stone of salivary gland or duct
Varices	Varicose veins
Volvulus	Twisted section of intestine

DIGESTIVE SYSTEM ANATOMY AND TERMINOLOGY QUIZ
(Quiz answers are located at the end of Unit 1)

1. This is NOT a part of the small intestine:
   a. ileum
   b. cecum
   c. duodenum
   d. jejunum

2. Term meaning "ring of muscles":
   a. pyloric
   b. parotid
   c. epiglottis
   d. sphincter

3. The throat is also known as the:
   a. larynx
   b. epiglottis
   c. esophagus
   d. pharynx

4. The three parts of the stomach:
   a. pyloric, rugae, fundus
   b. fundus, body, antrum
   c. antrum, pyloric, rugae
   d. ilium, fundus, pyloric

5. The projection at the back of the mouth:
   a. palate
   b. sublingual
   c. uvula
   d. parotid

6. Mucosal membrane that lines the stomach:
   a. cecum
   b. rugae
   c. frenulum
   d. fundus

7. The parts of the colon are:
   a. ascending, transverse, descending, sigmoid
   b. ascending, descending, sigmoid
   c. transverse, descending, sigmoid
   d. descending, sigmoid

8. Combining form meaning "abdomen":
   a. an/o
   b. cec/o
   c. celi/o
   d. col/o

9. Term that means connecting two ends of a tube:
   a. anastomosis
   b. amylase
   c. aphthous stomatitis
   d. atresia

10. Abbreviation that means a scope placed through the esophagus, into the stomach, and to the duodenum:
    a. ERCP
    b. EGD
    c. GERD
    d. PEG

DIGESTIVE SYSTEM—PATHOPHYSIOLOGY

Disorders of Oral Cavity

Cleft Lip and Cleft Palate (Orofacial Cleft) (Fig. 1-39)
Congenital defect

Cleft lip and palate

> Lip and palate do not properly join together

Causes feeding problems

- Infants cannot create sufficient suction for feeding

- Danger of aspirating food

- Results in speech defects

Treatment
> Surgical repair of defects

Ulceration
Canker sore—caused by herpes simplex virus

- Ulceration of oral mucosa

Also known as

- Aphthous ulcer (aphtha: small ulcer)

- Aphthous stomatitis

Heals spontaneously

Infections
Candidiasis
Candida albicans is naturally found in mouth

Thrush (oral candidiasis) is overarching infection

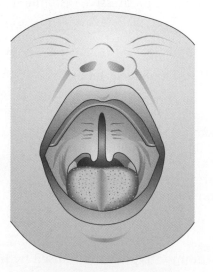

Figure **1-39** Cleft palate.

Causes

Antibiotic regimen

Chemotherapy

Glucocorticoids

Common in patients with diabetes and AIDS patients

Treatment

Nystatin (topical fungal agent)

Herpes simplex type 1

Herpetic stomatitis

- Viral cold sores and blisters

- Associated with herpes simplex virus type 1 (HSV-1)

Treatment

No cure

May be alleviated somewhat by antiviral medications

Cancer of Oral Cavity

Most common type is squamous cell carcinoma

Kaposi's sarcoma is type seen in AIDS patients

Increased in smokers

   Lip cancer also increased in smokers, particularly pipe smokers

Poor prognosis

Usually asymptomatic until later stages

Metastasis through lymph nodes

Esophageal Disorders

Scleroderma

Also known as progressive systemic sclerosis

Atrophy of smooth muscles of lower esophagus

Lower esophageal sphincter (LES) does not close properly

- Leads to esophageal reflux

- Strictures form

Symptom

Predominantly dysphagia

Esophagitis

Inflammation of esophagus

Types

Acute

Most common type is that caused by hiatal hernia

Infectious esophagitis is common in patients with AIDS

Ingestion of strong alkaline or acid substances

- Such as those in household cleaners

Inflammation leads to scarring

Chronic
Most common type is that caused by LES reflux

Cancer of Esophagus
Most common type is squamous cell or secondary adenocarcinoma

Usually caused by continued irritation

- Smoking

- Alcohol

- Hiatal hernia

- Chronic esophagitis/GERD

Poor prognosis

Hiatal Hernia (Diaphragmatic hernia)
Diaphragm goes over stomach

- Esophagus passes through diaphragm at natural opening (hiatus)

- Part of the stomach protrudes (herniates) through opening in diaphragm into thorax

Types (Fig. 1-40)
Sliding

- Stomach and gastroesophageal junction protrude through the hiatus

Paraesophageal/rolling hiatal

- Part of fundus protrudes

Symptoms
Heartburn

Reflux

Belching

Lying down causes discomfort

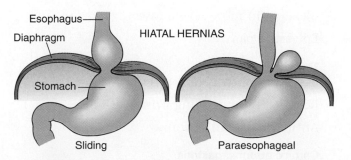

Figure **1-40** Sliding and paraesophageal hernias (hiatal hernias).

Dysphagia

Substernal pain after eating

Gastroesophageal Reflux Disease (GERD)
Associated with hiatal hernias

• Reflux of gastric contents

Lower esophageal sphincter does not constrict properly

Treatment
Reduce irritants, such as

  • Smoking

  • Spicy foods

  • Alcohol

Antacids

Elevate head of bed

Avoid tight clothing

Stomach and Duodenum Disorders

Gastritis
Inflammation of stomach mucosa

Acute superficial gastritis
Mild, transient irritation

Causes
Excessive alcohol

Infection

Food allergies

Spicy foods

Aspirin

H. pylori (Helicobacter pylori)

Symptoms
Nausea

Vomiting

Anorexia

Bleeding in more severe cases

Epigastric pain

Treatment
Usually spontaneous remission in 2 to 3 days

Removal of underlying irritation

Antibiotics for infection

Chronic atrophic gastritis
Progressive atrophy of epithelium

Types

Type A, atrophic or fundal

- Involves fundus of stomach
- Autoimmune disease
  - Decreases acid secretion
  - Results in high gastrin levels

Type B, antral

- Involves antrum region of stomach
- Often associated with elderly
  - May be associated with pernicious anemia
- Low gastrin levels
- Usually caused by infection
- Irritated by alcohol, drugs, and tobacco

Symptom abatement

- Bland diet
- Alcohol avoidance
- ASA avoidance
- Antibiotics for *H. pylori*

Peptic Ulcers

Erosive area on mucosa

- Extends below epithelium
- Chronic ulcers have scar tissue at base of erosive area

Ulcers can occur anywhere on gastrointestinal tract but typically are found on the

- Lower esophagus
- Stomach
- Proximal duodenum

Some causes

Alcohol

Smoking

Aspirin

Severe stress

Bacterial infection caused by *Helicobacter pylori (H. pylori)*, 90% of the time

Genetic factor

Constant use of anti-inflammatory drugs

Symptoms

Epigastric pain when stomach is empty

- Relieved by food or antacid

Burning

May include

- Vomiting blood
- Nausea
- Weight loss
- Anorexia

Severe cases may include

- Obstruction
- Hemorrhage
- Perforation

Treatment

Surgical intervention

Antacids

Dietary restrictions

Rest

Antibiotics

Gastric Cancer (malignant tumor of stomach)

Most often occurs in men over 40

Cause is unknown, but often associated with *Helicobacter pylori* (bacterial infection)

Predisposing Factors

Atrophic gastritis

Pernicious anemia

History of nonhealing gastric ulcer

Blood type A

Geographic factors

Environmental factors

Carcinogenic foods

- Smoked meats
- Nitrates
- Pickled foods

Symptoms

Usually asymptomatic in early stages

Treatment

Excision

Chemotherapy

Radiation (poor response)

Prognosis is poor

Pyloric Stenosis

Narrowing of the pyloric sphincter

Signs appear soon after birth

- Failure to thrive
- Projectile vomiting

Treatment
Surgery to relieve stenosis (pyloromyotomy)

Intestinal Disorders

■ Small Intestine

Malabsorption Conditions

Celiac disease
Most important malabsorption condition
Villi atrophy in response to food containing gluten and lose ability to absorb

- Gluten is a protein found in wheat, rye, oats, and barley

Symptoms
Malnutrition

Muscle wasting

Distended abdomen

Diarrhea

Fatigue

Weakness

Steatorrhea (excess fat in feces)

Treatment
Gluten-free diet

Steroids when necessary

Lactase deficiency
Enzyme deficiency

- Secondary to gastrointestinal damage, such as
  - Regional enteritis
  - Infection
- Common in African Americans, occurring in adulthood

Symptoms
Intolerance to milk

Intestinal cramping

Diarrhea

Flatulence

Treatment
Elimination of milk products

Crohn's disease (regional enteritis)
Inflammatory bowel disease (IBD)—affects terminal ileum and colon

Cause
Unknown

Symptoms
Vary greatly

Inflammation of GI tract

Diarrhea

Gas

Fever

Abdominal pain

Malaise

Anorexia

Weight loss

Treatment
No specific treatment

Palliative medications to control symptoms

Resection of affected section of intestine with anastomosis

Diet modifications

Duodenal Ulcers
Most common ulcer

Develop in younger population

Common in type O blood types

Appendicitis
Inflammation of vermiform appendix that projects from cecum

Obstruction of lumen leads to infection

- Appendix becomes hypoxic (decreased oxygen levels)
- May cause gangrene
- May rupture, causing peritonitis

Symptoms
Periumbilical (around umbilicus) pain, initially

Right lower quadrant (RLQ) pain as inflammation progresses

Nausea

Vomiting

Possible diarrhea

Treatment
Appendectomy

Management of any perforation or abscess

Meckel's Diverticulum
Appendage of ileum near cecum derived from an unobliterated yolk stalk in fetal development.

- Symptoms can mimic appendicitis.

Peritonitis
Inflammation of peritoneum (membrane that lines abdominal cavity)

Usually a result of

- Spread of infection from abdominal organ
- Puncture wound to abdomen
- Rupture of gastrointestinal tract—appendicitis or Meckel's diverticulum

Abscesses form, resulting in adhesions

- May result in obstruction

Types
Acute, chronic

Symptoms
Abdominal pain

Vomiting

Rigid abdomen

Fever

Leukocytosis (increased white cells in blood)

Treatment
Antibiotics

Suction of stomach and intestines

If possible, surgical removal of origin of infection, such as appendix

Fluid replacement

Bed rest

Obstruction
Any interference with passage of intestinal contents

May be

- Acute

- Chronic

- Partial

- Total

Types
Nonmechanical

- Paralytic ileus

- Result of trauma or toxin

Mechanical

- Result of tumors, adhesions, hernias

- Simple mechanical obstruction

  · One point of obstruction

- Closed-loop obstruction

  · At least two points of obstruction

- Diverticulosis

- Twisted bowel (volvulus)

- Telescoping bowel (intussusception)

Symptoms
Abdominal distention

Pain

Vomiting

Total constipation

Treatment
Surgical intervention

Symptomatic treatment

■ Large Intestine

Diverticulosis

Herniation of intestinal mucosa

- Forms sacs in lining, called diverticula

Diverticulitis

Sacs fill and become inflamed

- Common in aged

Symptoms

Diarrhea or constipation

Gas

Abdominal discomfort

Complications

Perforation

Bleeding

Peritonitis

Abscess

Obstruction

Treatment

Antimicrobials as necessary

High-fiber diet (greater than 20 g daily)

Stool softeners

Dietary restrictions of solid foods

Surgical intervention if necessary

Ulcerative Colitis (Fig. 1-41)

Inflammation of rectum that progresses to sigmoid colon

Intermittent exacerbations and remissions

May develop into toxic megacolon

- Leads to obstruction and dilation of colon

Increased risk for colorectal cancer

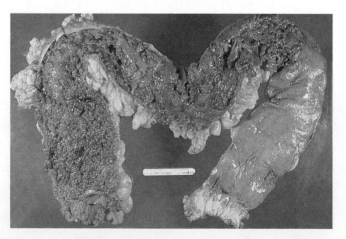

Figure **1-41** Ulcerative colitis.

Symptoms
Diarrhea

• Blood and mucus may be present

Cramping

Fever

Weight loss

Treatment
Remove physical or emotional stressors

Anti-inflammatory medications

Antimotility agents

Nutritional supplementation

Surgical intervention, if necessary

Colorectal Cancer
Usually develop from polyp

• In those 55 and older

Increased risks
Genetic factors

40 years of age and older

Diets high in

• Fat

• Sugar

• Red meat

Low-fiber diets

Symptoms
Asymptomatic until advanced

Some may experience

• Cramping

• Ribbon stools

• Feeling of incomplete evacuation

• Fatigue

• Weight loss

• Change in bowel habits

• Blood in stool

Treatment
Surgical excision

Radiation

Chemotherapy

Combination of above

Disorders of Liver, Gallbladder, and Pancreas

■ Disorders of Liver

Jaundice (Hyperbilirubinemia)
A sign of biliary disease, not a disease itself

- Results in yellow eyes (sclera) and skin

Types

Prehepatic

- Excess destruction of red blood cells
- Result of hemolytic anemia or reaction to transfusion

Intrahepatic

- Impaired uptake of bilirubin and decreased blending of bilirubin by hepatic cells
- Result of liver disease, such as cirrhosis or hepatitis

Posthepatic

- Excess bile flows into blood
- Result of obstruction
  - Due to conditions such as inflammation of liver, tumors, cholelithiasis

Treatment

Removal of cause

Cancer of Liver
Most commonly a metastasis; primary CA rare

Risk for primary liver CA

- Hepatitis B, C, and D
- Cirrhosis
- Myotoxins
- Heavy smoking/alcohol use

Treatment

Surgical resection if localized

Survival typically 3 or 4 months

Viral Hepatitis
Liver cells are damaged

Results in inflammation and necrosis

Damage can be mild or severe

Scar tissue forms in liver

- Leads to ischemia

Hepatitis A (HAV)

Infectious hepatitis—caused by hepatitis A virus

Transmission

- Most commonly fecal-oral route—contaminated food or water

Does not have a chronic state

Slow onset—complete recovery characteristic

Vaccine available for those who are traveling

Gamma globulin may be administered to those just exposed

Hepatitis B (HBV)
Serum hepatitis

Carrier state is common

Caused by hepatitis B virus

• Asymptomatic but contagious

Long incubation period

Transmission

• Intravenous drug users

• Transfusion

• Exposure to blood and bodily fluids

• Sexual transmission

• Mother-to-fetus transmission

• Immune globulin is temporary prophylactic

• Vaccine is now routine for children and is given to those at risk

Severe forms cause liver cell destruction, cirrhosis, death

Hepatitis C (HCV)
Transmission of virus

• Most commonly by transfusion

• IV drug users

Half of cases develop into chronic hepatitis

Increases risk of hepatocellular cancer

Carrier state may develop

Hepatitis D (HDV)
Transmission of hepatitis D virus

• Blood

• Intravenous drug users

Hepatitis B is present for this type to develop

Hepatitis E (HEV)
Transmission of hepatitis E virus

• Fecal-oral route

Does not develop into chronic or carrier

Hepatitis G
Transmission of hepatitis G virus

• IV drug use

• Sexual transmission

Symptoms of hepatitis
Stages
Preicteric

- Anorexia

- Nausea and vomiting

Liver enzymes may be elevated—indication of liver cell damage

- Fatigue

- Malaise

- Generalized pain with low-grade fever

- Cough

Icteric

- Jaundice

- Hepatomegaly (enlarged liver)

- Biliary obstruction

- Light-colored stools and dark urine

- Pruritus

- Abdominal pain

Posticteric (recovery)

- Reduction of symptoms

Treatment
None

In early stages gamma globulins may be used

Interferon may be used for cases of chronic hepatitis B and C

Nonviral hepatitis
Hepatitis that results from hepatotoxins

Symptoms

- Similar to viral hepatitis

Treatment

- Removal of hepatotoxin

Cirrhosis

Profuse liver damage

- Extensive fibrosis

  - Results in inflammation

Progressive disorder

Leads to liver failure

Types
Alcoholic liver

- Known as Laënnec's cirrhosis or portal cirrhosis

- Largest group

Biliary

- Associated with immune disorders

- Obstructions (intrahepatic or extrahepatic blood vessels) occur and disrupt normal function

Postnecrotic

- Associated with chronic hepatitis (A or C) and exposure to toxins

Symptoms
Asymptomatic in early stages

Nausea

Vomiting

Fatigue

Weight loss

Pruritus

Jaundice

Edema

Treatment
Symptomatic

Dietary restrictions

- Reduced protein and sodium

- Increased vitamins and carbohydrates

Diuretics

Antibiotics

Liver transplant

■ Disorders of Gallbladder

Cholecystitis
Inflammation of gallbladder and cystic duct

Cholangitis
Inflammation of bile duct

Cholelithiasis
Formation of gallstones (Fig. 1-42)

- Consists of cholesterol or bilirubin

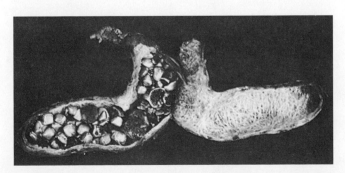

Figure **1-42** Resected gallbladder containing mixed gallstones.

- Occurs most often in those with high levels of cholesterol, calcium, or bile salts

Stones cause irritation and inflammation

- May lead to infection
- Obstruction
  - May result in pancreatitis
  - Rupture is possible

Symptoms
Often asymptomatic

Dietary intolerance particularly to fat

Right upper quadrant (RUQ) pain

Pain in back and/or shoulder

Epigastric discomfort

Bloating heartburn, flatulence

Treatment
Surgical intervention (laparoscopic cholecystectomy)

Lithotripsy

Medical management by use of drugs that break down stone

■ Disorders of Pancreas

Pancreatitis
Inflammation of pancreas resulting from digestive enzyme attack to pancreas

Acute and chronic forms

Commonly associated with alcoholism, biliary tract obstruction, drug toxicity, gallstone obstruction of common bile duct, and viral infections

Symptoms
Severe pain

Fever

Acute form is a medical emergency

Neurogenic shock

Septicemia

General sepsis

Complications
Adult respiratory distress syndrome (ARDS)

Renal failure

Treatment
No oral intake

- IV fluids given and carefully monitored

Analgesics

Stop process of autodigestion

Prevent systemic shutdown

Pancreatic Cancer
Increased risk
Cigarette smoking

Diet high in fat and protein

Symptoms
Weight loss

Jaundice

Anorexia

Most types of pancreatic cancer are asymptomatic until well advanced

Treatment
Surgery

Chemotherapy and radiation therapy

DIGESTIVE SYSTEM PATHOPHYSIOLOGY QUIZ
(Quiz answers are located at the end of Unit 1)

1. This type of hyperbilirubinemia is hallmarked by excess bile flow into the blood:
   a. intrahepatic
   b. prehepatic
   c. posthepatic
   d. jaundice

2. This type of hepatitis is transmitted by the fecal-oral route:
   a. A
   b. B
   c. C
   d. D

3. Which of the following is the recovery stage of hepatitis?
   a. prehepatic
   b. posthepatic
   c. preicteric
   d. posticteric

4. This type of cirrhosis is also known as portal cirrhosis:
   a. biliary
   b. alcoholic liver
   c. postnecrotic
   d. traumatic

5. This condition is the inflammation of the bile ducts:
   a. cholangitis
   b. cholecystitis
   c. cholelithiasis
   d. cholangioma

6. Formation of gallstones most often occurs with high levels of the following:
   a. bile salts and toxins
   b. cholesterol and toxins
   c. cholesterol and bile salts
   d. toxins

7. The primary factor that increases the risk of pancreatic cancer is:
   a. smoking
   b. alcohol
   c. intravenous drug use
   d. hepatitis

8. A potential complication of this condition is ARDS:
   a. hyperbilirubinemia
   b. hepatitis
   c. pancreatitis
   d. pancreatic cancer

9. The primary treatment for jaundice is:
   a. removal of cause
   b. antibiotics
   c. dialysis
   d. vaccine

10. This condition has as the largest group of those who abuse alcohol:
    a. cirrhosis
    b. hepatitis
    c. pancreatitis
    d. pancreatic cancer

■ MEDIASTINUM AND DIAPHRAGM

MEDIASTINUM AND DIAPHRAGM—ANATOMY AND TERMINOLOGY

Not an organ system

Mediastinum

That area between lungs that a median (partition) divides (Fig. 1-43) into

- Superior
- Anterior
- Posterior
- Middle

Space that houses heart, thymus gland, trachea, esophagus, nerves, lymph and blood vessels and major blood vessels

- Aorta
- Inferior vena cava

Diaphragm

A dome-shaped muscular partition that separates abdominal cavity from thoracic cavity

- Assists in breathing
  - Expands to assist lungs in exhalation/relaxation of diaphragm
  - Flattens out during inspiration/contraction of diaphragm
- Diaphragmatic hernia: esophageal hernia

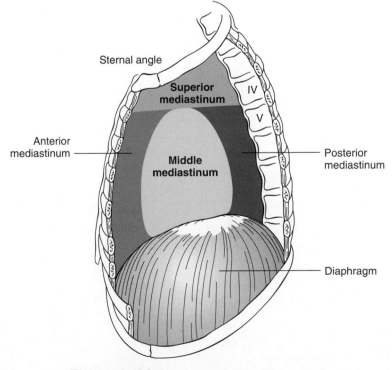

Figure **1-43** Mediastinum and diaphragm.

MEDIASTINUM AND DIAPHRAGM ANATOMY AND TERMINOLOGY QUIZ
(Quiz answers are located at the end of Unit 1)

1. The mediastinum is NOT an organ system.
   a. true
   b. false

2. The mediastinum is divided into:
   a. superior, anterior, posterior
   b. superior, anterior, posterior, middle
   c. anterior, posterior, middle
   d. middle, anterior, superior

3. During inspiration, the diaphragm:
   a. expands
   b. moves upward
   c. collapses
   d. flattens out

4. Term meaning "partition":
   a. middle
   b. aspect
   c. median
   d. diaphragm

5. The diaphragm is said to be this shape:
   a. square
   b. flat
   c. dome
   d. round

6. This separates the abdominal cavity from the thoracic cavity:
   a. mediastinum
   b. diaphragm
   c. superior
   d. inferior

7. This is the area between the lungs:
   a. mediastinum
   b. diaphragm
   c. superior
   d. inferior

8. This is an esophageal hernia:
   a. mediastinal
   b. diaphragmatic
   c. paraesophageal
   d. hiatal

9. A diaphragmatic hernia is also known as:
   a. esophageal
   b. epiglottis
   c. partitional
   d. medial

10. The diaphragm assists in:
    a. percussion
    b. auscultation
    c. contraction
    d. breathing

■ HEMIC AND LYMPHATIC SYSTEM
HEMIC AND LYMPHATIC SYSTEM—ANATOMY AND TERMINOLOGY

Hemic refers to blood

Lymphatic system removes excess tissue fluid

- Lymph tissue is scattered throughout body

- Composed of lymph nodes, vessels, and organs

Lymph

Colorless fluid containing lymphocytes and monocytes

Originates from blood and after filtering, returns to blood

Transports interstitial fluids and proteins that have leaked from blood system into venous system

Absorbs and transports fats from villi of small intestine to venous system

Assists in immune function

Lymph Vessels

Similar to veins

Organized circulatory system throughout body

Lymph Organs

Lymph nodes, spleen, bone marrow, thymus, tonsils, and Peyer's patches (lymphoid tissue on mucosa of small intestine)

Lymph nodes, areas of concentrated tissue (Fig. 1-44)

Spleen, located in left upper quadrant (LUQ) of abdomen

- Composed of lymph tissue

  - Function is to filter blood; activates lymphocytes and B cells to filter antigens

  - Stores blood

Thymus secretes thymosin, causing T cells to mature

- Larger in infants and shrinks with age

Tonsils

- Palatine tonsils

- Pharyngeal tonsils/adenoids

Hematopoietic Organ

Bone marrow, contains tissue that produces RBCs, WBCs, and platelets

- Produces stem cells

COMBINING FORMS

1.	aden/o	gland
2.	adenoid/o	adenoids

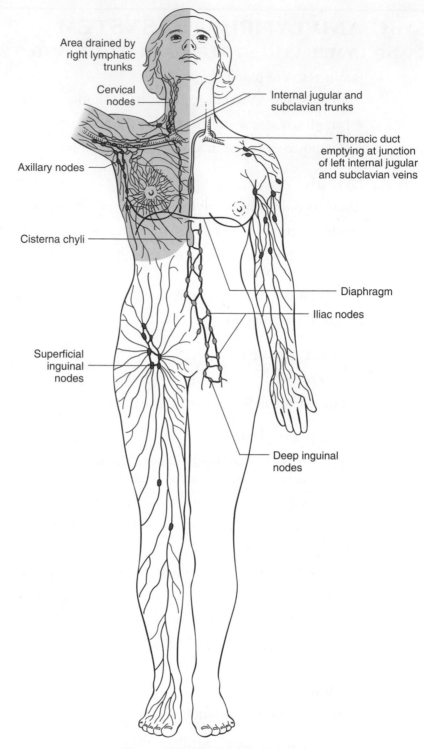

Area drained by
right lymphatic
trunks

Cervical
nodes

Internal jugular and
subclavian trunks

Thoracic duct
emptying at junction
of left internal jugular
and subclavian veins

Axillary nodes

Cisterna chyli

Diaphragm

Iliac nodes

Superficial
inguinal
nodes

Deep inguinal
nodes

Figure **1-44** Lymphatic system.

3.	axill/o	armpit
4.	cervic/o	neck/cervix
5.	immun/o	immune
6.	inguin/o	groin
7.	lymph/o	lymph
8.	lymphaden/o	lymph gland
9.	splen/o	spleen
10.	thym/o	thymus gland
11.	tonsill/o	tonsil
12.	tox/o	poison

PREFIXES

1.	hyper-	excess
2.	inter-	between
3.	retro-	behind

SUFFIXES

1.	-ectomy	removal
2.	-edema	swelling
3.	-itis	inflammation
4.	-megaly	enlargement
5.	-oid	resembling
6.	-oma	tumor
7.	-penia	deficient
8.	-pexy	fixation
9.	-phylaxis	protection
10.	-poiesis	production

MEDICAL TERMS

Axillary nodes	Lymph nodes located in armpit
Cloquet's node	Also called a gland; it is highest of deep groin lymph nodes
Inguinofemoral	Referring to groin and thigh
Jugular nodes	Lymph nodes located next to large vein in neck
Lymph node	Station along lymphatic system
Lymphadenectomy	Excision of a lymph node or nodes
Lymphadenitis	Inflammation of a lymph node
Lymphangiography	Radiographic recording of lymphatic vessels and nodes

Lymphangiotomy	Incision into a lymphatic vessel
Lymphangitis	Inflammation of lymphatic vessel or vessels
Parathyroid	Produces a hormone to mobilize calcium from bones to blood
Splenectomy	Excision of spleen
Splenography	Radiographic recording of spleen
Splenoportography	Radiographic procedure to allow visualization of splenic and portal veins of spleen
Stem cell	Immature blood cell
Thoracic duct	Largest lymph vessel; it collects lymph from portions of body below diaphragm and from left side of body above diaphragm
Transplantation	Grafting of tissue from one source to another

HEMIC AND LYMPHATIC SYSTEM ANATOMY AND TERMINOLOGY QUIZ

(Quiz answers are located at the end of Unit 1)

1. The spleen is located in this quadrant of the abdomen:
   a. RUQ
   b. LUQ
   c. LLQ
   d. LRQ

2. Produces RBCs and platelets:
   a. thymus
   b. tonsils
   c. lymph node
   d. bone marrow

3. Which of the following is NOT a lymph organ?
   a. adrenal
   b. spleen
   c. thymus
   d. tonsil

4. Lymph transports fluids and _____ that have leaked from the blood system back to veins.
   a. stem cells
   b. lymphocytes
   c. B cells
   d. proteins

5. This is largest in infants and shrinks with age:
   a. tonsils
   b. spleen
   c. thymus
   d. bone marrow

6. Combining form meaning "gland":
   a. axill/o
   b. thym/o
   c. aden/o
   d. tox/o

7. Prefix meaning "excess":
   a. hyper-
   b. hypo-
   c. inter-
   d. retro-

8. Suffix meaning "enlargement":
   a. -edema
   b. -poiesis
   c. -penia
   d. -megaly

9. Lymph node located on neck:
   a. thoracic
   b. jugular
   c. Cloquet's
   d. axillary

10. These cells originate in the bone marrow:
   a. B cells
   b. antigens
   c. erythrocytes
   d. stem cells

HEMIC AND LYMPHATIC SYSTEM—PATHOPHYSIOLOGY

Anemia

Reduction in number of erythrocytes or decrease in quality of hemoglobin

- Less oxygen is transported in the blood

Aplastic Anemia

Diverse group of anemias

Characterized by bone marrow failure with reduced numbers of red and white blood cells and platelets

Causes

Genetic or acquired (primary or secondary)

Toxins/chemical agents

    Benzene and antibiotics such as chloramphenicol

Irradiation

Immunologic

Idiopathic (unknown)

Treatment

Blood transfusion

Bone marrow transplant

Iron Deficiency Anemia

Characterized by small erythrocytes and a reduced amount of hemoglobin

Caused by low or absent iron stores or serum iron concentrations

- Blood loss
- Decreased intake of iron
- Malabsorption of iron

Symptoms

Pallor

Headache

Stomatitis

Oral lesions

Gastrointestinal complaints

Retinal hemorrhages

Thinning, brittle nails and hair

Treatment

Iron supplement

Pernicious Anemia

Megaloblastic anemia (large stem cells)

Inability to absorb vitamin B_{12} due to a lack of intrinsic factor (found in gastric juices)

Usually in older adults

Caused by impaired intestinal absorption of vitamin B_{12}

Symptoms
Pallor

Weakness

Neurologic manifestations

Gastric discomfort

Treatment
Injections of vitamin B_{12}

Transfusions

Hemolytic Anemia
May be acute or chronic

Shortened survival of mature erythrocytes—excessive destruction of RBC

• Inability of bone marrow to compensate for decreased survival of erythrocytes

Treatment
Treat cause

Sickle Cell Anemia
Occurs primarily in those of West African descent

Abnormal sickle-shaped erythrocytes (sickle cell) caused by an abnormal type of hemoglobin (Hemoglobin S)

Symptoms
Abdominal pain

Arthralgia

Ulceration of lower extremities

Fatigue

Dyspnea

Increased heart rate

Treatment
Symptomatic

Granulocytosis

Increase in granulocytes

• Neutrophils

• Eosinophils

• Basophils

Eosinophilia

Increase in number of eosinophilic granulocytes

Cause

Allergic disorders

Dermatologic disorders

Parasitic invasion

Drugs

Malignancies

Basophilia

Increase in basophilic granulocytes seen in leukemia

Monocytosis

Increased number of monocytes

Cause

Infection

Hematologic factors

Leukocytosis

Increased number of leukocytes

Cause

Acute viral infections, such as hepatitis

Chronic infections, such as syphilis

Leukocytopenia

Decreased number of leukocytes

Cause

Neoplasias

Immune deficiencies

Drugs

Virus

Radiation

Infectious Mononucleosis

Acute Infection of B Cells

Epstein-Barr virus most common cause

Symptoms

Fatigue

Fever

Weakness (asthenia)

Pharyngitis

Atypical lymphocytes in blood

Lymph node enlargement

Splenomegaly

Hepatomegaly

Transmission
Saliva

• Known as kissing disease

Treatment
Rest

Treatment of symptoms

Leukemia

Malignant disorder of blood and blood-forming organs

Leads to dysfunction of cells

• Primarily leads to proliferation of abnormal leukocytes—filling bone marrow and bloodstream

Acute Myelogenous Leukemia (AML)
Rapid onset

Short survival time

Symptoms
Abrupt onset

Fatigue

Lymphadenopathy

Bone pain and tenderness

Anemia

Bleeding

Fever

Infection

Anorexia

Splenomegaly

Hepatomegaly

Headache, vomiting, paralysis

Treatment
Chemotherapy

Bone marrow transplant following high-dose chemotherapy eradicating leukemic cells

Acute Lymphocytic Leukemia (ALL)
Immature lymphocytes (lymphoblasts)

Most cases occur in children and adolescents

Sudden onset

Treatment

Chemotherapy with drugs that suppress cell division and destroy rapidly dividing cells

Remission

Relapse—leukemia cells in bone marrow and blood requiring treatment

Chronic Myelogenous Leukemia (CML)

Mature and immature granulocytes in bone marrow and blood

Slow progressive disease (those over 55 years live many years without life threat)

Cells are more differentiated

Gradual onset with milder symptoms

• Majority of cases are in adults

Symptoms

Extreme fatigue

Weight loss

Splenomegaly

Night sweats

Fever

Infections

Treatment

Chemotherapy—target abnormal proteins

Bone marrow transplant—following high-dose chemotherapy

Chronic Lymphocytic Leukemia (CLL)

Increased numbers of mature lymphocytes in marrow, lymph nodes, spleen

Most common form seen in elderly

Slowly progressive

Treatment

Chemotherapy

Lymph

Lymphadenopathy

Any abnormality of lymph node

Enlargement of lymph node

Lymphangitis

Inflammation of lymphatic vessel

Lymphadenitis

Inflammation of lymph node

Localized inflammation associated with inflamed lesion

Generalized inflammation associated with disease

Inflammation can occur as result of

- Trauma

- Infection

- Drug reaction

- Autoimmune disease

- Immunologic disease

Malignant Lymphoma

Hodgkin Disease

Initial sign is a painless mass commonly located on neck

Giant Reed-Sternberg cells are present in lymphatic tissue

Presentation

Enlarged spleen (splenomegaly)

Abdominal mass

Mediastinal mass

Localized node involvement

- Orderly spreading of node involvement

- Cervical, axillary, inguinal, and retroperitoneal lymph node involvement

Symptoms

Night sweats

Fever

Weight loss

Itching (pruritus)

Anorexia

Weakness

Treatment

If localized: radiation therapy and chemotherapy

If systemic: chemotherapy alone

High probability of cure with new treatments

Non-Hodgkin Lymphoma

No giant Reed-Sternberg cells present

Involves multiple nodes scattered throughout body (follicular lymphoma)

Large cell lymphoma (large lymphocytes in diffuse nodes and lymph tissue)

- Noncontiguous spread of node involvement

- Not localized

Usually begins as a painless enlargement of node

Symptoms
Presents similar to Hodgkin disease

Treatment
Chemotherapy cures or stops disease progression

Burkitt's Lymphoma
Type of non-Hodgkin lymphoma

Usually found in Africa and New Guinea

Characterized by lesions in jaw and face

Epstein-Barr (herpes virus) has been found in Burkitt's lymphoma

Treatment
Radiation and chemotherapy for African type

Myeloma

Multiple Myeloma
B-cell cancer—lymphocytes that produce antibodies destroying bone tissue

• Also known as plasma cell myeloma

Increased plasma cells replace bone marrow

Overproduction of immunoglobulins—Bence Jones protein (found in urine)

Multiple tumor sites cause bone destruction

Results in weakened bone

Hypercalcemia

Anemia

Renal damage

Increased susceptibility to infections

Cause
Unknown

Treatment
Chemotherapy

Radiotherapy

Autologous bone marrow transplant (ABMT) prolongs remission—may be a cure

Palliative treatments

HEMIC AND LYMPHATIC SYSTEM PATHOPHYSIOLOGY QUIZ
(Quiz answers are located at the end of Unit 1)

1. This condition involves a reduced number of erythrocytes and decreased quality of hemoglobin:
   a. monocytosis
   b. eosinophilia
   c. anemia
   d. leukocytosis

2. This condition is hallmarked by a shortened survival of mature erythrocytes and inability of bone marrow to compensate for decreased survival:
   a. hemolytic anemia
   b. granulocytosis
   c. eosinophilia
   d. monocytosis

3. The most common cause of this disease is Epstein-Barr virus:
   a. leukocytopenia
   b. infectious mononucleosis
   c. leukocytosis
   d. hemolytic anemia

4. Inflammation of the lymphatic vessels is:
   a. lymphadenitis
   b. lymphoma
   c. lymphadenopathy
   d. lymphangitis

5. What giant cell is present in Hodgkin disease?
   a. B cell
   b. Reed-Sternberg
   c. T cell
   d. C cell

6. This condition increases plasma cells, which replace bone marrow:
   a. Burkitt's lymphoma
   b. Multiple myeloma
   c. Hodgkin disease
   d. leukemia

7. Injection of vitamin B may be prescribed for this type of anemia:
   a. pernicious
   b. aplastic
   c. sideroblastic
   d. sickle cell

8. These are large stem cells:
   a. megaloblasts
   b. leukocytes
   c. erythrocytes
   d. granulocytes

9. This is known as the kissing disease:
   a. monocytosis
   b. leukocytopenia
   c. infectious mononucleosis
   d. granulocytosis

10. This lymphoma is usually found in Africa:
    a. multiple
    b. Burkitt's
    c. B-cell
    d. T-cell

■ ENDOCRINE SYSTEM

ENDOCRINE SYSTEM—ANATOMY AND TERMINOLOGY

Regulates body through hormones (chemical messengers)

Ductless endocrine glands secrete hormones directly to bloodstream

Affects growth, development, and metabolism

Endocrine Glands (Fig. 1-45)

Pituitary (Hypophysis): Master Gland
Located at base of brain in a depression in skull (sella turcica)

Anterior pituitary (adenohypophysis)

- Adrenocorticotropic hormone (ACTH)—stimulates adrenal cortex and increases production of cortisol

- Follicle-stimulating hormone (FSH)—males, stimulates sperm and testosterone production; females, with luteinizing hormone (LH) stimulates secretion of estrogen and follicle development and ovulation

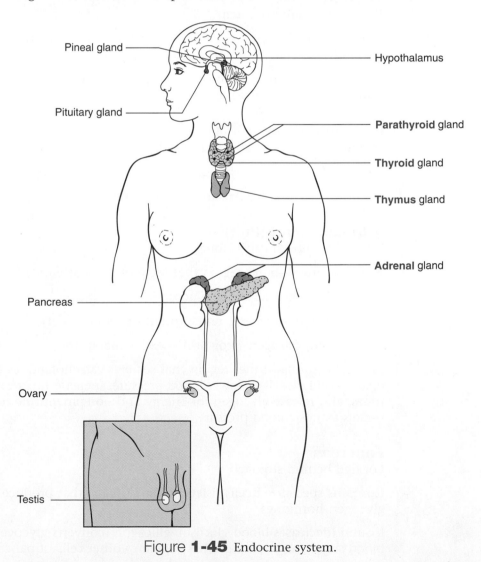

Figure **1-45** Endocrine system.

- Growth hormone (GH or somatotropin STH)—stimulates protein processing resulting in growth of bones, muscle, and fat metabolism, and maintains blood glucose levels

- Luteinizing hormone (LH)—males, stimulates testosterone production; females, stimulates secretion of progesterone and estrogen

- Melanocyte-stimulating hormone (MSH)—increases skin pigmentation

- Prolactin (PRL)—secreted by anterior pituitary, stimulates milk production and breast development

- Thyroid-stimulating hormone (TSH or thyrotropin)—stimulates thyroid gland

Posterior pituitary (neurohypophysis)—stores and releases hormones

- Antidiuretic hormone (ADH) or vasopressin—stimulates reabsorption of water by kidney tubules and increases blood pressure by constricting arterioles

- Oxytocin (OT)—stimulates contractions during childbirth, production and release of milk

Thyroid
Two lobes overlying trachea

Secretes two hormones that increase cell metabolism—thyroxine (T_4) and triiodothyronine (T_3)—synthesized from iodine

Secretes one hormone that decreases blood calcium—thyrocalcitonin (nasal spray used to treat osteoporosis)

Parathyroid Glands (4)
Located on posterior side of thyroid

Secretes PTH (parathyroid hormone) or parathoromone

Promotes calcium homeostasis in bloodstream

Adrenal Gland (Pair)
Located on top of each kidney

Adrenal cortex—outer region that secretes corticosteroids

- Cortisol—increases blood glucose

- Aldosterone—increases reabsorption of sodium (salt)

- Androgen, estrogen, progestin—sexual characteristics

Adrenal medulla—inner region that secretes catecholamines (epinephrine to dilate blood vessels to lower blood pressure, increase heart rate, dilate bronchial tubes, and release glycogen for energy and norepinephrine to constrict blood vessels to raise blood pressure)

Pancreas
Located behind stomach

Contains specialized cells (islets of Langerhans) that produce insulin and glycogen hormones

Insulin (decreases blood glucose), glucagon (converts glycogen to glucose, raising blood sugar), and somatostatin (regulates other cells of pancreas)

Thymus

Located behind sternum

Atrophies during adolescence

Produces thymosin—stimulates T-lymphocytes, effecting a positive immune response

Hypothalamus (Part of Brain)

Located below thalamus and above pituitary gland

Stimulates anterior pituitary to release hormones and posterior hypothalamus to store and release horomones

Pineal

Located between two cerebral hemispheres and above third ventricle

Secretes melatonin—more so at night, which affects sleep cycle

Also responsible for delaying sexual maturation in children

Also has neurotransmitters such as somatostatin, norepinephrine, seratonin, and histamine

Ovaries (Pair, Females)

Estrogen production stimulates ova production and secondary female sex characteristics

Progesterone—prepares the uterus for and maintains pregnancy

Placenta

Produces HCG (human chorionic gonadotropin) to sustain a pregnancy

Testes (Pair, Males)

Testosterone—male sex characteristics

COMBINING FORMS

1.	aden/o	in relationship to a gland
2.	adren/o	adrenal gland
3.	adrenal/o	adrenal gland
4.	andr/o	male
5.	calc/o, calc/i	calcium
6.	cortic/o	cortex
7.	crin/o	secrete
8.	dips/o	thirst
9.	estr/o	female
10.	gluc/o	sugar
11.	glyc/o	sugar
12.	gonad/o	ovaries and testes
13.	home/o	same
14.	hormon/o	hormone

15. kal/i	potassium
16. lact/o	milk
17. myx/o	mucus
18. natr/o	sodium
19. pancreat/o	pancreas
20. parathyroid/o	parathyroid gland
21. phys/o	growing
22. pituitar/o	pituitary gland
23. somat/o	body
24. ster/o, stere/o	solid, having three dimensions
25. thry/o	thyroid gland
26. thyroid/o	thyroid gland
27. toc/o	childbirth
28. toxic/o	poison
29. ur/o	urine

PREFIXES

1. eu-	good/normal
2. oxy-	sharp, oxygen
3. pan-	all
4. tetra-	four
5. tri-	three
6. tropin-	act upon

SUFFIXES

1. -agon	assemble
2. -drome	run, relationship to conducting, to speed
3. -emia	blood condition
4. -in	a substance
5. -ine	a substance
6. -tropin	act upon
7. -uria	urine

MEDICAL TERMS

Adrenals	Glands, located at top of kidneys, that produce steroid hormones (cortex) and catecholamines (medulla)
Contralateral	Opposite side
Hormone	Chemical substance produced by body's endocrine glands

Isthmus	Connection of two regions or structures
Isthmus, thyroid	Tissue connection between right and left thyroid lobes
Isthmusectomy	Surgical removal of isthmus
Lobectomy	Removal of a lobe
Thymectomy	Surgical removal of thymus
Thymus	Gland that produces hormones important to immune response
Thyroglossal duct	A duct in embryo between thyroid and posterior tongue which occasionally persists into adult life and causes cysts, fistulas, or sinuses
Thyroid	Part of endocrine system that produces hormones that regulate metabolism
Thyroidectomy	Surgical removal of thyroid

ENDOCRINE SYSTEM ANATOMY AND TERMINOLOGY QUIZ
(Quiz answers are located at the end of Unit 1)

1. Which of the following is NOT affected by the endocrine system?
   a. digestion
   b. development
   c. progesterone
   d. metabolism

2. Gland that overlies the trachea:
   a. parathyroid
   b. adrenal
   c. pancreas
   d. thyroid

3. Gland that is located on the top of each kidney:
   a. parathyroid
   b. adrenal
   c. pancreas
   d. thyroid

4. The outer region of the adrenal gland that secretes corticosteroids:
   a. cortex
   b. medulla
   c. sternum
   d. medullary

5. Located on the thyroid:
   a. hypophysis
   b. thymus
   c. pineal
   d. parathyroid

6. Located at the base of the brain in a depression in the skull:
   a. pituitary
   b. thymus
   c. adrenal
   d. pineal

7. Stimulates contractions during childbirth:
   a. cortisol
   b. PTH
   c. ADH
   d. oxytocin

8. Produced only during pregnancy by the placenta:
   a. estrogen and progesterone
   b. melatonin
   c. thymosin
   d. adrenocorticotropic hormone

9. Combining form meaning "secrete":
   a. dips/o
   b. crin/o
   c. gluc/o
   d. kal/i

10. Prefix meaning "good":
   a. tri-
   b. tropin-
   c. pan-
   d. eu-

ENDOCRINE SYSTEM—PATHOPHYSIOLOGY

Diabetes Mellitus

Caused by a deficiency in insulin production or poor use of insulin by body cells

Islets of Langerhans (pancreatic cells) secrete glucagon and insulin to regulate fat, carbohydrate, and protein metabolism

Types of Diabetes Mellitus

Type 1, IDDM (insulin-dependent diabetes mellitus), immune mediated
Onset before age 30—peak onset age 12

Includes beta islet cell destruction, insulin deficiency

Acute onset

Positive family history

Requires insulin

Ketoacidosis (fats improperly burned leads to ketones and acids circulating)

Type 2, NIDDM (non–insulin-dependent diabetes mellitus)
Adult onset, after age 30, but it is now occurring earlier

Insidious onset/asymptomatic

Positive in immediate family

Dietary management and/or oral hypoglycemics and/or insulin

Most common type—85% are obese at onset

Insulin is present

Ketoacidosis does not occur

Symptoms
Polyuria

Polydipsia

Glycosuria

Hyperglycemia

Polyphagia

Unexplained weight loss

Acute complications
Hypoglycemia

Hyperglycemia with coma

Diabetic ketoacidosis

Chronic complications
Diabetic neuropathy (Fig. 1-46)

Retinopathy

Coronary artery disease (atherosclerosis)

Stroke

Peripheral vascular disease

Infection

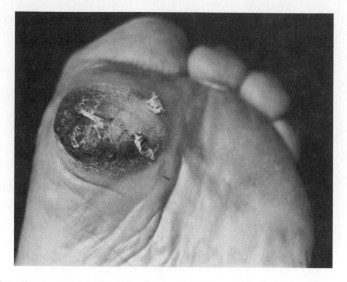

Figure **1-46** Patient with diabetes mellitus and neuropathy had severe claw toes, and shear forces across plantar surface of first metatarsal head caused recurrent ulceration.

Gestational diabetes mellitus—predisposition to diabetes
Most often recognized in second trimester

Glucose intolerance may be temporary, occurring only during pregnancy

Many will develop diabetes mellitus within 15 years

Pituitary Disorders

Tumors

    Most common cause of pituitary disorders

    May secrete hormone

        Such as prolactin or ACTH

Anterior Pituitary
Dwarfism (hypopituitarism)
Can be caused by deficiency of somatotrophin (growth hormone)

Gigantism (Fig. 1-47) (hyperpituitarism)
Can be caused by excess of somatotrophin (growth hormone) in childhood

Treatment
Resection of tumor or irradiation of pituitary

Acromegaly (hyperpituitarism)
Increased GH in adulthood

Enlargement of facial bones, feet, and hands

Treatment
Pituitary adenoma is irradiated or removed

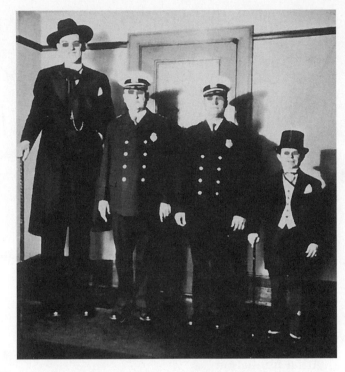

Figure **1-47** Gigantism. A pituitary giant and dwarf contrasted with normal-size men.

Posterior Pituitary
Diabetes insipidus
Insufficient antidiuretic hormone—kidney tubules fail to retain needed water and salts

Causes polyuria, polydipsia, and dehydration

ADH or SIADH—syndrome of inadequate antidiuretic hormone

Excessive secretion of antidiuretic hormone

Causes excessive water retention

Treatment
Some types have no treatment

Others can be controlled with vasopressin (drug)

Thyroid Disorders
Goiter (Fig. 1-48)
Enlargement of thyroid gland in the neck

Cause
Hypothyroid disorders

Hyperthyroid disorders

Hyperthyroidism—Thyrotoxicosis
Excessive thyroid hormone production

Most common form: Graves' disease (familial)—results of autoimmune process

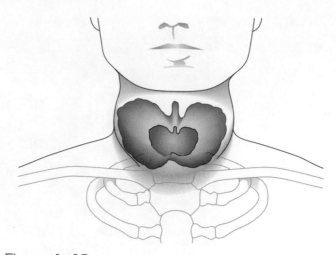

Figure **1-48** Goiter is an enlargement of thyroid gland.

Characterized by
Goiter

Tachycardia

Atrial fibrillation

Dyspnea

Palpitations

Fatigue

Tremor

Nervousness

Weight loss

Exophthalmos (protruding eyes)

• Decreased blinking

Treatment
Medication (antithyroid drugs)

Radioactive iodine

Surgical excision

Thyrotoxicosis Storm/Crisis
Thyroid storm/crisis is an acute, life-threatening hypermetabolic state induced by excessive release of thyroid horomones

• Most extreme state of thyrotoxicosis

Hypothyroidism
Primary: inadequate thyroid hormone production

   Resulting in increasing levels of thyroid-stimulating hormone (TSH) production

Secondary: inadequate amounts of thyroid-stimulating hormone synthesized

Types
Cretinism

- Congenital
- Occurs in children
- If not treated, it will cause a severe delay in physical/mental development

Myxedema

- Severe form
- Occurs in adults
  - Atherosclerosis
- Symptoms
  - Cold intolerance
  - Weight gain
  - Mental sluggishness
  - Fatigue

Hashimoto's thyroiditis

- Autoimmune disorder

Treatment
Medication (levothyroxine synthetic hormone replacement)

Parathyroid Disorders

Hyperparathyroidism—Excessive Parathyroid Hormone (PTH)
Leads to hypercalcemia

- Affects heart and bones and damages kidneys

Symptoms
Brittle bones

Kidney stones

Cardiac disturbances

Treatment
Surgical excision

Hypoparathyroidism—Abnormally Low PTH
Leads to hypocalcemia

Symptoms
Nerve irritability—twitching or spasms

Muscle cramps

Tingling and burning (paresthesias) of fingertips, toes, and lips

Anxiety, nervousness

Tetany (constant muscle contraction)

Treatment
Calcium and vitamin D

Adrenal Gland Disorders

Cushing Syndrome—Hypercortisolism
Excess levels of adrenocorticotropic hormone (ACTH)

Causes
Hyperfunction of adrenal cortex

Long-term use of steroid medications

Symptoms
Weight gain

- Fat deposits on face (moonface) and trunk (buffalo hump)

Glucose intolerance

- Diabetes may develop (20%)

Hypernatremia

Hypokalemia

Virilization

Hypertension

Muscle wasting

Osteoporosis

Change in mental status

Delayed healing

Treatment
Medication

Radiation therapy

Surgical intervention

Addison's Disease—Primary Adrenal Insufficiency
Deficiency of adrenocortical hormones resulting from destruction of adrenal glands
- Glucocorticoids

- Mineralocorticoids

Causes
Tumors

Autoimmune disorders

Viral

Tuberculosis

Infection

Symptoms
Decreased blood glucose levels

Elevated serum ACTH

Fatigue

Lack of ability to handle stress

Weight loss

Infections

Hypotension

Decreased body hair

Hyperpigmentation

Treatment
Hormone (glucocorticoid) replacement

Hyperaldosteronism
Excess aldosterone secreted by adrenal cortex

Types
Primary hyperaldosteronism (Conn's syndrome)

- Caused by an abnormality of adrenal cortex
  - Usually an adrenal adenoma

Secondary hyperaldosteronism

- Caused by other than adrenal stimuli

Symptoms
Hypertension

Hypokalemia

Neuromuscular disorders

Treatment
Treat the underlying condition that caused hyperaldosteronism

- Such as adrenal adenoma

Adrenal Medulla
Hypersecretion

Pheochromocytoma—benign tumor of medulla

Excessive production of epinephrine and norepinephrine

Symptoms
Severe headaches

Sweating

Flushing

Hypertension

Muscle spasms

Treatment
Antihypertensive drugs

Remove tumor

Androgen and Estrogen Hypersecretion

Androgen, male characteristic hormone

- Virilization, development of male characteristics

Hypersecretion of estrogen, female characteristic hormone

- Feminization

Causes

Underlying condition

- Adrenal tumor

- Cushing syndrome

- Adenomas or carcinomas

- Defects in steroid metabolism

Treatment

Surgical intervention for tumor

Underlying condition

ENDOCRINE SYSTEM PATHOPHYSIOLOGY QUIZ
(Quiz answers are located at the end of Unit 1)

1. This type of diabetes typically occurs before age 30:
   a. type 1
   b. type 2

2. The acronym that indicates that insulin is not required is:
   a. IDDM
   b. NIDDM
   c. PIDDM
   d. NDDMI

3. The most common cause of pituitary disorders is:
   a. hypersecretion
   b. hyposecretion
   c. tumor
   d. infection

4. In excess, this hormone can cause gigantism:
   a. somatotrophin
   b. thyroid
   c. mineralocorticoids
   d. adrenocortical

5. Goiter can be caused by which of the following:
   a. hypothyroidism
   b. parathyroidism
   c. hyperthyroidism
   d. both a and c

6. This type of hypothyroidism is an autoimmune disorder:
   a. myxedema
   b. Hashimoto's
   c. cretinism
   d. hypokalemia

7. Tetany can be caused by:
   a. hypoparathyroidism
   b. hyperthyroidism
   c. hyperparathyroidism
   d. hyperaldosteronism

8. Conn's syndrome is also known as:
   a. primary hypoparathyroidism
   b. primary hyperthyroidism
   c. primary hyperparathyroidism
   d. primary hyperaldosteronism

9. Development of male characteristics is known as:
   a. virilization
   b. feminization
   c. hypertrophy
   d. hyperaldosteronism

10. The treatment for Addison's disease is often:
    a. chemotherapy
    b. radiation
    c. hormone replacement
    d. all of the above

■ NERVOUS SYSTEM

NERVOUS SYSTEM—ANATOMY AND TERMINOLOGY

Controlling, regulating, and communicating system

Organization

- Central nervous system (CNS), brain and spinal cord
- Peripheral nervous system (PNS), cranial and spinal nerves
  - Autonomic nervous system—motor and sensory nerves of viscera (involuntary)
  - Somatic nervous system—motor and sensory nerves of skeletal muscles

Cells of the Nervous System (Fig. 1-49)

Neurons—Primary Cells of Nervous System

Classified according to function (afferent [sensory], efferent [motor], interneurons [associational])

- Dendrites (receive signals)
- Cell body (nucleus, within cell body)
- Axon (carries signals from cell body)
- Myelin sheath (insulation around axon)

Glia

Astrocytes

Star shaped—transport water and salts between capillaries and neurons

Microglia

Multiple branching processes—protect neurons from inflammation

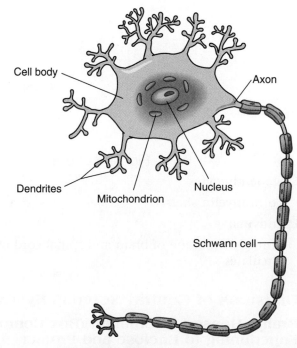

Figure **1-49** Myelinated axon.

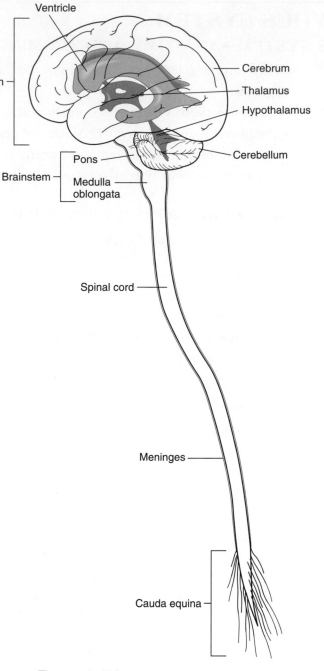

Figure **1-50** Brain and spinal cord.

Oligodendrocytes

   Form myelin sheath

Ependymal

   Lining membrane of brain and spinal cord where central spinal fluid
   circulates

Divisions of Central Nervous System (CNS) (Fig. 1-50)

Brain—Housed in Cranium (Box Comprised of 8 Bones)— Functioning to Enclose and Protect
Listing from inferior to superior

Brainstem

Medulla oblongata—crossover area left to right and center of respiratory and cardiovascular systems

Pons—connection of nerves (face and eyes)

Midbrain

Diencephalon

Hypothalamus controls autonomic nervous system, body temperature, sleep, appetite, and control of pituitary

Thalamus relays impulses to cerebral cortex for sensory system (pain)

Cerebellum

Controls voluntary movement and balance

Cerebrum

Largest part of brain

Functions

Mental processes, personality, sensory interpretation, movements, and memory

Two hemispheres

Right controls left side of body

Left controls right side of body

Divided into five lobes

- Frontal

- Parietal

- Temporal

- Occipital

- Insula

Vertebral Column—33 Vertebrae

7 cervical

12 thoracic

5 lumbar

5 sacrum (fused)

4 coccygeal (fused)—tailbone

Spinal Cord—housed within vertebrae from medulla oblongata to second lumbar

Spinal and brain meninges (coverings—dura mater [external], arachnoid, pia mater [internal])

Spine and brain spaces bathed by cerebrospinal fluid (CSF) (subarachnoid space)

Cavities within brain contain cerebrospinal fluid (ventricles)

Peripheral Nervous System (PNS)

Cranial nerves, 12 pair

Spinal nerves, 31 pair

Autonomic Nervous System (ANS)—Housed within Both PNS and CNS

Two divisions

- Sympathetic system—functions in fight and flight (stress)
- Parasympathetic system—functions to restore and conserve energy

COMBINING FORMS

1.	cephal/o	head
2.	cerebell/o	cerebellum
3.	cerebr/o	cerebrum
4.	crani/o	cranium
5.	dur/o	dura mater
6.	encephal/o	brain
7.	gangli/o	ganglion
8.	ganglion/o	ganglion
9.	gli/o	glial cells
10.	lept/o	slender
11.	mening/o	meninges
12.	meningi/o	meninges
13.	ment/o	mind
14.	mon/o	one
15.	myel/o	bone marrow, spinal cord
16.	neur/o	nerve
17.	phas/o	speech
18.	phren/o	mind
19.	poli/o	gray matter
20.	pont/o	pons
21.	psych/o	mind
22.	quadr/i	four
23.	radic/o	nerve root
24.	radicul/o	nerve root
25.	rhiz/o	nerve root
26.	vag/o	vagus nerve

PREFIXES

1.	hemi-	half
2.	per-	through

3. quadri-   four

4. tetra-   four

SUFFIXES

1. -algesia   pain sensation

2. -algia   pain

3. -cele   hernia

4. -esthesia   feeling

5. -iatry   medical treatment

6. -ictal   pertaining to

7. -kines/o   movement

8. -paresis   incomplete paralysis

9. -plegia   paralysis

MEDICAL ABBREVIATIONS

1. ANS   autonomic nervous system

2. CNS   central nervous system

3. CSF   cerebrospinal fluid

4. CVA   stroke/cerebrovascular accident

5. EEG   electroencephalogram

6. LP   lumbar puncture

7. PNS   peripheral nervous system

8. TENS   transcutaneous electrical nerve stimulation

9. TIA   transient ischemic attack

MEDICAL TERMS

Burr	Drill used to create an entry into the cranium
Central nervous system	Brain and spinal cord
Craniectomy	Permanent, partial removal of skull
Craniotomy	Opening of the skull
Cranium	That part of the skeleton that encloses the brain
Discectomy	Removal of a vertebral disc
Electroencephalography	Recording of the electric currents of the brain by means of electrodes attached to the scalp
Laminectomy	Surgical excision of posterior arch of vertebra—includes spinal process
Peripheral nerves	12 pairs of cranial nerves, 31 pairs of spinal nerves, and autonomic nervous system; connects peripheral receptors to the brain and spinal cord

Shunt	An artificial passage
Skull	Entire skeletal framework of the head
Somatic nerve	Sensory or motor nerve
Stereotaxis	Method of identifying a specific area or point in the brain
Sympathetic nerve	Part of the peripheral nervous system that controls automatic body function and sympathetic nerves activated under stress
Trephination	Surgical removal of a disk of bone
Vertebrectomy	Removal of vertebra

NERVOUS SYSTEM ANATOMY AND TERMINOLOGY QUIZ
(Quiz answers are located at the end of Unit 1)

1. Portion of nervous system that contains cranial and spinal nerves:
   a. central
   b. peripheral
   c. autonomic
   d. parasympathetic

2. Part of neuron that receives signals:
   a. dendrites
   b. cell body
   c. axon
   d. myelin sheath

3. NOT associated with glia:
   a. monocytes
   b. astrocytes
   c. microglia
   d. oligodendrocytes

4. Largest part of brain:
   a. cerebellum
   b. cerebrum
   c. cortex
   d. pons

5. Divided into two hemispheres:
   a. cerebellum
   b. cerebrum
   c. cortex
   d. pons

6. Number of pairs of cranial nerves:
   a. 10
   b. 11
   c. 12
   d. 13

7. Controls right side of body:
   a. left cerebrum
   b. right cerebrum
   c. right cortex
   d. left cortex

8. Combining form that means "brain":
   a. mening/o
   b. mon/o
   c. esthesi/o
   d. encephal/o

9. Prefix that means "four":
   a. per-
   b. tetra-
   c. para-
   d. bi-

10. Combining form that means "speech":
    a. phas/o
    b. rhiz/o
    c. poli/o
    d. myel/o

NERVOUS SYSTEM—PATHOPHYSIOLOGY

Dementias—Classified by Causative Factor

Cognitive deficiencies

Causes

Alzheimer's disease

Vascular disease

Head trauma

Tumors

Infection

Toxins

Substance abuse

AIDS

Alzheimer's Disease

Most common type of dementia

Progressive intellectual impairment

- Results in damage to neurons (neurofibrillary tangles)

- Fatal within 3 to 20 years

Causes

Mostly unknown

Perhaps genetic defect, autoimmune reaction, or virus

Symptoms

Behavior change

Memory loss

Confusion

Disorientation

Restlessness

Speech disturbances

Personality change—anxiety, depression

Irritability

Inability to complete activities of daily living

Treatment

- No cure

- Aricept (drug has modest effect in early stages)

- Symptomatic treatment

- Support for family

Vascular Dementia

Result of brain infarctions (vascular occlusion resulting in loss of brain function)

Nutritional Degenerative Disease
Deficiency

- B vitamins

- Niacin

- Pantothenic acid

Associated with alcoholism

Amyotrophic Lateral Sclerosis (ALS)
Motor neuron disease (MND)

Also known as Lou Gehrig's disease

- Baseball player who died of ALS

Deterioration of neurons of spinal cord and brain

Results in atrophy of muscles and loss of fine motor skills

Difficulty walking, talking, and breathing

Mental functioning remains normal

Survival is 2 to 5 years after diagnosis

Genetic cause/familial chromosome 21 aberration

- Death usually results from respiratory failure

Treatment
Symptomatic only

Emotional support

No cure

Huntington's Disease—Chorea
Inherited progressive atrophy of cerebrum

Symptoms
Restlessness

Rapid, jerky movements in arms and face (uncontrollable jerking and facial grimacing)

Rigidity

Intellectual impairment/bradyphrenia/apathy

Treatment
Genetic defect of chromosome 4

No cure

Symptomatic

Parkinson's Disease (Parkinsonism)
Decreased secretion of dopamine

Typically occurs after age 40

Cause unknown

Symptoms

Muscle rigidity and weakness

Bradykinesia—slow voluntary movements

Postural instability, stooped

Shuffling gait

Tremors at rest

Masklike facial appearance

Depression

Treatment

Medications to reduce symptoms

Dopamine replacement

Multiple Sclerosis (MS)

Common neurologic condition

• Demyelination of central nervous system—replaced by sclerotic tissue

Diagnosed in young adults 20–40 years old

Results in myelin destruction and gliosis of white matter of central nervous system

Speculation that it is an autoimmune condition or result of a virus

Exacerbations and remission patterns

Symptoms

Precipitated by "an event," e.g., infection, pregnancy, stress

Loss of feeling (paresthesias)

Vision problems

Bladder disorder

Mood disorders

Weakness of limbs—unsteady gait and paralysis

Treatment

Symptomatic

Management of relapses

Reducing relapses and disease progression—disease-modifying drugs (DMDs)

Myasthenia Gravis (MG)

Means grave muscle weakness

Autoimmune neuromuscular condition—antibodies block neurotransmission to muscle cells

Most have pathologic changes of thymus

Symptoms

Insidious

Muscle weakness and fatigability

May be localized or generalized

Often affects

- Swallowing
- Breathing
- Compromised swallowing and breathing may lead to crisis

Treatment
Anticholinesterase drugs

- Restores normal muscle strength and recoverability after fatigue

Corticosteroids (prednisone) and immunosuppressive drugs

Thymectomy

Tourette syndrome

Symptoms

Spasmodic, twitching movements, uncontrollable vocal sounds, inappropriate words

Begins with twitching eyelids and facial muscles (tics)

Verbal outbursts

Causes

Unknown

Excess dopamine or hypersensitivity to dopamine

Treatment

Antipsychotic drugs

Antidepressant drugs

Mood-elevating drugs

Poliomyelitis
Contagious viral disease

Affects motor neurons

Causes paralysis and respiratory failure

Prevent with vaccination

Postpolio Syndrome (PPS)
Also known as postpoliomyelitis neuromuscular atrophy

Progressive muscle weakness

- Past history of paralytic polio

Symptoms
Muscle weakness and fatigability

- May include atrophy and muscle twitching

Treatment
Symptomatic

Maintenance of respiratory function

Guillain-Barré Syndrome

Also known as

- Idiopathic polyneuritis
- Acute inflammatory polyneuropathy
- Landry's ascending paralysis

Demyelination of peripheral nerves—acquired disease

Symptoms

Primary ascending motor paralysis

Variable sensory disturbances

Treatment

Supportive

Congenital Neurologic Disorders

Hydrocephalus

Excessive amounts of circulating cerebrospinal fluid in ventricles of brain

Circulation is impaired in brain or spinal cord

Compresses brain

Treatment

Surgical placement of a shunt

Spina Bifida (Fig. 1-51)

Developmental birth defect that causes incomplete development of spinal cord and its coverings

Vertebrae overlying open portions of spinal cord do not fully form and remain unfused and open

- Spina bifida occulta—may not be noticed, no protrusion through defect
- Spina bifida manifesta, which includes:
  - Myelomeningocele (spina bifida cystica)
    - Meninges and spinal cord protrude through defect
  - Meningocele
    - Meninges herniated through defect

Results in neurologic deficiencies

Treatment

Surgical repair

Mental, Behavioral and Neurodevelopmental Disorders

Schizophrenia

Variety of syndromes

Results in changes in brain

Hereditary factors are considered a cause

- Also, fetal brain damage caused by viral infections, complications of pregnancy, nutritional deficiences

Stress usually precipitates onset

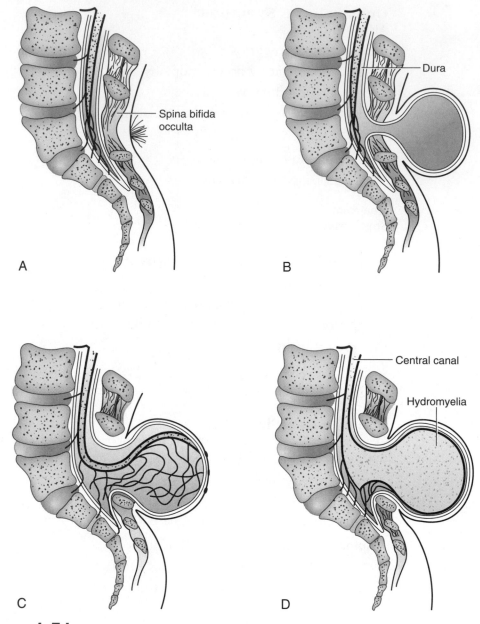

Figure **1-51** **A.** Spina bifida occulta. **B.** Meningocele. **C.** Myelomeningocele. **D.** Myelocystocele or hydromyelia.

Symptoms

Delusions of persecution and/or grandeur

Disorganized thought

Repetitive behaviors

Behavior issues

Decreased speech

Decreased ability to solve problems

Loss of emotions/flat affect

Hallucinations

Types are based on characteristics

Treatment
Antipsychotic drugs

Drugs have very unpleasant side effects, such as tardive dyskinesia, with symptoms as follows:

- Excessive movement
- Grimacing
- Jerking
- Tremors
- Shuffling gait
- Dry mouth
- Blurred vision

Depression
Mood (sustained emotional state) disorder

Exact cause is unknown

Symptoms
Sadness

Hopelessness

Lethargy

Insomnia

Anorexia

Treatment
Antidepressant drugs

Electroconvulsive therapy

Central Nervous System (CNS) Disorders
■ Vascular Disorder

Transient Ischemic Attack (TIA)
Temporary reduction of blood flow to brain that produces strokelike symptoms but no lasting damage

Often a warning sign before cerebrovascular accident

Symptoms
Depend on location of ischemia

- Usual recovery within 24 hours

No loss of consciousness

Slurred, indiscernible speech

May display muscle weakness in legs/arms

Paresthesia (numbness) of face

Mental confusion may be present

Repeated attacks common in the presence of atherosclerotic disease

Cerebrovascular Accident (CVA) or Stroke
Infarction of brain due to lack of blood/oxygen flow

Necrosis of tissue with total occlusion of vessel

Causes
Atherosclerotic disease—thrombus formation

Embolus

Hemorrhage—arterial aneurysm

Symptoms
Depend on location of obstruction

- Thrombus
  - Gradual onset
  - Often occurs at rest
  - Intracranial pressure (ICP) minimal
  - Localized damage
- Embolus
  - Sudden onset
  - Occurs anytime
  - ICP minimal
  - Localized damage unless multiple emboli
- Hemorrhage
  - Sudden onset
  - Occurs most often with activity
  - ICP high
  - Widespread damage
  - May be fatal

Treatment
Anticoagulant drugs (clot dissolving) if caused by thrombus or embolus—tissue plasminogen activator (tPA)

Carotid endarterectomy (removes artherosclerotic plaque)

Oxygen treatment

Underlying condition treated, such as

- Hypertension
- Atherosclerosis
- Thrombus

Aneurysm—Cerebral
Dilation of artery

- May be localized or multiple

Rupture possible, often on exertion

- Fatal if rupture is massive

Symptoms

May display visual effects, such as

- Loss of visual fields

- Photophobia

- Diplopia

Headache

Confusion

Slurred speech

Weakness

Stiff neck (nuchal rigidity)

Treatment

Dependent on diagnosis prior to rupture

Surgical intervention

Encephalitis

Infection of parenchymal tissue of brain or spinal cord

- Often viral

Accompanying inflammation

Usually results in some permanent damage

Symptoms

Stiff neck

Headaches

Vomiting

Fever

May have seizure

Lethargy

Some types of encephalitis

Herpes simplex

Lyme disease

West Nile fever

Western equine

Treatment

Symptomatic

Supportive

Reye's Syndrome

Associated with viral infection

- Especially when aspirin has been administered

Changes occur in brain and liver

- Leads to increased intracranial pressure

Symptoms
Headaches

Vomiting

Lethargy

Seizures

Treatment
Symptomatic treatment

Brain Abscess
Localized infection

Necrosis of tissue

Usually spread from infection elsewhere, such as ears or sinus

Symptoms
Neurologic deficiencies

Increased intracranial pressure

Treatment
Antibiotics for bacterial infections

Surgical drainage

■ Epilepsies
Chronic seizure disorder

Types
Partial seizures (focal)
State of altered focus but conscious—simple

Impaired consciousness—complex

Specialized epileptic seizures

Aura

- Auditory or visual sign that precedes a seizure

Generalized seizures
Absence seizures—petit mal

- Brief loss of awareness

- Most common in children (febrile causation)

Tonic-clonic—grand mal or ictal event

- Loss of consciousness

- Alternate contraction and relaxation

- Incontinence

- No memory of seizure

Causes
Tumor

Hemorrhage

Trauma

Edema

Infection

Excessive cerebrospinal fluid

High fever

Treatment

Correct cause

Anticonvulsant drugs

Neurosurgery

Postictal event—after seizure—neurologic symptoms (weakness, etc.)

■ Trauma

Head Injury—Traumatic Brain Injury (TBI)
Concussion
Mild blow to head

Temporary axonal disturbances

Grade 1: temporary confusion and amnesia (brief)

Grade 2: memory loss for very recent events and confusion

Grade 3: amnesia for recent events and disorientation (longer duration)

Results in reversible interference with brain function

• Recovery within 24 hours with no residual damage

Contusion
Bruising of brain

Force of blow determines outcome

Hematomas—blood accumulation (clot)
Compresses surrounding structures

Classified based on location

• Epidural

   • Develops between dura and skull

• Subdural

   • Develops between dura and arachnoid

      · Development within 24 hours is acute

      · Development within a week is subacute

   • ICP increases with enlargement of hematoma

• Subarachnoid

   • Develops between pia and arachnoid

   • Blood mixes with cerebrospinal fluid

      · No localized hematoma forms

- Intracerebral
  - As a result of a contusion

Symptoms
Increased ICP

Others dependent on location and severity of injury

Treatment
Identification of the location of hematoma

Medications to decrease edema

Antibiotics

Surgical intervention—burr hole if necessary to decrease the ICP

Spinal Cord Injury
Result of trauma to vertebra, cord, ligaments, intervertebral disc

Vertebral injuries classified as
- Simple—affects spinous or transverse process

- Compression—anterior fracture of vertebrae

- Comminuted—vertebral body is shattered

- Dislocation—vertebrae are out of alignment

- Flexion injury in which hyperflexion compresses vertebra

Dislocation

Rotation

Symptoms
Depend on vertebral level and severity

Paralysis

Loss of sensation

Drop in blood pressure

Loss of bladder and rectal control

Decreased venous circulation

Treatment
Identification of area of injury

Immobilization

Corticosteroids to decrease edema

Bladder and bowel management

Rehabilitation

■ Tumors of Brain and Spinal Cord

Increases ICP

Life threatening

Rarely metastasize outside of central nervous system

Secondary brain tumors are common

Metastasis from lung or breast

Gliomas Common Type

Primary malignant tumor—encapsulated and invasive

Types based on cell from which tumor arises and location of tumor

Glioblastoma
Located in cerebral hemispheres (deep in white matter)

Highly aggressive

Oligodendrocytoma
Usually located in frontal lobes

Oligodendroblastoma, more aggressive form

Ependymoma
Located in ventricles

Most often occurs in children

Ependymoblastoma, more aggressive form

Astrocytoma
Located anywhere in brain and spinal cord

Invasive but slow growing

Pineal Region
Germ cell tumors
Usually in adolescents

Rare

Variable growth rate

Several other pineal tumors
Pineocytoma

Teratoma

Germinoma

Blood Vessel
Angioma
Usually located in posterior cerebral hemispheres

Slow growing

Hemangioblastoma
Located in cerebellum

Slow growing

Medulloblastoma
Aggressive tumor

Located in posterior cerebellar vermis (fourth ventricle roof)

Meningioma
Originates in arachnoid

Slow growing

Pituitary Tumor
Related to aging

Slow growing

- Such as macroadenomas

Cranial Nerve Tumors
Neurilemmomas most common location: cranial nerve VIII

Slow growing

Metastatic

Spinal Cord Tumors
Symptoms are based on location of spinal compression

Intramedullary

- Originates in neural tissue

Extramedullary

- Originates outside the spinal cord

Metastatic tumors of spinal cord are more common

- Myeloma—marrow
- Lymphoma—lymph
- Carcinomas—lung, breast, prostate

Most common type of primary extramedullary tumor

- Meningiomas—anyplace in spine
- Neurofibromas—common in thoracic and lumbar regions

NERVOUS SYSTEM PATHOPHYSIOLOGY QUIZ
(Quiz answers are located at the end of Unit 1)

1. Most common dementia is:
   a. Alzheimer's disease
   b. secondary
   c. nutritional degenerative disease
   d. Lou Gehrig's disease

2. MND stands for:
   a. maximal neuron disorder
   b. migrating niacin disorder
   c. motor neuron disease
   d. motor neuropathic disorder

3. Dopamine replacement is useful in treating:
   a. multiple sclerosis
   b. Parkinson's disease
   c. Huntington's disease
   d. CVA

4. Condition in which primary symptoms are muscle weakness and fatigability:
   a. amyotrophic lateral sclerosis
   b. multiple sclerosis
   c. dyskinesis
   d. myasthenia gravis

5. Another name for idiopathic polyneuritis is:
   a. Guillain-Barré syndrome
   b. multiple sclerosis
   c. amyotrophic lateral sclerosis
   d. postpolio syndrome

6. This condition is thought to be caused by genetic factors and, possibly, fetal brain damage:
   a. Parkinson's
   b. schizophrenia
   c. spina bifida
   d. Guillain-Barré syndrome

7. This condition is associated with viral infection, especially when aspirin has been administered:
   a. Reye's syndrome
   b. Guillain-Barré syndrome
   c. Lou Gehrig's disease
   d. Conn's syndrome

8. Concussion is a mild blow to the head in which recovery is expected within

   _____.
   a. 12 hours
   b. 24 hours
   c. 48 hours
   d. 1 week

9. ICP means:
   a. intercranial pressure
   b. intracranial pressure
   c. interior cranial pressure
   d. intensive cranial pressure

10. In this type of hematoma, blood mixes with cerebrospinal fluid:
    a. epidural
    b. subdural
    c. subarachnoid
    d. intracerebral

■ SENSES

SENSES—ANATOMY AND TERMINOLOGY

Sight	Eyes
Hearing	Ears
Smell	Nose
Taste	Tongue
Touch	Skin

Sight: Three Layers of Eye (Fig. 1-52)

Cornea (Outer Layer)

Fibrous, transparent layer that extends over dome of eye

Refracts (bends) light to focus on receptor cells (posterior eye)

Avascular (nourished by aqueous humor and tears)

Sclera (Extension of Outer Layer)

White of eye

Extends from edge of cornea (anterior surface) to optic nerve (posterior surface)

• Lies over choroid

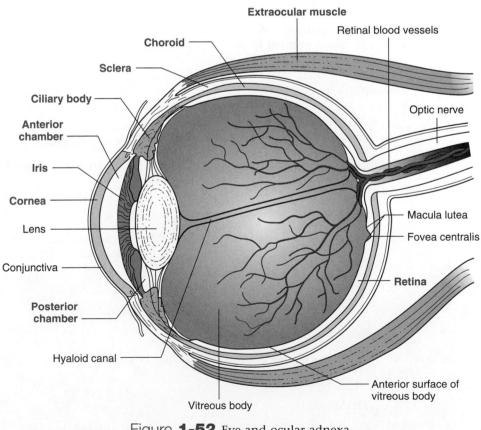

Figure **1-52** Eye and ocular adnexa.

Choroid (Middle Layer)
Vascular layer between sclera and retina

- Supplies nutrients

Retina (Inner Layer)
Contains rods and cones

- Rods provide night and peripheral vision

- Cones provide day and color vision and are stimulated by primary colors of red, green, and blue

Conjunctiva
Covers anterior sclera and lines eyelid (contiguous layer)

Lens
Behind pupil

Lens is connected by zonules to ciliary body

Ciliary body muscles cause lens to change shape to refract light rays (accommodation)

Fluids
Aqueous humor (front of lens)—watery substance secreted by ciliary body

    Maintains shape of front portion of eye

    Refracts light

    Nourishes cornea

Vitreous humor (behind lens)—gel-like substance (not readily re-formed) filling large space behind lens

    Maintains shape of eyeball

    Refracts light

Optic Nerve
Light rays from rods and cones travel from eye to brain via optic nerve

Optic nerve meets retina in optic disc (no light receptors)—blind spot

Pathway of light ray

    Cornea—refraction site

    Anterior chamber (aqueous humor)—refraction site

    Pupil

    Lens—refraction site

    Posterior chamber (vitreous humor)—refraction site

    Retina (rods and cones)

    Optic nerve fibers—nerve cells act as a cable connecting the eye with the brain

    Optic chiasm

    Thalamus

    Cerebral cortex (occipital lobe)—light is interpreted

Hearing, Three Divisions of Ear

External Ear
Auricle (pinna)—sound waves enter ear

External auditory canal—tunnel from auricle to middle ear

Middle Ear
Begins with tympanic membrane (eardrum)

Ossicles—small bones conducting sound waves from middle to inner ear

- Malleus

- Incus

- Stapes

Eustachian tube—leads to pharynx

Inner Ear (Labyrinth)
Vestibule

Semicircular canals/vestibular apparatus

Cochlea contains perilymph and endolymph (liquids through which sound waves are conducted)

- Organ of Corti—auditory receptor area

Auditory nerve—electrical impulse is conducted to cerebral cortex for interpretation (hearing)

Pathway of sound vibration (exterior to brain)

Pinna

External auditory canal

Tympanic membrane

Malleus

Incus

Stapes

Oval window

Cochlea

Auditory fluid/receptors in organ of Corti

Auditory nerve

Cerebral cortex

Smell

Olfactory Sense Receptors
Located in nasal cavity

Closely related to sense of taste

Cranial nerve I

Taste

Gustatory sense—sweet, salty, and sour differentiated

Taste buds located on anterior portion of tongue

Cranial nerves VII and IX

Touch

Mechanoreceptors
Widely distributed throughout body

React to touch and pressure

- Meissner corpuscles (touch)

- Pacinian corpuscles (pressure)

Proprioceptors
Position and orientation

Dysfunctions

- Vestibular nystagmus—involuntary movement of eyes

- Vertigo—sense of spinning/dizziness

Thermoreceptors
Under skin

Sense temperature changes

Nociceptors
Pain sensors

In skin and internal organs

COMBINING FORMS

1.	ambly/o	dim, dullness
2.	aque/o	water
3.	audi/o	hearing
4.	blephar/o	eyelid
5.	conjunctiv/o	conjunctiva
6.	cor/o, core/o	pupil
7.	corne/o	cornea
8.	cycl/o	ciliary body
9.	dacry/o	tear
10.	essi/o, esthesi/o	sensation
11.	glauc/o	gray
12.	ir/o	iris
13.	irid/o	iris

14.	kerat/o	cornea
15.	lacrim/o	tear
16.	mi/o	smaller
17.	myring/o	eardrum
18.	ocul/o	eye
19.	ophthalm/o	eye
20.	opt/o	eye, vision
21.	optic/o	eye
22.	ot/o	ear
23.	palpebr/o	eyelid
24.	papill/o	optic nerve
25.	phac/o	eye lens
26.	phak/o	eye lens
27.	phot/o	light
28.	presby/o	old age
29.	pupill/o	pupil
30.	retin/o	retina
31.	scler/o	sclera
32.	scot/o	darkness
33.	staped/o	stapes
34.	tympan/o	eardrum
35.	uve/o	uvea
36.	vitre/o	glassy
37.	xer/o	dry

PREFIXES

1.	audi-	hearing
2.	eso-	inward
3.	exo-	outward

SUFFIXES

1.	-opia	vision
2.	-omia	smell
3.	-tropia	to turn

MEDICAL ABBREVIATIONS

1.	AD	right ear
2.	AS	left ear
3.	AU	both ears

4.	H or E	hemorrhage or exudate
5.	IO	intraocular
6.	IOL	intraocular lens
7.	OD	right eye
8.	OS	left eye
9.	OU	each eye
10.	PERL	pupils equal and reactive to light
11.	PERRL	pupils equal, round, and reactive to light
12.	PERRLA	pupils equal, round, and reactive to light and accommodation
13.	REM	rapid eye movement
14.	TM	tympanic membrane

MEDICAL TERMS

Anterior segment	Those parts of eye in the front of and including lens (cornea, iris, ciliary body, aqueous humor)
Apicectomy	Excision of a portion of temporal bone
Astigmatism	Condition in which refractive surfaces of eye are unequal
Aural atresia	Congenital absence of external auditory canal
Blepharitis	Inflammation of eyelid
Cataract	Opaque covering on or in lens
Chalazion	Granuloma around sebaceous gland
Cholesteatoma	Tumor that forms in middle ear
Conjunctiva	The lining of eyelids and covering of anterior sclera
Dacryocystitis	Blocked, inflamed infection of nasolacrimal duct
Dacryostenosis	Narrowing of lacrimal duct
Ectropion	Eversion (outward sagging) of eyelid
Entropion	Inversion of eyelid (lashes rubbing cornea)
Enucleation	Removal of an organ or organs from a body cavity
Episclera	Connective covering of sclera
Exenteration	Removal of an organ all in one piece, commonly used to describe radical excision
Exophthalmos	Protrusion of eyeball
Exostosis	Bony growth
Fenestration	Creation of a new opening in inner wall of middle ear
Glaucoma	Eye diseases that are characterized by an increase of intraocular pressure
Hordeolum	Stye—infection of sebaceous gland (nodule on lid margin)
Hyperopia	Farsightedness, eyeball is too short from front to back
Keratomalacia	Softening of cornea associated with a deficiency of vitamin A

Keratoplasty	Surgical repair of the cornea
Labyrinth	Inner connecting cavities, such as internal ear
Labyrinthitis	Inner ear inflammation
Lacrimal	Related to tears
Mastoidectomy	Removal of mastoid bone
Ménière's disease	Condition that causes dizziness, ringing in ears, and deafness
Myopia	Nearsightedness, eyeball too long from front to back
Myringotomy	Incision into tympanic membrane
Ocular adnexa	Orbit, extraocular muscles, and eyelid
Ophthalmoscopy	Examination of the interior of eye by means of a scope, also known as fundoscopy
Otitis media	Noninfectious inflammation of middle ear; serous otitis media produces liquid drainage (not purulent), and suppurative otitis media produces purulent (pus) matter
Otoscope	Instrument used to examine ear
Papilledema	Swelling of optic disc (papilla)
Posterior segment	Those parts of eye behind lens
Ptosis	Drooping of upper eyelid
Sclera	Outer covering of eye
Strabismus	Extraocular muscle deviation resulting in unequal visual axes
Tarsorrhaphy	Suturing together of eyelids
Tinnitus	Ringing in the ears
Transmastoid	Creates an opening in mastoid for drainage antrostomy
Tympanolysis	Freeing of adhesions of the tympanic membrane
Tympanometry	Test of the inner ear using air pressure
Tympanostomy	Insertion of ventilation tube into tympanum
Uveal	Vascular tissue of the choroid, ciliary body, and iris
Vertigo	Dizziness
Xanthelasma	Yellow plaque on eyelid (lipid disorder)

SENSES ANATOMY AND TERMINOLOGY QUIZ
(Quiz answers are located at the end of Unit 1)

1. The middle layer of the eye:
   a. sclera
   b. retina
   c. episclera
   d. choroid

2. The covering of the anterior sclera and lining of eyelid:
   a. aqueous humor
   b. ossicles
   c. vitreous
   d. conjunctiva

3. Which of the following is NOT a bone of the middle ear?
   a. cochlea
   b. stapes
   c. malleus
   d. incus

4. This cranial nerve controls the sense of smell:
   a. I
   b. II
   c. III
   d. IV

5. Which of the following is NOT part of the inner ear?
   a. pinna
   b. vestibule
   c. semicircular canals
   d. cochlea

6. These receptors react to touch:
   a. nociceptors
   b. mechanoreceptors
   c. proprioceptors
   d. thermoreceptors

7. These receptors react to position and orientation:
   a. nociceptors
   b. mechanoreceptors
   c. proprioceptors
   d. thermoreceptors

8. Combining form meaning "eyelid":
   a. aque/o
   b. blephar/o
   c. optic/o
   d. uve/o

9. Combining form meaning "eye lens":
   a. cor/o
   b. irid/o
   c. ocul/o
   d. phak/o

10. Abbreviation meaning the pupils are equal, round, and reactive to light and accommodation:
    a. PERRLA
    b. PERRL
    c. PERL
    d. PURL

SENSES—PATHOPHYSIOLOGY

Eye

Visual Disturbances

Astigmatism

Irregular curvature of refractive surfaces (cornea or lens) of eye

Can be congenital or acquired (as a result of disease or trauma)

Image is distorted

Treatment

Corrected with cylindrical lens

Diplopia

Double vision

Amblyopia

Dimness of vision—impairment of vision without detectable organic lesion of eye

Hyperopia

Farsightedness

Shortened eyeball

- Can see objects in distance, not close up

Treatment

Corrected with convex lens

Presbyopia

Age-related farsightedness

Treatment

Magnification (reading glasses or bifocals)

Myopia

Nearsightedness

Elongated eyeball

- Can see objects up close, not in distance

Treatment

Corrected with concave lens thicker at periphery

Nystagmus—unilateral or bilateral

Rapid, involuntary eye movements

Movements can be

- Vertical
- Horizontal
- Rotational
- Combination of above

Cause
> Brain tumor or inner ear disease

Normal in newborns

Due to underlying condition or adverse effect of drug

Various types, such as

- Vestibular nystagmus

- Rhythmic eye movements

Strabismus
Cross-eyed

Due to muscle weakness or neurologic defect

Forms of strabismus

- Hypotropia (downward deviation of one eye)

- Hypertropia (upward deviation of one eye)

- Estropia (one eye turns inward)

- Exotropia (one eye turns outward)

Treatment
- Eye exercises/patching of normal eye

- Surgery to establish muscle balance

Infections
Conjunctivitis (pink eye)
Inflammation of conjunctival lining of eyelid or covering of sclera

Due to

- Infection

- Allergy

- Irritation

Treatment
- Varies with cause

- Antibiotic eye drops

Hordeolum (stye)
Bacterial infection of eyelid hair follicle

- Usually *Staphylococcus*

Results in mass on eyelid

Treatment
- Antibiotics

- Incision and drainage may be necessary

Keratitis
Corneal inflammation

May be caused by herpes simplex virus, contact lens issue, or exposure

Causes tearing and photophobia, pain

Macular Degeneration
Destruction of fovea centralis

- Fovea centralis is small pit in center of retina (fovea centralis retinae)

Usually age related—leading cause of blindness in elderly

Results from exposure to ultraviolet rays or drugs

- Also may have a genetic component

Central vision is lost

Two types of macular degeneration

- Wet—development of new vascularization and leaking blood vessels near macula

- Dry (85% of cases)—atrophy and degeneration of retinal cells and deposits of drusen (clumps of extracellular waste)

Treatment
None for "dry" macular degeneration

Surgical intervention with laser for "net" macular degeneration to coagulate leaking vessels; success is limited

Medications

Detached Retina
Retinal tear—two layers of retina separate from each other

- Vitreous humor then leaks behind retina

- Retina then pulls away from choroid

Results in increasing blind spot in visual field

Condition is painless

Pressure continues to build if left unattended

Final result is blindness

Treatment
Surgical intervention with laser to repair tear (emergency/urgency)—photocoagulation for small tears

Scleral buckle for large retinal detachments

Pneumatic retinopexy for medium to large retinal detachment. Gas bubble is injected into vitreous cavity; pressure to tear resulting in retinal reattachment.

Cataracts
Lens becomes opaque with protein aggregates

Classified by morphology
Size

Shape

Location

Also may be classified by etiology (cause) or time cataract occurs

Examples of classification
Congenital cataract

- Bilateral opacity present at birth

- Also known as developmental cataract

Heat cataract

- Also known as glassblowers' cataract

- Caused by exposure to radiation

Traumatic cataract (Fig. 1-53)

- Result of injury to eye

Senile cataract

- Age related

- Usually forms on anterior lens

Symptoms
　Blurring of vision

　Halos around lights

Treatment
　Removal of cataract with intraocular lens implantation

If no intraocular lens implant, then glasses or contact lenses for refraction

Glaucoma

Excess accumulation of intraocular aqueous humor

- High pressure results in decreased blood flow and edema

- Damages retinal cells and optic nerve

Narrow-angle glaucoma
Acute type of glaucoma

Rapid onset is painful

Chronic glaucoma
Also known as

　　- Wide-angle glaucoma

　　- Open-angle glaucoma

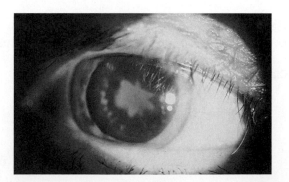

Figure **1-53** A concussion injury that resulted in a traumatic cataract.

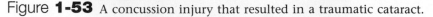

Asymptomatic

Diagnosed in eye examination using tonometry to test anterior chamber pressure

Treatment

Medications that decrease output of aqueous humor and decrease intraocular pressure (IOP)

Laser treatment to provide drainage

Ear

■ Infections

Otitis Media

Infection or inflammation of middle ear cavity

Chronic infection produces adhesions

Results in loss of hearing

Often occurs in children in combination with URI (upper respiratory infection)

Causes severe ear pain (otalgia)

Treatment

Antibiotics

Surgical intervention with placement of tubes to allow for drainage

• Useful in patients with recurrent infection

Otitis Externa

Also known as swimmer's ear

Infection of external auditory canal and pinna (exterior ear)

Caused by bacteria or fungus

Results in pain and discharge

Treatment

Antibiotic

Encouraged to keep ear dry

■ Hearing Loss

Conductive Hearing Loss

Due to a defect of sound-conducting apparatus

• Accumulation of wax

• Scar tissue on tympanic membrane

Also known as:

• Transmission hearing loss

• Conduction deafness

Treatment

• Hearing aids

Sensorineural

Due to a lesion of cochlea or central neural pathways

Also known as

- Perceptive deafness

May be divided into

- Cochlear hearing loss
  - Due to a defect in receptor or transducing mechanisms of cochlea
- Retrocochlear hearing loss
  - Due to defect located proximal to cochlea (vestibulocochlear nerve or auditory area of brain)

Presbycusis is age-related sensorineural hearing loss

Treatment
- Medication, implant, surgery

Ototoxic Hearing Loss

Caused by ingestion of toxic substance

Also known as toxic deafness

Ménière's Disease

Inner ear disturbance

Also known as idiopathic endolymphatic hydrops

Cause unknown

Common cause of vertigo (dizziness)

Other symptoms include hearing loss and tinnitus

SENSES PATHOPHYSIOLOGY QUIZ
(Quiz answers are located at the end of Unit 1)

1. This condition can be acquired or congenital and results in an irregular curvature of the refractive surfaces of the eye:
   a. diplopia
   b. hyperopia
   c. nystagmus
   d. astigmatism

2. In this condition, the eyeball is shorter than normal and results in being able to see objects in the distance but not close up:
   a. diplopia
   b. hyperopia
   c. nystagmus
   d. astigmatism

3. Rapid, involuntary eye movement is the predominant symptom of this condition:
   a. diplopia
   b. hyperopia
   c. nystagmus
   d. astigmatism

4. Age-related farsightedness is:
   a. presbyopia
   b. hyperopia
   c. diplopia
   d. myopia

5. Another name for a stye is:
   a. keratitis
   b. hordeolum
   c. hyperopia
   d. strabismus

6. An inflammation of the cornea that is caused by herpes simplex virus is:
   a. keratitis
   b. hordeolum
   c. hyperopia
   d. strabismus

7. In this condition there is destruction of the fovea centralis:
   a. macular degeneration
   b. detached retina
   c. glaucoma
   d. cataract

8. This is an infection that occurs in the middle ear cavity:
   a. otitis media
   b. otitis externa
   c. ototoxic hearing loss
   d. retrocochlear hearing loss

9. The hearing loss that can be due to a lesion on the cochlea is:
   a. conductive
   b. sensorineural
   c. ototoxic
   d. transmission

10. This condition is also known as perceptive deafness:
   a. conductive
   b. sensorineural
   c. otitis media
   d. transmission

UNIT 1 QUIZ ANSWERS

Integumentary System

Anatomy and Terminology Quiz

1. c	6. c
2. d	7. d
3. a	8. b
4. b	9. c
5. d	10. c

Pathophysiology Quiz

1. c	6. c
2. c	7. d
3. a	8. b
4. d	9. d
5. b	10. a

Musculoskeletal System

Anatomy and Terminology Quiz

1. b	6. d
2. c	7. b
3. a	8. d
4. c	9. a
5. a	10. c

Pathophysiology Quiz

1. d	6. d
2. c	7. a
3. b	8. c
4. a	9. b
5. d	10. d

Respiratory System

Anatomy and Terminology Quiz

1. b	6. c
2. d	7. c
3. c	8. b
4. a	9. d
5. a	10. d

Pathophysiology Quiz

1. b	6. a
2. a	7. c
3. d	8. b
4. d	9. a
5. d	10. c

Cardiovascular System

Anatomy and Terminology Quiz

1. d	6. b
2. a	7. d
3. c	8. a
4. a	9. d
5. d	10. d

Pathophysiology Quiz

1. b	6. a
2. c	7. c
3. c	8. c
4. c	9. a
5. d	10. d

Female Genital System and Pregnancy

Anatomy and Terminology Quiz

1. d	6. a
2. a	7. b
3. a	8. b
4. b	9. c
5. c	10. d

Pathophysiology Quiz

1. b	6. a
2. d	7. a
3. a	8. c
4. c	9. b
5. b	10. c

Male Genital System

Anatomy and Terminology Quiz

1. c	6. a
2. a	7. a
3. d	8. d
4. b	9. d
5. a	10. b

Pathophysiology Quiz

1. a	6. b
2. b	7. d
3. d	8. b
4. a	9. a
5. c	10. b

Urinary System

Anatomy and Terminology Quiz

1. c	6. d
2. d	7. c
3. a	8. b
4. c	9. d
5. b	10. a

Pathophysiology Quiz

1. c	6. c
2. d	7. a or c
3. d	8. c
4. c	9. b
5. b	10. c

Digestive System

Anatomy and Terminology Quiz

1. b	6. b
2. d	7. a
3. d	8. c
4. b	9. a
5. c	10. b

Pathophysiology Quiz

1. c	6. c
2. a	7. a
3. d	8. c
4. b	9. a
5. a	10. a

Mediastinum and Diaphragm

Anatomy and Terminology Quiz

1. a	6. b
2. b	7. a
3. d	8. b
4. c	9. a
5. c	10. d

Hemic and Lymphatic System

Anatomy and Terminology Quiz

1. b	6. c
2. d	7. a
3. a	8. d
4. d	9. b
5. c	10. d

Pathophysiology Quiz

1. c	6. b
2. a	7. a
3. b	8. a
4. d	9. c
5. b	10. b

Endocrine System

Anatomy and Terminology Quiz

1. c	6. a
2. d	7. d
3. b	8. a
4. a	9. b
5. d	10. d

Pathophysiology Quiz

1. a	6. b
2. b	7. a
3. c	8. d
4. a	9. a
5. d	10. c

Nervous System

Anatomy and Terminology Quiz

1. b	6. c
2. a	7. a
3. a	8. d
4. b	9. b
5. b	10. a

Pathophysiology Quiz

1. a	6. b
2. c	7. a
3. b	8. b
4. d	9. b
5. a	10. c

Senses

Anatomy and Terminology Quiz

1. d	6. b
2. d	7. c
3. a	8. b
4. a	9. d
5. a	10. a

Pathophysiology Quiz

1. d	6. a
2. b	7. a
3. c	8. a
4. a	9. b
5. b	10. b

Reimbursement Issues

Some of the CPT code descriptions for physician services include physician extender services. Physician extenders, such as nurse practitioners, physician assistants, and nurse anesthetists, etc., provide medical services typically performed by a physician. Within this educational material the term "physician" may include "and other qualified health care professionals" depending on the code. Refer to the official CPT® code descriptions and guidelines to determine codes that are appropriate to report services provided by non-physician practitioners.

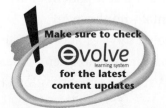

Make sure to check **evolve** learning system **for the latest content updates**

■ REIMBURSEMENT ISSUES

Your Responsibility

Ensure accurate coding based upon services provided and documented

Obtain correct reimbursement for services rendered

Recognize upcoding (maximizing) or downcoding is never appropriate

Stay abreast of current and changing

- Reimbursement policies
- Coding guidelines

Health **I**nsurance **P**ortability and **A**ccountability **A**ct of 1996 (HIPAA)

- HIPAA changes are based on various resources such as
  - Centers for Medicare and Medicaid Policy Manuals
  - National Correct Coding Guidelines

Population Changing = Reimbursement Change

In 2010, the Administration on Aging (AOA) of Department of Health and Human Services published a population survey

- In 1900 persons 65 and older were only 4.1% of population in United States
- In 2010 that same group had grown to 13%
- By 2050, elderly will be over 20% of the population

Medicare primarily for elderly

Medicare

Getting Bigger All the Time!

- In 2010, 21% of federal spending went to Medicare and Medicaid
- By 2020, federal spending for Medicare and Medicaid is expected to reach 31%
- By 2018, national health spending expected to reach $4.4 trillion

Health care will continue to expand to meet enormous future demands

- Job security for coders!

Those Covered

Originally established for those 65 and older, and implemented in 1966

Later disabled and permanent renal disease (end-stage renal disease or transplant) added in 1972

Persons covered are called "beneficiaries"

Basic Structure

Medicare program established in 1965

Part A: Hospital and Institutional Care Coverage

- This is the part that most inpatient coders will work with

Part B: Supplemental—nonhospital

   Example: Physician services and medical equipment

- This is the part that most outpatient coders will work with

Part C: Medicare Advantage Organizations (MAO) plans—combines part A and B (added later)

Plans include

Health Maintenance Organization (HMO)

Preferred Provider Organization (PPO)

Private Fee-for-Service (PPFS)

Special Needs Plans (SNPs)

Medical Savings Account (MSA)

HMO Point of Service (HMOPOS)

Part D: Prescription Drug Plan (PDP) (added January 1, 2006)

Plans include

- Medicare Advantage Plan (MA-PD)
- Private prescription drug plans (PDPs)
- Premium paid by beneficiary

Officiating Office

Department of Health and Human Services (DHHS) (www.dhhs.gov)

Delegated to Centers for Medicare and Medicaid Services (CMS) (formerly HCFA)

- CMS runs Medicare and Medicaid
- CMS delegates daily operation to Medicare Administrative Contractors (MACs)
- MACs are usually insurance companies
- The Medicare Prescription Drug Improvement and Modernization Act of 2003 allowed CMS to reduce the current 48 Fiscal Intermediaries to 19 Medicare Administrative Contractors (MACs); originally, there were 15 Part A and B, and 4 DME
    - The final 19 MACs were replaced with 10 MACs

Funding for Medicare

Social security taxes

Equal match from government

CMS sends money to MACs

MACs handle paperwork and pay claims

Medicare Covers

Medical necessity and frequency limitations
Defined in

- LCDs (Local Coverage Determinations)
- NCDs (National Coverage Determinations)

Beneficiary pays
20% of Medicare-approved amount after deductible is met

Part A and B annual deductible

Medicare pays
Part A all covered costs except deductible

Part B 80% of Medicare-allowed amount of covered services after deductible is met

Participating Providers

Signed Quality Improvement Organization (QIO) agreement with MACs to accept assignment on Medicare claims

Provider agrees to accept the Medicare Fee Schedule amount as payment in full

- Accepting assignment

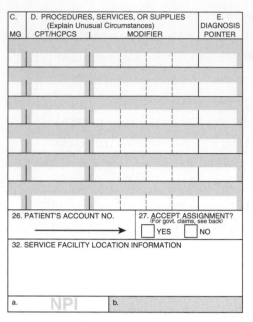

Figure **2-1** Block 27, Accept Assignment on the CMS-1500 (02/12), Health Insurance Claim Form. (Courtesy U.S. Department of Health and Human Services, Centers for Medicare and Medicaid Services.)

Block 27 on CMS-1500 (Fig. 2-1)

National Provider Identification (NPI)
10-digit number assigned to all covered healthcare providers

- Designed to provide one unique identifier for all providers as part of HIPAA

- Eliminates the need for additional numbers by other carriers

Good reasons to participate
- Significant decrease in reimbursement amount for nonparticipating providers

Participating providers receive approximately 5% more from Medicare than non-PAR providers

Check sent directly from MACs to QIO providers

Faster claims processing

Provider names listed in QIO directory

- Sent to all beneficiaries

Part A, Hospital Inpatient
Hospitals submit charges electronically or, if an exempt facility, on CMS-1450 (UB-04) form

MS-DRG basis for payment for Medicare patients

- Using principal diagnosis or principal procedure

Covered in-hospital expenses
Semiprivate room

Meals and special diets in hospital

All medically necessary services

Noncovered in-hospital expenses
Personal convenience items

Example: Slippers, TV

Any service or procedure determined to be "not medically necessary"

Types of covered expenses
Rehabilitation

Skilled nursing

Some personal convenience items for long-term illness or disabilities

Home health visits

Hospice care

- Not automatically covered

- Must meet certain criteria

Part B, Supplemental
Part B pays services and supplies not covered under Part A

Not automatic

Beneficiaries purchase

- Pay monthly premiums

Types of items covered in part B
Physician services

Outpatient hospital services

Ambulatory surgical services

Home health care

Medically necessary supplies and equipment

Coding for Medicare Part B services
Three coding systems used to report Part B

- CPT (procedures and service)

- HCPCS (drugs, supplies, equipment, and special services)

- ICD-9-CM (diagnosis codes)

Electronic Transactions

HIPAA

- Created to govern health care portability

- Electronic data interchange (EDI)

Transactions

- Activities involving transfer of health care information

Transmission

- Movement of electronic data between two entities

Today 99% Part A and 95% Part B claims filed electronically

- Using Electronic Remittance Advice (ERA)

The software that supports electronic transmissions

- 5010 version

NATIONAL CORRECT CODING INITIATIVE (NCCI)

Developed by the Centers for Medicare and Medicaid Services to

- Promote national correct coding methods

- Control improper coding that results in inappropriate payment of Part B claims (physician) and hospital outpatient claims

- Complete list may be found at http://www.cms.gov/NationalCorrectCodInitEd/

Unbundling

CMS defines unbundling as

- Billing multiple procedure codes for a group of procedures that are covered by a single comprehensive code

  Example: Dividing one service into parts and coding for each part separately, such as:

  - Reporting bilateral procedures unilaterally

    Reporting 31231, bilateral or unilateral diagnostic nasal endoscopy, with Modifier -50 (bilateral procedure), rather than correctly as 31231

  - Downcoding to use an additional code

    Reporting one of two lacerations of the same complexity and site with a lesser code to enable reporting two separate repairs

  - Separating the surgical approach from the major surgical service

    Coding separately for a thoracic approach during an anterior spine procedure

FEDERAL REGISTER

Government publishes updates, revisions (changes), deletions in laws (Fig. 2-2) (www.gpo.gov/fdsys/)

November and December issues contain major outpatient facility updates

QUALITY IMPROVEMENT ORGANIZATIONS (QIO)

Social Security Act (SSA) was amended to establish QIO

Purpose:

- To ensure quality of patient care

- Protect beneficiaries by addressing complaints

- Ensure Medicare pays only for reasonable and necessary services

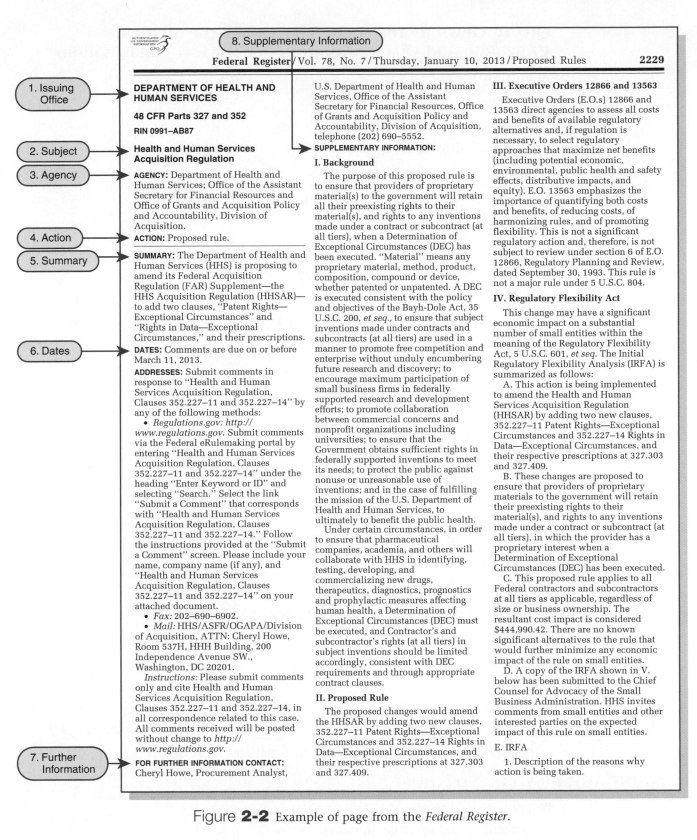

Figure **2-2** Example of page from the *Federal Register*.

QIO Reviews (Formerly Referred to as the Medicare Utilization and Quality Control Peer Review Organization)

Admission

Discharge

Quality of care

MS-DRG (Medicare Severity Diagnosis-Related Groups) validation

Coverage

Procedure

The Review

Begins with nurse who screens records based on QIO guidelines

Out-of-compliance cases forwarded to physician reviewer

Violations can result in severe sanctions

RESOURCE-BASED RELATIVE VALUE SCALE (RBRVS)

Physician payment reform implemented in 1992

Prior to reform, physicians were paid lowest of

- Physician's charge for service
- Physician's customary charge
- Prevailing charge in locality

National Fee Schedule (NFS)

RBRVS payment method

Termed Medicare Fee Schedule (MFS)

Payment 80% of MFS, after patient deductible

Used for physicians and suppliers

Relative Value Units (RVUs)

Assigns national unit values to each CPT code

Local adjustments made

- Work and skill required
- Overhead costs
- Malpractice costs

Often referred to as fee schedule

Annually, CMS updates RVU based on national and local factors

MEDICARE FRAUD AND ABUSE

Program established by Medicare

- To decrease and eliminate fraud and abuse

Beneficiary signatures on file

- Service, charges submitted without need for patient signature

Presents opportunity for fraud

Fraud

Intentional deception to benefit

Example: Submitting for services not provided

Anyone who submits for Medicare services can be violator

- Physicians
- Hospitals
- Laboratories
- Billing services
- YOU

Fraud Can Be

Billing for services not provided

Misrepresenting diagnosis or CPT/HCPCS codes

Kickbacks

Unbundling services

Falsifying medical necessity

Systematic waiver of copayment or deductible

Office of the Inspector General (OIG)

Develops and publishes Work Plan annually

Outlines Medicare monitoring program

MACs monitor those areas identified in plan

Complaints of Fraud or Abuse

Submitted orally or in writing to MACs or OIG

Allegations made by anyone against anyone

Allegations followed up by MACs or OIG
http://oig.hhs.gov/reports-and-publications/workplan/index.asp

Abuse

Generally involves

- Impropriety
- Lack of medical necessity for services reported

Review takes place after claim submitted

- MACs do historical review of claims

Kickbacks

Bribe or rebate for referring patient for any service covered by Medicare

Any personal-gain kickback

A felony

- $25,000 fine or
- 5 years in jail or
- Both

Protect Yourself

Use your common sense

Submit only truthful and accurate claims

• Stay current with all coding changes

If you are unsure about charges, services, or procedures

• Check with physician or supervisor

MANAGED HEALTH CARE

Network health care providers that offer health care services under one organization

Group hospitals, physicians, or other providers

Majority of people with health care coverage are covered by a Managed Health Care Organization (e.g., HMO, PPO, POS)

Managed Care Organizations

Responsible for health care services to an enrolled group or person

Coordinate various health care services

Negotiate with providers and groups

Preferred Provider Organization (PPO)

Providers form network to offer health care services as group

Enrollees who seek health care outside PPO pay more

Point of Service (POS)

In-network or out-of-network providers may be used

Benefits are paid at a higher rate to in-network providers

Subscribers are not limited to providers, but to amount covered by plan

Health Maintenance Organization (HMO)

Total package health care

Out-of-pocket expenses minimal

Assigned physician acts as gatekeeper to refer patient to outside organization

REIMBURSEMENT TERMINOLOGY

Advance Beneficiary Notice	ABN, notification in advance of services that Medicare probably will not pay for and the estimated cost to patient (Fig. 2-3)
Ancillary Service	A service that is supportive of care of a patient, such as laboratory services
Assignment	A legal agreement that allows the provider to receive direct payment from a payer and the provider to accept payment as payment in full for covered services

---

A. Notifier:

B. Patient Name: **C. Identification Number:**

Advance Beneficiary Notice of Noncoverage (ABN)

<u>NOTE:</u> If Medicare doesn't pay for **D.** —————— below, you may have to pay.
Medicare does not pay for everything, even some care that you or your health care provider have good reason to think you need. We expect Medicare may not pay for the **D.** —————— below.

D.	E. Reason Medicare May Not Pay:	F. Estimated Cost

WHAT YOU NEED TO DO NOW:
- Read this notice, so you can make an informed decision about your care.
- Ask us any questions that you may have after you finish reading.
- Choose an option below about whether to receive the **D.** —————— listed above.
  Note: If you choose Option 1 or 2, we may help you to use any other insurance that you might have, but Medicare cannot require us to do this.

G. OPTIONS: Check only one box. We cannot choose a box for you.

☐ **OPTION 1.** I want the **D.** —————— listed above. You may ask to be paid now, but I also want Medicare billed for an official decision on payment, which is sent to me on a Medicare Summary Notice (MSN). I understand that if Medicare doesn't pay, I am responsible for payment, but **I can appeal to Medicare** by following the directions on the MSN. If Medicare does pay, you will refund any payments I made to you, less co-pays or deductibles.

☐ **OPTION 2.** I want the **D.** —————— listed above, but do not bill Medicare. You may ask to be paid now as I am responsible for payment. **I cannot appeal if Medicare is not billed**.

☐ **OPTION 3.** I don't want the **D.** —————— listed above. I understand with this choice I am **not** responsible for payment, and **I cannot appeal to see if Medicare would pay.**

H. Additional Information:

This notice gives our opinion, not an official Medicare decision. If you have other questions on this notice or Medicare billing, call **1-800-MEDICARE** (1-800-633-4227/**TTY:** 1-877-486-2048).
Signing below means that you have received and understand this notice. You also receive a copy.

I. Signature:	J. Date:

Form CMS-R-131 (03/11)   Form Approved OMB No. 0938-0566

Figure **2-3** Centers for Medicare and Medicaid Services Advance Beneficiary Notice of Noncoverage (ABN).

Attending Physician	The physician legally responsible for oversight of an inpatient's care (in residency programs, the teaching physician that monitors the resident's work)
Beneficiary	The person who benefits from insurance coverage; also known as subscriber, dependent, enrollee, member, or participant
Birthday Rule	When both parents have insurance coverage, the parent with the birthday earlier in the year carries the primary coverage for a dependent

Certified Registered Nurse Anesthetist	CRNA, an individual with specialized training and certification in nursing and anesthesia
"Clean Claim"	A properly completed claim submitted to a payer with all data fields containing current and accurate information and submitted within the timely filing period required by the insurer
Coinsurance	Cost-sharing of covered services
Compliance Plan	Written strategy developed by medical facilities to ensure appropriate, consistent documentation within the medical record and ensure compliance with third-party payer guidelines and the Office of the Inspector General (OIG) Workplan guidelines
Concurrent Care	More than one physician providing care to a patient at the same time
Coordination of Benefits	COB, management of multiple third-party payments to ensure overpayment does not occur
Co-payment	Cost-sharing between beneficiary and payer
Deductible	That portion of covered services paid by the beneficiary before third-party payment begins
Denial	Statement from a payer that coverage is denied
Documentation	Detailed chronology of facts and observations, procedures, services, and diagnoses relative to the patient's health
Durable Medical Equipment	DME, medically related equipment that is not disposable, such as wheelchairs, crutches, and vaporizers
Electronic Data Interchange	EDI, computerized submission of health care insurance information exchange
Employer Identification Number	EIN, Internal Revenue Service (IRS)–issued identification number used on tax documents
Encounter Form Superbill	Medical document that contains information regarding a patient visit for health care services, can serve as a billing and/or coding document
Explanation of Benefits	EOB or EOMB, written, detailed listing of medical service payments by third-party payer to inform beneficiary and provider of payment
Fee Schedule	List of established payment for medical services arranged by CPT and HCPCS codes
Follow-up Days	FUD, established by third-party payers and listing the number of days after a procedure for which a provider must provide services to a patient for no fee. Also known as *global days*, *global package*, and *global period*
Group Provider Number	GPN, a numeric designation for a group of providers that is used instead of the individual provider number
HMO	Health Maintenance Organization
Invalid Claim	Claim that is missing necessary information and cannot be processed or paid

Medical Record	Documentation about the health care of a patient to include diagnoses, services, and procedures rendered
National Provider Identifier	NPI, 10-digit number assigned to provider by CMS and National Plan and Provider Enumeration System (NPPES) and used for identification purposes when submitting services to third-party payers
Noncovered Services	Any service not included by a third-party payer in the list of services for which payment is made
Point of Service	POS, a plan in which either an in-network or out-of-network provider may be used with a higher rate paid to in-network providers
Preferred Provider Organization	PPO, providers form a network to offer health care services to a group
Prior Authorization	Also known as preauthorization, which is a requirement by the payer to receive written permission prior to patient services in order to be considered for payment by the payer
Provider Identification Number	PIN, a number assigned by a third-party payer to providers to be used for identification purposes when submitting claims
Reimbursement	Payment from a third-party payer for services rendered to a patient covered by the payer's health care plan
Rejection/Denial	A claim that did not pass the edits and is returned to the provider as rejected
Resource-Based Relative Value Scale	RBRVS, a list of physician services with assigned units of monetary value
State License Number	Identification number issued by a state to a physician who has been granted the right to practice in that state
UPIN	Unique provider identification number was replaced by the NPI
Usual, Customary, and Reasonable	UCR, used by some third-party payers to establish a payment rate for a service in an area with the usual (standard fee in area), customary (standard fee by the physician), and reasonable (as determined by payer) fee amounts

REIMBURSEMENT QUIZ
(Quiz answers are located at the end of Unit 2)

1. Any person who is identified as receiving life or medical benefits:
   a. primary
   b. beneficiary
   c. participant
   d. recipient

2. According to the Birthday Rule, if both parents are covered by an employer-provided health policy, the insurance policy that would be primary for reporting their child's health services is:
   a. parent with the birthday earlier in the year
   b. parent with the birthday later in the year
   c. either parent
   d. parent whose birthday is closer to the child's

3. Abbreviation for reusable medical equipment is:
   a. DRG
   b. CRN
   c. DME
   d. DIM

4. Management of multiple third-party payments to ensure that overpayment does not occur:
   a. PRO
   b. COB
   c. DME
   d. FUD

5. CMS delegates the daily operation of the Medicare program to:
   a. DHHS
   b. QIO
   c. RVU
   d. MACs

6. A QIO provider is one who:
   a. signs an agreement with the MACs
   b. submits charges directly to CMS
   c. receives 5% less than some other physicians
   d. can bill the patient the total remaining balance after payment from Medicare

7. This part of Medicare covers the inpatient portion of covered costs after the deductible has been paid:
   a. Part A
   b. Part B
   c. Part C
   d. Part D

8. This issue of the *Federal Register* contains major outpatient facility changes for CMS programs for the coming year:
   a. October/November
   b. November/December
   c. December/October
   d. November/August

9. This is the RBRVS payment method:
   a. RAI
   b. OPPS
   c. APC
   d. NFS

10. Entity responsible for development of the plan that outlines monitoring of the Medicare program:
    a. MACs
    b. OIG
    c. DHSS
    d. HEW

REIMBURSEMENT QUIZ ANSWERS

1. b	6. a
2. a	7. a
3. c	8. b
4. b	9. d
5. d	10. b

Overview of CPT, ICD-9-CM, and HCPCS Coding

Some of the CPT code descriptions for physician services include physician extender services. Physician extenders, such as nurse practitioners, physician assistants, and nurse anesthetists, etc., provide medical services typically performed by a physician. Within this educational material the term "physician" may include "and other qualified health care professionals" depending on the code. Refer to the official CPT® code descriptions and guidelines to determine codes that are appropriate to report services provided by non-physician practitioners.

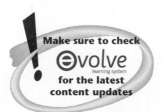

■ INTRODUCTION TO MEDICAL CODING

Translates services/procedures/supplies/drugs into CPT/HCPCS codes

Translates diagnosis(es) into ICD-9-CM codes

Two Levels of Service Codes

1. Level I CPT

2. Level II HCPCS, National Codes

Diagnosis Codes, ICD-9-CM

ICD-9-CM, Volumes 1 and 2, *International Classification of Diseases,* 9th ed., Clinical Modification

Volume 1, Tabular

- Classification system

- Translates diagnosis(es) (dx) into standardized codes that explain why service was provided

- Very specific in nature

- May be up to five numeric or alphanumeric places

- Example: Diabetes becomes 250.--

Volume 2, Index

Volume 3, Index and Tabular of Procedures (hospital version)

■ CPT

Developed by the AMA in 1966

Five-digit codes to report services provided to patients

Updated each November for use January 1

Resequencing was a 2010 new initiative for CPT

- Historically in numerical order

- Not the case for more than 100 codes

- Pound symbol (#) appears before the resequenced codes

    Example: In the 51725-51798 range, code 51797 follows 51729 (in numeric order). Code 51797 also appears in correct numeric order in the CPT, but next to the code a note states "Code is out of numerical sequence. See 51725-51798."

See Appendix N of the CPT for a complete list of the resequenced codes.

Types of CPT Codes

- Medical
- Surgical
- Diagnostic services
- Anesthesia
- Evaluation and Management

CPT Codes

Allow communication that is both effective and efficient

Inform third-party payers of services/procedures provided

Used as a basis of payment

Incorrect Coding

Results in providers being paid inappropriately (either overpayment or underpayment)

Outpatient Physician (Non-Hospital) Services

Reported on standardized insurance form

CMS-1500 example (Fig. 3-1)

CPT Format

Symbols. Used to convey information

- Bullet = New code symbol

▲ Triangle = Revised code

►◄ Right and left triangles = Beginning and ending of text change

+ Plus = Add-on code

  • Full list in Appendix D of CPT

⊘ Circle with line = Modifier -51 exempt code

  • Modifier -51 cannot be used with these codes

  • Full list in Appendix E of CPT

⊙ Bullseye = Codes that include moderate (conscious) sedation

  • Such as 45391, flexible colonoscopy

  • Full list in Appendix G of CPT

⚡ Lightning bolt symbol = Codes for which the FDA status pending

  • Full list in Appendix K of CPT

Number sign = Resequenced CPT codes

  • Such as 21552, excision of tumor, 3 cm or greater, resequenced code in 2010

  • Full text in Appendix N

○ Circle = Recycled/reinstated code

CPT Sections

1. Evaluation & Management (E/M)
2. Anesthesia
3. Surgery
4. Radiology
5. Pathology and Laboratory
6. Medicine

> **TIP:** During your examination, the front section of the CPT (Introduction and Illustrations) is an excellent resource on the format, definitions of terms, medical terms, and instructions in the CPT. Review these well before the examination to familiarize yourself with where to find the information that is contained in the front section.
>
> Also, flag the different sections of the CPT for easy access during the examination—for example, the list of illustrations section, E/M Guidelines, Appendices, and other major sections of the manual.

Categorized by

Sections

Subsections

HEALTH INSURANCE CLAIM FORM

APPROVED BY NATIONAL UNIFORM CLAIM COMMITTEE (NUCC) 02/12

CARRIER →

	PICA						PICA	

1. MEDICARE MEDICAID TRICARE CHAMPVA GROUP HEALTH PLAN FECA BLK LUNG OTHER
☐(Medicare#) ☐(Medicaid#) ☐(ID#DoD#) ☐(Member ID#) ☐(ID#) ☐(ID#) ☐(ID#)

1a. INSURED'S I.D. NUMBER   (For Program in Item 1)

2. PATIENT'S NAME (Last Name, First Name, Middle Initial)

3. PATIENT'S BIRTH DATE SEX
MM   DD   YY   M☐   F☐

4. INSURED'S NAME (Last Name, First Name, Middle Initial)

5. PATIENT'S ADDRESS (No., Street)

6. PATIENT RELATIONSHIP TO INSURED
Self☐ Spouse☐ Child☐ Other☐

7. INSURED'S ADDRESS (No., Street)

CITY   STATE

8. RESERVED FOR NUCC USE

CITY   STATE

ZIP CODE   TELEPHONE (Include Area Code)
(   )

ZIP CODE   TELEPHONE (Include Area Code)
(   )

9. OTHER INSURED'S NAME (Last Name, First Name, Middle Initial)

10. IS PATIENT'S CONDITION RELATED TO:

11. INSURED'S POLICY GROUP OR FECA NUMBER

a. OTHER INSURED'S POLICY OR GROUP NUMBER

a. EMPLOYMENT? (Current or Previous)
☐YES   ☐NO

a. INSURED'S DATE OF BIRTH   SEX
MM   DD   YY   M☐   F☐

b. RESERVED FOR NUCC USE

b. AUTO ACCIDENT?   PLACE (State)
☐YES   ☐NO

b. OTHER CLAIM ID (Designated by NUCC)

c. RESERVED FOR NUCC USE

c. OTHER ACCIDENT?
☐YES   ☐NO

c. INSURANCE PLAN NAME OR PROGRAM NAME

d. INSURANCE PLAN NAME OR PROGRAM NAME

10d. CLAIM CODES (Designated by NUCC)

d. IS THERE ANOTHER HEALTH BENEFIT PLAN?
☐YES   ☐NO   *If yes,* complete items 9, 9a, and 9d.

READ BACK OF FORM BEFORE COMPLETING & SIGNING THIS FORM.

12. PATIENT'S OR AUTHORIZED PERSON'S SIGNATURE I authorize the release of any medical or other information necessary to process this claim. I also request payment of government benefits either to myself or to the party who accepts assignment below.

SIGNED _____ DATE _____

13. INSURED'S OR AUTHORIZED PERSON'S SIGNATURE I authorize payment of medical benefits to the undersigned physician or supplier for services described below.

SIGNED _____

14. DATE OF CURRENT ILLNESS, INJURY, or PREGNANCY(LMP)
MM   DD   YY   QUAL.

15. OTHER DATE   QUAL.   MM   DD   YY

16. DATES PATIENT UNABLE TO WORK IN CURRENT OCCUPATION
FROM   MM   DD   YY   TO   MM   DD   YY

17. NAME OF REFERRING PROVIDER OR OTHER SOURCE

17a.
17b. NPI

18. HOSPITALIZATION DATES RELATED TO CURRENT SERVICES
FROM   MM   DD   YY   TO   MM   DD   YY

19. ADDITIONAL CLAIM INFORMATION (Designated by NUCC)

20. OUTSIDE LAB? $ CHARGES
☐YES   ☐NO

21. DIAGNOSIS OR NATURE OF ILLNESS OR INJURY Relate A-L to service line below (24E)   ICD Ind.

A. |_____   B. |_____   C. |_____   D. |_____

E. |_____   F. |_____   G. |_____   H. |_____

I. |_____   J. |_____   K. |_____   L. |_____

22. RESUBMISSION CODE   ORIGINAL REF. NO.

23. PRIOR AUTHORIZATION NUMBER

24. A. DATE(S) OF SERVICE						B. PLACE OF SERVICE	C. EMG	D. PROCEDURES, SERVICES, OR SUPPLIES (Explain Unusual Circumstances) CPT/HCPCS MODIFIER	E. DIAGNOSIS POINTER	F. $ CHARGES	G. DAYS OR UNITS	H. EPSDT Family Plan	I. ID. QUAL.	J. RENDERING PROVIDER ID. #
From MM	DD	YY	To MM	DD	YY									
1														NPI
2														NPI
3														NPI
4														NPI
5														NPI
6														NPI

25. FEDERAL TAX I.D. NUMBER   SSN☐ EIN☐

26. PATIENT'S ACCOUNT NO.

27. ACCEPT ASSIGNMENT? (For govt. claims, see back)
☐YES   ☐NO

28. TOTAL CHARGE $

29. AMOUNT PAID $

30. Rsvd for NUCC Use $

31. SIGNATURE OF PHYSICIAN OR SUPPLIER INCLUDING DEGREES OR CREDENTIALS
(I certify that the statements on the reverse apply to this bill and are made a part thereof.)

SIGNED _____ DATE _____

32. SERVICE FACILITY LOCATION INFORMATION

a. NPI   b.

33. BILLING PROVIDER INFO & PH # (   )

a. NPI   b.

NUCC Instruction Manual available at: www.nucc.org   *PLEASE PRINT OR TYPE*   APPROVED OMB-0938-1197 FORM 1500 (02-12)

PHYSICIAN OR SUPPLIER INFORMATION ↕
PATIENT AND INSURED INFORMATION ↕

Figure **3-1** The CMS-1500 (02/12) Health Insurance Claim Form was revised from the CMS-1500 form to accommodate reporting of ICD-10-CM codes. The CMS-1500 (02/12) version was mandated for use on October 1, 2013. (Courtesy U.S. Department of Health and Human Services, Centers for Medicare and Medicaid Services.)

Subheadings

Categories

   Anatomy

      Knee or Shoulder

   Procedure

      Incision or Excision

   Condition

      Fracture or Dislocation

   Description

      Cast or Strap

   Surgical approach

      Anterior Cranial Fossa or Middle Cranial Fossa

Guidelines

Section-specific information begins each section

Provides instruction pertinent to entire section

Notes

Located throughout CPT

Provides instruction pertinent to specific subsection

Two Types of Code Descriptions

1. **Stand-alone:** Full description

   Example: 10080 Incision and drainage of pilonidal cyst; simple

2. **Indented:** Dependent on preceding stand-alone for meaning

   Example: 10080 Incision and drainage of pilonidal cyst; simple

         10081   complicated

Semicolon

- Description preceding semicolon is the common part of the description and applies to any indented codes under it

- You must return to stand-alone for full description

   Example: 10081 Incision and drainage of pilonidal cyst; complicated

Modifiers Add Information

CPT Modifier

Appended to the end of the CPT/HCPCS code

Some modifiers are informational; others affect reimbursement

   Example: 43820 gastrojejunostomy

- -62 two primary surgeons

- 43820-62 two surgeons performed a gastrojejunostomy

- Only used if both surgeons submit same CPT code and both surgeons dictate a separate operative report

Level II HCPCS Modifiers

"-AS" physician's assistant

"-F1" Left hand, second digit

All modifiers used on CPT or HCPCS codes

All HCPCS modifiers begin with a letter

Modifiers are placed in Block D. Modifier (Fig. 3-1)

Unlisted Services

Codes usually end in "99" = "no specific code" in Category I or Category III

Used when a more specific code cannot be assigned

Written report must accompany claim form indicating

- Nature
- Extent
- Need
- Time
- Effort
- Equipment used

Category II Codes—Supplemental Tracking Codes

Used for performance measurements

- Optional unless practice participating in Physician Quality Reporting System (PQRS), formerly the PQRI (Physician Quality Improvement Reporting Initiative)

These codes collect data concerning the quality of care and test results

Alphanumeric and end in the letter "F" (0005F)

Located after the Medicine section in CPT

- On CPC exam

Category III Codes—New Technology

Temporary codes—may be included in this section up to 5 years

Identify emerging technology, services, and procedures

Located after Category II codes

Alphanumeric and end in the letter "T" (0055T)

- May or may not receive future Category I code status
- Category I codes (00100-99607)
- Approved by AMA and the Food and Drug Administration (FDA)
- Proven clinical effectiveness (efficacy)
- Category III has not been approved and has no proven clinical effectiveness (efficacy)
- Use Category III code instead of unlisted code if no Category I code appropriate
- Use unlisted code if no Category III code exists
- On CPC exam

The Index

Used to locate service/procedure terms and codes

Speeds up code location

Uses dictionary format

- First entries and last entries on top of page
- Code display in index
  - Single code: 38115
  - Multiple codes: 26645, 26650
  - Range of codes: 22305-22325

Location Methods

Service/procedure: Repair, excision

Anatomic site: Meniscus, knee

Condition or disease: Cleft lip, clot

Synonym: Toe and interphalangeal joint

Eponym: Jones procedure, Heller operation

Abbreviation: ECG, PEEP (positive end-expiratory pressure)
"See" in index

Cross-reference terms: "Look here for code"

Index: Stem, Brain: *See* Brainstem

Appendices of CPT

Appendix A: Modifiers

Appendix B: Summary of Additions, Deletions, and Revisions

Appendix C: Clinical Examples (E/M Codes)

Appendix D: Summary of CPT Add-on Codes

Appendix E: Summary of CPT Codes Exempt from Modifier -51

Appendix F: Summary of CPT Codes Exempt from Modifier -63

Appendix G: Summary of CPT Codes That Include Moderate (Conscious) Sedation

Appendix H: Alphabetical Clinical Topics Listing (moved to AMA website)

Appendix I: Genetic Testing Code Modifiers (Deleted)

Appendix J: Electrodiagnostic Medicine Listing of Sensory, Motor, and Mixed Nerves

Appendix K: Product Pending FDA Approval

Appendix L: Vascular Families

Appendix M: Deleted CPT Codes

Appendix N: Summary of Resequenced CPT Codes

Appendix O: Multianalyte Assays with Algorithmic Analyses

Review information in the CPT appendices prior to examination

■ EVALUATION AND MANAGEMENT (E/M) SECTION (99201-99499)

> Your job is to code only from what is documented in medical record
> Optimize—never maximize
> Accurately report documented services
> Coding for services not provided is a punishable CRIME

Subsections by type of service

Types of service

- Consultation

- Office Services

- Hospital Services, etc.

Integral Factors When Selecting E/M Codes

1. Place of Service
Explains setting of service

- Office

- Emergency Department

- Nursing Home

2. Type of Service
Physicians provide many types of service

- Consultations (not reported for Medicare)

- Admissions

- Office visits

3. Patient Status
The four status types are

1. New patient

2. Established patient

3. Outpatient

4. Inpatient

New patient
Has not received any professional service in last 3 years from the same physician or another physician of the same specialty and in the same group

New patients are more labor-intensive for physician, medical staff, and clerical staff

Established patient
Has received professional services in last 3 years from the same physician or another physician of the same specialty in the same group

Medical record available with current, relevant information

Outpatient

One who has not been formally admitted to a health care facility

> *Example:* Patient receives services at clinic or same-day surgery center

Inpatient

One who has been formally admitted to a health care facility

> *Example:* Patient admitted to a hospital or nursing home

Physician dictates:

- Admission orders

- H&P (history and physical)

- Requests for consultations

Levels of E/M Service Based on

Skill required to provide service

Time spent

Level of knowledge necessary to treat the patient

Effort required

Responsibility required/assumed

E/M Levels Divided Based on

Key Components (KC)
- History (Hx)

- Physical examination (PE)

- Medical decision making (MDM)

Contributory Factors (CF)
- Counseling

- Coordination of care

- Nature of presenting problem

Every Encounter Contains Varying Amount of KC and CF
More extensive component/factor

- Higher level of service

  - Less extensive component/factor

- Lower level of service

KEY COMPONENTS

Four Elements of a History

1. Chief Complaint (CC)

2. History of Present Illness (HPI)

3. Review of Systems (ROS)

4. Past, Family, or Social History (PFSH)

Chief Complaint (CC)—Subjective

Reason for encounter or presenting problem: Patient's current complaint in patient's own words

Documented in medical record for each encounter

History of Present Illness (HPI)—Subjective

Description of development of current illness, e.g., date of onset

Patient describes HPI

Provider must personally document

PHYSICIAN AND PATIENT DIALOGUE

Development of a CC of Abdominal Pain (HPI):

"Started Thursday night and was mild. During the night, it got worse. Friday morning I went to work but had to leave because the pain got so bad."

Location. Specific source of pain

"Pain was in lower left-hand side, a little toward back."

Quality. Is pain sharp, intermittent, burning?

"Pain is really sharp and constant."

Severity. Is pain intense, moderate, mild?

"Pain is terrible, worst pain I have ever had." (intensity of pain or on a scale of 1 to 10)

*Duration. How long has pain been present?

"Pain has been going on now for 3 days."

Timing. Is pain constant or does it come and go?

"Pain just continues. It just doesn't go away."

Context. When does it hurt most?

"Pain is just there, it doesn't matter what I am doing."

Modifying factors. Does anything make it better or worse?

"Nothing I do makes it any better or any worse."

Associated signs and symptoms. Does anything else feel different when pain is present?

"Yes, I have nausea when pain is worst."

---

*Duration not listed in CPT as HPI element

Review of Systems (ROS)—Subjective

Questions posed to the patient to identify signs and symptoms that have been or are being experienced relating to the HPI

Organ systems (OS), e.g., respiratory system, cardiovascular system

Extent of ROS depends on CC and patient status (new, established, inpatient, outpatient)

ROS Elements
Constitutional—General, fever, weight loss or gain

Eyes—Organ System (OS)

Ears, Nose, Mouth, Throat (OS)

Cardiovascular (OS)

Respiratory (OS)

Gastrointestinal (OS)

Genitourinary (OS)

Musculoskeletal (OS)

Integumentary (OS)

Neurological (OS)

Psychiatric (OS)

Endocrine (OS)

Hematologic/Lymphatic (OS)

Allergic/Immunologic (OS)

Past, Family, and Social History (PFSH)

Past
Contains relevant information about past illness, injury, or treatment, including

- Major illnesses/injuries

- Operations

- Hospitalizations

- Allergies

- Immunizations

- Dietary status

- Current medications

Family History
Health status or cause of death of family members

- Parents

- Siblings

- Children

Family history items related to CC

- Hereditary diseases

Social History
Review of past and current activities

- Marital status

- Employment

- Occupational history

- Use of drugs/alcohol/tobacco

- Educational activities

- Sexual history

- Other relevant or contributory factors

Four History Levels

1. Problem Focused (PF)

2. Expanded Problem Focused (EPF)

3. Detailed (D)

4. Comprehensive (C)

Problem-Focused History
CC

Brief HPI

No ROS

No PFSH

Expanded Problem-Focused History
CC

Brief HPI

Problem focused ROS

No PFSH

Detailed History
CC

Extended HPI

Problem pertinent ROS, extended to include a limited number of additional systems

Pertinent PFSH directly related to problem

Comprehensive History
CC

Extended HPI

Complete ROS directly related to CC, plus review of 10+ systems

Complete PFSH

Summary of elements required for each level of history (Fig. 3-2)

History Elements

Chief Complaint (CC)
Reason for the encounter in the patient's words

History of Present Illness (HPI)
Location
Quality
Severity
Duration*
Timing
Context
Modifying factors
Associated signs and symptoms

Review of Systems (ROS)
Constitutional symptoms (fever, weight loss, etc.)
Ophthalmologic (eyes)
Otolaryngologic (ears, nose, mouth, throat)
Cardiovascular
Respiratory
Gastrointestinal
Genitourinary
Musculoskeletal
Integumentary (skin and/or breast)
Neurologic
Psychiatric
Endocrine
Hematologic/Lymphatic
Allergic/Immunologic

Past, Family, and/or Social History (PFSH)
Past major illnesses, operations, injuries, and treatments
Family medical history for heredity and risk
Social activities, both past and current

Elements Required for Each Level of History

		Problem Focused	Expanded Problem Focused	Detailed	Comprehensive
History	HPI	Brief 1-3	Brief 1-3	Extended 4+	Extended 4+
	ROS	None	Problem-pertinent 1	Extended 2-9	Complete 10+
	PFSH	None	None	Pertinent 1	Complete 2-3

*Duration is not listed in the CPT E/M Guidelines, but is listed in the DGs.

Figure **3-2** History elements required for each level of history.

Four Examination Levels (Objective)

Problem-Focused Examination (1995 Documentation Guidelines [DG])

Limited examination of affected body area or organ system

Expanded Problem-Focused Examination (1995 DG)

Limited examination of affected body area or organ system

Other related body area(s) or organ system(s)

Detailed Examination (1995 DG)

Extended examination of affected body area(s) and other symptomatic or related organ system(s)

Examination Elements

General (OS)
Constitutional

Body Areas (BA)
Head (including the face)
Neck
Chest (including breasts and axillae)
Abdomen
Genitalia, groin, buttocks
Back
Each extremity

Organ System (OS)
Ophthalmologic (eyes)
Otolaryngologic (ears, nose, mouth, throat)
Cardiovascular
Respiratory
Gastrointestinal
Genitourinary
Musculoskeletal
Integumentary
Neurologic
Psychiatric
Hematologic/Lymphatic/Immunologic

Elements Required for Each Level of Examination

	Problem Focused	Expanded Problem Focused	Detailed	Comprehensive
Examination	Limited to affected BA or OS	Limited to affected BA or OS and other related OS(s)	Extended of affected BA(s) and other related OS(s)	General multi-system (OSs only)

Figure **3-3** Examination elements required for each level of examination.

Comprehensive Examination (1995 DG)
Eight or more organ systems

Summary of elements required for each level of examination (Fig. 3-3)

Medical Decision Making Complexity (MDM)

Management Options
Based on number of possible diagnoses

Levels: Minimal, limited, multiple, or extensive

Data Reviewed
Laboratory, radiology; any test/procedure results are documented along with the data reviewed and the identity of the reviewer in medical record

- "Hemoglobin within normal limits."

- "Chest x-ray, negative."

Old medical records (data) from others may be requested and reviewed

Levels: Minimal, limited, moderate, or extensive

Risks

Risks of morbidity (poor outcome), complications, or mortality (death) associated with problem, diagnostic procedure

Other diseases or factors (co-morbidities)

- Diabetes

- Extreme age

Urgency relates to risks

- Myocardial infarction

- Ruptured appendix

Levels: Minimal, low, moderate, or high

See Fig. 3-4, CMS Table of Risk

Four Levels of MDM Complexity

1. Straightforward MDM

Number of diagnoses or management options: Minimal

Amount or complexity of data: Minimal/None

Risk of complications or death: Minimal

2. Low-complexity MDM

Number of diagnoses or management options: Limited

Amount or complexity of data: Limited

Risk of complications or death: Low

3. Moderate-Complexity MDM

Number of diagnoses or management options: Multiple

Amount or complexity of data: Moderate

Risk of complications or death: Moderate

4. High-Complexity MDM

Number of diagnoses or management options: Extensive

Amount or complexity of data: Extensive

Risk of complications or death: High

Summary of elements required for each level of MDM (Fig. 3-5)

The diagnosis or management options, amount or complexity of data, and risk are totaled to arrive at the level of MDM

- Only two of three categories must meet or exceed each other in any level to assign the MDM

Example: Moderate complexity for diagnosis or management options and moderate complexity of amount or complexity of data, but only a low risk would be assigned a moderate level MDM

Example: Low risk of death, moderate diagnosis or management options, and high amount or complexity of data: Assign the moderate level of MDM

TABLE OF RISK
(Total = highest risk in any one category)

Level of risk	Presenting problem(s)	Diagnostic procedure(s) ordered	Management options selected
Minimal	• One self-limited or minor problem, e.g., cold, insect bite, tinea corpus	• Laboratory tests requiring venipuncture • Chest x-rays • EKG/EEG • Urinalysis • Ultrasound, e.g., echocardiography • KOH prep	• Rest • Gargles • Elastic bandages • Superficial dressings
Low	• Two or more self-limited or minor problems • One stable chronic illness, e.g., well-controlled hypertension or non–insulin-dependent diabetes, cataract, BPH • Acute uncomplicated illness or injury, e.g., cystitis, allergic rhinitis, simple sprain	• Physiologic tests not under stress, e.g., pulmonary function tests • Non-cardiovascular imaging studies with contrast, e.g., barium enema • Superficial needle biopsies • Clinical laboratory tests requiring arterial puncture • Skin biopsies	• Over-the-counter drugs • Minor surgery with no identified risk factors • Physical therapy • IV fluids without additives
Moderate	• One or more chronic illnesses with mild exacerbation, progression, or side effects of treatment • Two or more stable chronic illnesses • Undiagnosed new problem with uncertain prognosis, e.g., lump in breast • Acute illness with systemic symptoms, e.g., pyelonephritis, pneumonitis, colitis • Acute complicated injury, e.g., head injury with brief loss of consciousness	• Physiologic tests under stress, e.g., cardiac stress test, fetal contraction stress test • Diagnostic endoscopies with no identified risk factors • Deep needle or incisional biopsy • Cardiovascular imaging studies with contrast and no identified risk factors, e.g., arteriogram, cardiac catheterization • Obtain fluid from body cavity, e.g., lumbar puncture, thoracentesis, culdocentesis	• Minor surgery with identified risk factors • Elective major surgery (open, percutaneous, or endoscopic) with no identified risk factors • Prescription drug management • Therapeutic nuclear medicine • IV fluids with additives • Closed treatment of fracture or dislocation without manipulation
High	• One or more chronic illnesses with severe exacerbation, progression, or side effects of treatment • Acute or chronic illnesses or injuries that pose a threat to life or bodily function, e.g., multiple trauma, acute MI, pulmonary embolus, severe respiratory distress, progressive severe rheumatoid arthritis • Psychiatric illness with potential threat to self or others • Peritonitis • Acute renal failure • An abrupt change in neurologic status, e.g., seizure, TIA, weakness, or sensory loss	• Cardiovascular imaging studies with contrast with identified risk factors • Cardiac electrophysiological tests • Diagnostic endoscopies with identified risk factors • Discography	• Elective major surgery (open, percutaneous, or endoscopic) with identified risk factors • Emergency major surgery (open, percutaneous or endoscopic) • Parenteral controlled substances • Drug therapy requiring intensive monitoring for toxicity • Decision not to resuscitate or to de-escalate care because of poor prognosis

Figure **3-4** Centers for Medicare and Medicaid Services (CMS) Table of Risk.

Medical Decision Making Elements

Number of Diagnoses or Management Options
Minimal
Limited
Multiple
Extensive

Amount or Complexity of Data to Review
Minimal/None
Limited
Moderate
Extensive

Risk of Complications or Death If Condition Goes Untreated
Minimal
Low
Moderate
High

Elements Required for Each Level of Medical Decision Making

	Straightforward	Low	Moderate	High
Number of diagnoses or management options	Minimal	Limited	Multiple	Extensive
Amount or complexity of data to review	Minimal/None	Limited	Moderate	Extensive
Risk	Minimal	Low	Moderate	High

Figure **3-5** Elements required for each level of medical decision making.

Contributory Factors

Counseling

Provided to patient or family members (synopsis must be stated in medical record)

Discussion of diagnosis, test results, impressions, recommendations, prognosis, risks/benefits of treatment options or lack thereof, and risk factor reduction

Coordination of Care
Work done on behalf of patient by physician to provide care

Nature of Presenting Problem
Type of problem patient presents to physician with or reason for encounter

Levels of Presenting Problem

Minimal Presenting Problem
May not require a physician

Example: A dressing change or removal of an uncomplicated suture

Self-limiting or Minor Presenting Problem
Self-limiting problems are minor and with a good outcome and no complications predicted

> *Example:* Sore throat or a slightly irritated skin tag

Low-Severity Presenting Problem
Without treatment, low risk

> *Example:* A middle-aged, healthy male with an upper respiratory infection

Moderate-Severity Presenting Problem
Without treatment, moderate risk

> *Example:* An elderly male with bacterial pneumonia

High-Severity Presenting Problem
Without treatment, high risk

> *Example:* An elderly male in very poor health with diabetic ketoacidosis

Time
Direct or face-to-face: Physician or other qualified health care professional and patient together

> *Example:* Clinic visit or at bedside in hospital

Calculated for code assignment beginning and ending times documented in medical record

Unit/Floor: Time spent by physician on patient's floor or unit, also at patient's bedside

> *Example:* Reviewing patient records or at chart desk and then with patient

---

Over 50% of the total time should include counseling and/or coordination of care, and the documentation must reflect the total time of the visit and the time spent counseling and/or in coordination of care to qualify to assign the code based on time.

Use of E/M Code
Codes are grouped by type of service and place of service

- Consultation

- Office visit

- Hospital admission

Different codes are required for various levels of service assignment

New patient (99201-99205) services to new patient in office or other outpatient setting

Selection of Level of E/M Services
For the following categories/subcategories, all three of the key components must meet or exceed the level stated in the code description:

- Office or Other Outpatient Services, New Patient

- Hospital Observation Services

- Initial Hospital Care

- Observation or Inpatient Care Services

- Office or Other Outpatient Consultations

- Inpatient Consultations
- Emergency Department Services
- Initial Nursing Facility Care
- Other Nursing Facility Services
- Domiciliary, Rest Home (e.g., Boarding Home), or Custodial Care Services, New Patient
- Home Services, New Patient

For the following categories/subcategories, two of the three key components must meet or exceed the level stated in the code description:

- Office or Other Outpatient Services, Established Patient
- Subsequent Observation Care
- Subsequent Hospital Care
- Subsequent Nursing Facility Care
- Domiciliary, Rest Home (e.g., Boarding Home), Established Patient
- Home Services, Established Patient

New Patient (99201-99205)
All new patients must be seen by physician

Established Patient (99211-99215)
99211 may not require a physician's presence

No such code in New Patient category; all new patients are seen by physician

Hospital Observation Status (99217-99220, 99224-99226, 99234-99236)
Not officially admitted to "inpatient status"

Patient not ill enough to admit but is too ill not to be monitored or discharged

Read notes at beginning of subsection

Observation services are not codes for "inpatient" services

Observation admission can be reported only for first day of service

When patient admitted on observation status and discharged on same day:

- Assign code from 99234-99236 (Observation or Inpatient Care Services category including admission and discharge)

Patient in hospital overnight for observation but less than 48 hours:

- **First day:** 99218-99220 (Initial Observation Care)
- **Second day:** 99217 (Observation Care Discharge Services)

If observation stay longer than 48 hours:

- **First day:** 99218-99220 (Initial Observation Care)
- **Second day:** 99224-99226 (Subsequent Observation Care)
- **Third day:** 99217 (Observation Care Discharge Services)

Initial Observation Care

- Beginning of observation care service
- Does not require a specific hospital unit; can be a regular bed on a floor or in emergency department (ED)
- Status specified as "observation"

E/M services immediately prior to admission bundled into observation service

> *Example:* Office visit prior to observation, bundled into observation service

Hospital Inpatient Services (99221-99239)
Officially admitted to a hospital setting

Total (all day and night)

Partial (all day and no night, all night and no day, or a variation)

- Time in and out must be specified in medical record

Types of Physician Status
Attending: Primary or admitting physician

Consultant: Physician whose opinion and advice requested by attending physician

Referring: Physician requesting a consultation from another physician regarding a patient's health status

Types of Care
Concurrent care given to patient by more than one physician each of different specialties

> *Example:* Pulmonologist and cardiologist both treating patient for different conditions at same time

Three Types of Hospital Inpatient Services
Initial Hospital Care (99221-99223)
First service includes admission

Initial paperwork

Initial treatment plans and orders

Used only once for each admission

- Only one admission by the attending or admitting physician billable per hospitalization

Subsequent Hospital Care (99231-99233)
After initial service

Physician reviews patient's progress using documentation, information received from nursing staff, examination of patient

- May be reported by multiple physicians of different specialties managing different conditions (concurrent care); only one per day per physician per specialty

Hospital Discharge Services (99238, 99239)
Final day of hospital stay when patient in hospital more than 1 day

Documentation indicates final patient status

Time based

- Total time

- Does not need to be continuous time

Beginning and ending time or total time spent must be documented to assign the extended discharge code or use lowest level code

Final Status of Patient
Summary of stay (Discharge)
Condition (final examination)

Medications

Plan for return (follow-up care) to physician

How hospital stay progressed

Discharged destination (to home, nursing facility, etc.)

Only attending physician can use discharge code (only one discharge per admission)

Code based on time spent in service

Beginning and ending time or total time spent must be documented to assign the extended discharge code or must use lowest level code

Consultation Services (99241-99255)
One physician or appropriate source requests another physician's opinion or advice

Either inpatient or outpatient; outpatient consultations include those provided in ED

Outpatient consultations (99241-99245)

Inpatient consultations (99251-99255)

Effective January 1, 2010, CMS no longer recognized CPT consultation codes (ranges 99241-99245 and 99251-99255) for inpatient facility and office/outpatient settings.

Consultation services reported with

- New patient office/outpatient (99201-99205)

- Established patient office/outpatient (99212-99215)

- Initial hospital codes (99221-99223)

Third-Party-Payer Consultations
Request consult for

- Past medical treatment

- Current condition

- Payers may request prior to approving procedure

- Report services with -32, mandated services

Emergency Department Services (99281-99288)
No distinction between new and established patients

Must be open 24 hours a day to qualify as ED (ER)

ED services often require additional codes from Critical Care Services

- Typically billed by ED physicians

Other Emergency Services (99288) reports two-way communication for emergency care

Critical Care Services (99291, 99292)

Example: Vital organ failure

Critical care services are provided to patients over 71 months of age in life-threatening (critically ill/injured) situations

Time-based codes

- Total time under 30 minutes reported with appropriate E/M code (e.g., ED)

Critical Care Services (99291, 99292)
Time must be documented in medical record to select from this code range; does not need to be continuous

- Over 71 months of age

99291 and 99292 reports total length of time a physician spends caring for critically ill patient

- 99291: 30-74 minutes

- 99292: Each additional 30 minutes

Nursing Facility Services (99304-99318)
Non-hospital settings with professional staff

- Provide continuous health care services to patients who are not acutely ill

Formerly known as Skilled Nursing Facility (SNF), Intermediate Care Facility (ICF), and Long-Term Care Facility (LTCF)

Various levels of nursing facility services

Initial Nursing Facility Assessment (99304-99306)
Provided at time of patient's initial admission/readmission

Subsequent Nursing Facility Care codes (99307-99310)
99307 stable, recovering, or improving

99308 not responding or minor complication

99309 significant complication or new problem

99310 significant new problem requiring immediate physician attention

Nursing Facility Discharge Services (99315, 99316)
For final discharge service

Time-based

- Total time, does not need to be continuous

Other Nursing Facility Services (99318)

- Annual Nursing Facility Assessment

Domiciliary, Rest Home, or Custodial Care Services (99324-99337)
Health care services are not available on site

Types of services provided are lodging, meals, supervision, personal care, leisure activities

Residents cannot live independently

Codes for either new or established patients

Domiciliary, Rest Home, or Home Care Plan Oversight Services (99339, 99340)
Read notes at beginning of subsection

Reports individual physician supervision of patient in home or domiciliary rest home

Services not face-to-face

Time-based

- 99339 15-29 minutes

- 99340 30 minutes or more

Reported once per 30-day period

Home Services (99341-99350)

Care provided in patient's home

Services based on key components and contributory factors

Codes for new or established patients

Prolonged Services (99354-99359)

Time codes for direct and non-direct contact

Report time beyond the usual E/M service

- Time must be documented in medical record

Codes for first 30-74 minutes and each additional 30 minutes thereafter

If less than 30 minutes, do not report service as prolonged

Standby Services (99360)

Not caring for other patient(s) to use these codes

Standing by only for that patient, if needed

Standby requested by another physician

- Must be documented in medical record

Report in 30-minute increments

Less than 30 minutes—do not report

Can report for subsequent 30 minutes only if a full 30 minutes

Carriers have strict policies regarding reimbursement for this service

Case Management Services (99363-99368)

Anticoagulant Management Services, 99363 and 99364

- Anticoagulants such as warfarin
  - Thins the blood
- By physician or another qualified health care professional
- Provided in an outpatient setting for period of
  - 60 days or more
  - 60 days or less is not reported

Medical Team Conferences (99366-99368)

Codes for with or without face-to-face patient/family contact

- Minimum of 3 health care professionals, different specialties/disciplines participate in team
- Each member must have performed face-to-face evaluation in past 60 days
- Documentation must reflect member's contribution of information and treatment recommendation
- Not reported for organization or facility contracted services

Time-based

  Begins and ends at start and conclusion of review

Care Plan Oversight Services (99374-99380)
Used to report supervision of patient care in home health agency, hospice, domiciliary, or equivalent environment

Patient not present

Codes are time-based

- 15-29 minutes 30 minutes or more

- Time must be documented in medical record

Reported once for each 30-day period

Preventive Medicine Services (99381-99429)
Used to report services when patient is not currently ill

  Example: Annual checkup

Codes divided by new or established and age

If significant problem is encountered during preventive examination

- E/M code also reported, append modifier -25

Counseling Risk Factor Reduction and Behavior Change Intervention (99401-99429)
Patient is seen specifically to promote health and/or wellness

  Example: Diet, exercise program

Patient without symptoms or an established diagnosis to use these codes

Codes based on

- Time, individual or group, physician review of assessment data

Non-Face-to-Face Services (99441-99449)
Physician E/M services using telephone/online

- 99441-99443 telephone E/M services

  Established patient, family member of the patient, or a guardian

- 99444 online E/M services

  Established patient, family member of the patient, or a guardian

- 99446-99449 report interprofessional telephone/internet consultations

  - Usually provided on urgent/emergency basis

  - No face-to-face, based on total time

Special E/M Services (99450-99456)
- 99450 is reported for services provided for insurance or disability assessments

Involves no treatment; any treatment provided would be coded separately

99455-99456 report work related or medical disability evaluation

Codes divided

- 99455: Assessment by treating physician
- 99456: Assessment by nontreating physician

Newborn Care (99460-99465)
Initial and subsequent care in/other than hospital or birthing center

For normal newborn infant

Per day, for E/M services

99463, initial hospital/birthing center when admission and discharge is same day

Delivery/Birthing Room Attendance and Resuscitation Services (99464-99465)
99464, attendance at delivery

Documented request by attending in medical record

Provides initial stabilization

99465, resuscitation and ventilation

Inpatient Neonatal Intensive Care Services and Pediatric and Neonatal Critical Care Services (99466-99486)
Pediatric Critical Care Patient Transport
Critically ill or injured patient

24 months or younger

99466, 99467, first 30-74 minutes

Each additional 30 minutes

Reports face-to-face interfacility transport

99485, 99486, supervision by a control physician

First 30 minutes (#99485) and each additional 30 minutes (#99486)

Inpatient Neonatal and Pediatric Critical Care
99468-99482

Divided by

Initial day

Subsequent day

Divided by age

Neonatal (Age 28 days or younger)

Pediatric (29 days through 24 months)

Pediatric (2 through 5 years)

Initial and Continuing Intensive Care Services
99477-99480

Hospital Care

99477 for neonate 28 days of age or younger

99478-99480 divided by birth weight

very low birth weight (VLBW) ≤1500 grams (≤3.3 pounds)

low birth weight (LBW) 1501-2500 grams (3.3-5.5 pounds)

normal birth weight 2501-5000 grams (5.51-11.01 pounds)

Subdivided on day

Initial

Subsequent

Complex Chronic Care Coordination Services (99487-99489)

• Codes 99487-99489 report complex chronic care coordination

Based on whether the service was provided face-to-face or no face-to-face contact

Reported for the first hour of service and each additional 30 minutes of service

Clinical management of patients with multiple, complex medical conditions

• Codes 99495 and 99496 are transitional care management codes

Based on:

○ Number of days after discharge from a medical facility

○ Medical decision making complexity (moderate or high)

Involves management of various available care options for the patient

Transitional Care Management Services (99495, 99496)

• Patient is transitioning from a clinical setting to a community setting

Requires face-to-face visit with patient

○ 99495 within 14 days of discharge

○ 99496 within 7 days of discharge

Other Evaluation and Management Services (99499)

• 99499 reports unlisted E/M services

Accompanied by a special report

■ PRACTICE EXERCISES

Practice Exercise 3-1: Progress Note, Acute and Chronic Renal Failure

PROGRESS NOTE

LOCATION: Inpatient, Hospital

PATIENT: Mike Lumbardi

ATTENDING PHYSICIAN: George Orbitz, MD

NEPHROLOGY PROGRESS NOTE: Mike had no major events. He tolerated the angiogram very well. He had peripheral vascular disease, but nothing to bypass, unfortunately. The patient denies any chest pain, shortness of breath. He has no nausea or vomiting. He has no leg edema and no GI symptoms.

PHYSICAL EXAMINATION: His vital signs were stable this morning. Temperature 36.9°C. Blood pressure 165/85. Heart rate 52 per minute. Respirations 16 per minute. Sats were 96% on room air. The patient was not in any respiratory, cardiac, or neurologic distress. He had no increase in jugulovenous pressure; regular rate and rhythm. The lungs were clear bilaterally without any crackles. The abdomen was soft and nontender; no organomegaly. No edema, with decreased pulses bilaterally, with signs of chronic venous and arterial insufficiency.

Intake/output in the past 8 hours: 1286 in, 1050 out.

Labs are pending from this morning, but his creatinine yesterday was 1.3.

IMPRESSION
1. Acute on top of chronic renal failure related to intravascular volume depletion, with creatinine coming down from 1.6 to 1.3.
2. Peripheral vascular disease.
3. Hypertension.

RECOMMENDATIONS
1. Basic metabolic panel is pending today.
2. If his creatinine goes up over time, he might need to have a renal MRA to look for renal artery stenosis.
3. Since patient is making urine, I don't think that his creatinine will go up acutely after his angiogram yesterday.

CPT Code(s): _____

ICD-9-CM Code(s): _____

Abstracting Questions

1. Are all three key elements (history, examination, and MDM complexity) documented? _____

2. How many key elements are required for this type of service? _____

3. Should both acute and chronic renal failure be reported, and if so, which is reported first? _____

4. Is the volume depletion reported? _____

Practice Exercise 3-2: Clinic Visit, Diarrhea

CLINIC NOTE

FOLLOW-UP CLINIC VISIT

SUBJECTIVE: This is a $3\frac{1}{2}$-year-old girl who presents today. Mother states that patient has had diarrhea over the past 3-4 days. Yesterday she had about 4-5 stools. They have been mustard colored, real runny, sometimes in little slivers. No blood has been present. She threw up 3-4 days ago, but this has since ended. Her eating is down, although she is drinking a lot. She will complain of her stomach hurting. Her temperature was as high as 103°F, and that was about 3 days ago. She is taking Motrin.

OBJECTIVE: On general appearance: She is alert and does not appear to be in any acute distress. Temperature is 97.2°F. Weight is 42 pounds. HEENT: Eyes are clear. The right TM has some increased erythema present. Landmarks are still seen. The left TM is nice and clear with good landmarks. Oropharynx is unremarkable. Neck is supple. Heart reveals a regular rate and rhythm without murmur. GU: Normal female genitalia.

ASSESSMENT
1. Viral gastroenteritis.
2. Possibly early right otitis media.

PLAN: I did discuss with mother that we could put her daughter on an antibiotic now, but we also could wait to see if she starts complaining of right ear pain or if her fever comes back. If that is the case, I did give mother a prescription for Amoxicillin to have her daughter take 375 mg p.o. t.i.d. × 10 days, and I would want to recheck her ear in 3 weeks. If she does not have any complaints or fever, mother will hold off just so Amoxicillin does not worsen her diarrhea. Mother was in agreement with this plan.

CPT Code(s): _____

ICD-9-CM Code(s): _____

Abstracting Questions

1. What category of E/M codes is used to report this service? _____

2. What body system is reviewed in the statement "right TM"? _____

Practice Exercise 3-3: Vomiting

Dr. Sutton is an employee of the hospital.

LOCATION: Outpatient, Hospital

PATIENT: Penny Karlin

PRIMARY CARE PHYSICIAN: Ronald Green, MD

ED PHYSICIAN: Paul Sutton, MD

SUBJECTIVE: This is a 50-year-old female who is presenting to the emergency department today with a complaint of vomiting.

HISTORY OF PRESENT ILLNESS: This patient has quite significant recent medical history; recently diagnosed with grade IV esophageal cancer. She has been to the Lato Clinic and evaluated there, as well as in Los Angeles with endoscopy, and eventually to the Lato Clinic for further workup. With her workup there they found that she had quite extensive cancer with metastatic disease to the bones as well as to the stomach and thought that palliative oncologic treatment was all that could be offered and she should return to the area for this. She is scheduled to have a central line placed tomorrow and also considerations to nutritional needs. She stated that over the past several days she has had some fundraisers and some events for her and she really wanted to attend even though she was not able to keep foods and fluids down. She has been taking only small sips at a time. It seems like her ability to swallow is getting quite impaired, and as a result she cannot swallow her pain pill, so she is having severe pain in her back, hip, and abdomen. She has had increasing fatigue, has vomited several times, and just is not doing well and comes in for this at this time.

PAST MEDICAL HISTORY: Remarkable for esophageal cancer grade IV adenocarcinoma, noted with pelvic mets.

MEDICATIONS: Oxycodone and promethazine.

ALLERGIES: NKA, other than latex.

SOCIAL HISTORY: No smoking or alcohol.

REVIEW OF SYSTEMS: Negative for fever or chills. No shortness of breath. No headache. Patient's got nausea and abdominal and lower chest pain as positives on her review of systems.

On admission to the emergency department today, the patient's vital signs show a temperature of 36.8, pulse of 99, respiratory rate at 18, and blood pressure 132/84. General: This is a 50-year-old female who is awake, alert, and cooperative. HEENT: Head is normocephalic and atraumatic. Pupils are reactive to light. Conjunctivae clear. Nares patent. TMs are clear. Mouth reveals a somewhat dry oropharynx with some chapping of the lips, which appear parched. Neck is supple. Trachea is midline. Examination of lungs reveals clear breath sounds. Cardiovascular: S1 and S2 without murmur, click, or rub. Abdomen is soft. There is mild tenderness to palpation in the epigastric region. No mass, guarding, or rigidity. Extremities are without deformity or edema. Skin exam shows no rash. Cranial nerves 2 through 12 grossly intact. No gross motor or sensory deficits noted at this time.

SUMMARY OF EMERGENCY DEPARTMENT COURSE: The patient is seen and evaluated for the above-mentioned complaint. Orthostatic blood pressures were obtained: lying 112/87 with a pulse of 78, sitting 108/74 with a pulse of 98, and standing 102/80 with a pulse of 116. So she had quite an increase in her heart rate with standing, which I believe is significant. I did start an IV here in the department with normal saline; I gave her a liter of normal saline and 4 mg of morphine for her pain, which did help her pain significantly. It came down from an 8 to a 3. Checked some blood counts and metabolic panel as well as giving her some Phenergan for nausea, and this did help take away the nausea. Her CBC shows a hemoglobin level of 9.1, white count is okay, and her electrolytes are normal. So I think she is on the cusp of dehydration; certainly some anemia present here. I spoke with Dr. Green, who is covering for Dr. White, the patient's oncologist here, and he agreed to come in and evaluate the patient and did admit the patient to his service for further evaluation and treatment.

ASSESSMENT
1. Acute nausea and vomiting and dehydration.
2. Adenocarcinoma of the esophagus with metastatic disease.

PLAN: As above, the patient will be admitted for further evaluation and treatment per Dr. Green, certainly to control her pain, and it looks to me that the patient is going to have to change her pain regimen from oral to either parenteral or transdermal delivery system. She is going to have a line placed tomorrow, and further evaluation and treatment will be based on Dr. Green's plan for the patient. These plans as mentioned above were reviewed with the patient, who was in agreement. She will be admitted in fair condition with poor prognosis.

CPT Code(s): _____

ICD-9-CM Code(s): _____

Abstracting Questions

1. What level of history was documented? _____

2. What level of examination was documented? _____

3. What level of medical decision making was documented? _____

4. This case began in the emergency department, but what was the ultimate disposition of this patient? _____

5. Why is a neoplasm code not the first-listed diagnosis? _____

Practice Exercise 3-4: Well-Child Check

CLINIC NOTE

LOCATION: Outpatient, Hospital

PATIENT: Bradley Wellingstone

PHYSICIAN: Rolando Ortez, MD

SUBJECTIVE: This is a 3-week-old former 32-week gestational male infant who was in RNICU from birth. He did have some mild respiratory difficulties, oxygen requirements that resolved without further sequelae. He was also there for sepsis and feeding difficulties as well as apnea. He was discharged home on caffeine citrate, home apnea monitoring. He did return 2 days ago to get his first dose of Synagis. He is here for general checkup otherwise.

OBJECTIVE: He is on 24-calorie Enfamil and is taking that well without difficulty, taking almost 2 ounces at feeding; urinating and stool schedule is normal. No other complaints from his mother.

ASSESSMENT: On exam, alert, in no distress, and afebrile. His weight is up to 2341 grams, which is up 150 grams. Fontanelle, eyes, ears, nose, and pharynx are clear. Neck is supple. Lungs are clear to auscultation. Heart is regular rate and rhythm without murmur. Abdomen benign. Extremities: Full range of motion. No hip abnormalities. Skin is without rash. Neurologic exam without defect.

IMPRESSION: Thriving former 32-weeker. Now 3 weeks old.

PLAN: Anticipatory guidance discussed. We talked about feeding issues, accident prevention, car seat use, sleeping position on the side or the back. We will see them back in 1 month for his next Synagis dose as well as a recheck. We will have him on caffeine citrate 10 mg/day along with home apnea monitoring with plans to stop the caffeine in 1 month. With any problems, they need to give us a call or come back in sooner for re-evaluation.

CPT Code(s): _____

ICD-9-CM Code(s): _____

Abstracting Questions

1. From what CPT section would a code be located to report this? _____

2. From what CPT subcategory would this service be reported? _____

3. Was the patient a new or established patient with the provider? _____

4. Does the age of the patient affect code assignment? _____

5. What type of diagnosis code was reported? _____

Practice Exercise 3-5: NICU Progress Note, Ventilator Assist

Dr. Ortez has been following this infant since birth.

LOCATION: Inpatient, Hospital

PATIENT: Loren Black

ATTENDING PHYSICIAN: Rolando Ortez, MD

SUBJECTIVE: Baby is currently 2 days old, slightly under 48 hours.

OBJECTIVE: Weight today is 1716 kg (decreased by 135 grams). He is down 5.1% of his weight since birth. OFC is 30 cm (decreased 0.5 cm). Intake yesterday was 152 cc, 82 cc/kg/day. Output was 170 cc, 3.8 cc/kg/hour. He has had no stools since birth. Vital signs reveal his temperature to be acceptable while on an open, radiant warmer. Heart rate is generally in the 110s-120s. Respiratory rate has generally been equal to the IMV (60). Mean blood pressures have generally been in the 40s-50s. Oxygen saturations have remained in the high 90s.

PHYSICAL EXAMINATION: In general, he is pink, on current ventilator settings. He does have slightly dysmorphic features with wide-set eyes and slightly down-slanting palpebral fissures. Ears are low set and posteriorly rotated. Endotracheal tube was in place. Neck was without masses. Chest reveals symmetric expansion and lungs are clear to auscultation on current ventilator settings. Cardiac Exam: Regular rate without murmur or click. Peripheral pulses are 2+ and symmetric. Abdominal Exam: UAC in place. Liver is palpable 1 cm below the right costal margin. No splenomegaly or masses were noted. Genital Exam: Normal male. Testes are not palpable. Extremity Exam: No fixed decreased range of motion, deformity, or joint abnormality. Neurologic Exam: Mild, diffuse hypotonia. No focal deficits are appreciated.

CURRENT MEDICATIONS
1. Ampicillin 90.4 mg IV q12h.
2. Gentamicin 5.4 mg IV q18h.
3. Morphine sulfate 0.18 mg IV q6h and q1h p.r.n.
4. Dopamine 5 mcg/kg/min.
5. Vecuronium 0.18 mg IV q1-2h p.r.n.

LABORATORY STUDIES: Last arterial blood gas was obtained on ventilator setting of IMV 60, pressures of 24/4, and FIO_2 of 0.5 revealed pH 7.27, Pco_2 51.1, Po_2 66.5, and bicarbonate 22.5. Chemistry panel this morning reveals sodium of 134, potassium of 4.9, chloride of 102, glucose of 111, BUN of 18, creatinine of 1.0, calcium of 7.5, magnesium of 3.8, phosphorus of 7.7, bilirubin of 7.8. CBC reveals a white count of 6190. Platelet count was 98,000. Chest x-ray continues to show significant evidence of hyaline membrane disease. Endotracheal tube is near the carina and has been withdrawn somewhat.

IMPRESSION/RECOMMENDATIONS
1. Two-day-old infant who was born at 30 weeks' gestation. He does have clinical features suggestive of Noonan syndrome.
2. Respiratory: Continues to show evidence of hyaline membrane disease with respiratory failure. He has received three doses of surfactant therapy. He does have echocardiographic evidence of PDA, and we will be treating this at this time. We will attempt to decrease his ventilator settings based on serial clinical examination, pulse oximetry, arterial blood gas determinations, and chest x-ray.
3. Cardiovascular: Status is acceptable at this time while on dopamine at 5 mcg/kg/min. Echocardiogram shows a patent ductus arteriosis. There also

appears to be a slight abnormality to the pulmonary valve, which could be associated with his possible Noonan syndrome. He is going to receive indomethacin therapy.

4. Gastrointestinal: Abdominal exam remains benign. He is NPO. He does have mild hyperbilirubinemia. Direct antibody test was negative. We will begin phototherapy at this time.

5. Hematologic: Serial CBCs have been acceptable except for mild thrombocytopenia. We will continue to monitor, especially in light of the indomethacin therapy. He has not required any blood product transfusions since birth.

6. Infectious Disease: Blood culture remains negative at this time. We have discontinued his gentamicin, and he is being placed on cefotaxime because of the indomethacin.

7. Neurologic: Exam remains acceptable given his extreme prematurity. He will require screening intracranial ultrasound and long-term neurodevelopmental follow-up.

8. Renal/Metabolic: Urine output remains adequate and renal function studies are acceptable. Previous metabolic parameters are acceptable. We will repeat in the morning.

9. Fluids/Electrolytes/Nutrition: Weight loss is acceptable and electrolytes are in the more normal range today. We will adjust his TPN accordingly.

10. Apnea/Bradycardia: None since birth.

11. Health Care Maintenance: None yet.

SOCIAL HISTORY: Mom and dad are being kept up to date with regard to the patient's condition. Their questions have been answered, and they are in agreement with the outlined management plan.

CPT Code(s): _____

ICD-9-CM Code(s): _____

Abstracting Questions

1. The surfactant therapy was given for which diagnosis? _____

2. What does PDA mean? _____

■ ANESTHESIA SECTION (00100-01999)

Anesthesiologist

Doctor of medicine specializing in anesthesia

Usually outside practices, e.g., Anesthesia Associates, Inc., or Pain Clinic, Ltd.

Professional services reported separately

CRNA

Certified Registered Nurse Anesthetist

Uses of Anesthesia

Manage unconscious patients, life functions, and resuscitation

Analgesia

Relieve pain

Some Methods of Anesthesia

Endotracheal: Through mouth (general anesthesia)

Local: Application to area (injection or topical)

Epidural: Between vertebral spaces—injection into epidural space

Regional: Field or nerve block

MAC: Monitored anesthesia care (service provided by an anesthesiologist or CRNA)

Patient is monitored, and if necessary, sedation (including general anesthesia) may be provided

Spinal: Anesthesia applied to the spinal cord area, outside the dura mater

General: State of unconsciousness accomplished through drug administration or by inhalation

Patient-Controlled Analgesia (PCA)

Patient self-administers drug

Used to relieve chronic pain or temporarily for severe pain following surgery

Moderate (Conscious) Sedation

Codes in Medicine Section of CPT

99143-99145 assigned when surgeon administers sedation

99148-99150 assigned when another physician administers sedation

• No anesthesia personnel are present

Decreased level of consciousness

Not reported by physician if provided in nonfacility setting

Anesthesia Formula

$(B + T + M) \times$ conversion factor = Anesthesia payment

B is for Base Units

Published in *Relative Value Guide (RVG)* by American Society of Anesthesiologists

National unit values for anesthesia services based on complexity of service

T Is for Time
Patient record indicates time, e.g., 60 minutes

Usually, 15 minutes = 1 unit

   Example: 60 minutes = 4 units

Some payers may indicate 1 unit = 1 minute

Begins: Anesthesiologist begins to prepare patient for induction—preoperative

Continues throughout procedure—intraoperative

Ends: Patient no longer under care of anesthesiologist—postoperative

M Is for Modifying Unit
Additional units based on physical status of patient (see modifiers that follow)

Physical Status Modifiers, P1-P6
Located in Anesthesia Guidelines

Not reported to Medicare

Help to show complexity of service

- P1 Normal healthy
- P2 Mild systemic disease
- P3 Severe systemic disease
- P4 Severe systemic disease is constant threat to life
- P5 Not expected to survive without the operation
- P6 Clinically brain dead

Qualifying Circumstances Codes (99100-99140)
Anesthesia services provided under difficult circumstances

Located in both Anesthesia Guidelines and Medicine section

Listed in addition to primary anesthesia code

More than one may be reported

Summing Up Formula
Base units (from *RVG*) based on CPT codes

Time units (usually 15 min is a unit)

- Total time ÷ 15 = time units

Modifiers [Qualifying Circumstances (99100-99140) and/or Physical Status (P1-P6)]

Conversion Factors
CMS anesthesia conversion factors

Sum of money allocated by payer, per unit for payment of anesthesia services

Anesthesia for Multiple Surgical Procedures
Once anesthetized, length of time, not number of procedures performed during session

Report highest relative value guide (RVG) valued CPT code

   Example: Two procedures during same session

- One, 10 base units; the other, 5 base units
- Report only 10 base units and combined time for all procedures

Anesthesia Modifiers
Anesthesia code reported twice

- Once for anesthesiologist
- Once for CRNA

Each reports service on separate claim form

- One claim for anesthesiologist's service
- One claim for CRNA's service

Anesthesia modifiers report supervision/direction circumstances

- AA, anesthesia services performed personally by anesthesiologist
- AD, medical supervision >4 concurrent procedures
- QK, medical direction of 2-4 concurrent procedures
- QX, CRNA service with medical direction
- QY, medical direction of 1 CRNA
- QZ, CRNA service without medical

Anesthesia modifier always precedes the physical status modifier

■ PRACTICE EXERCISES

Practice Exercise 3-6: Perforated Appendicitis

Assign anesthesia code(s) and any necessary modifiers. Do not assign surgery codes. Do not assign diagnosis codes. During this procedure the anesthesiologist was medically directing two CRNAs providing anesthesia for concurrent procedures. The patient's physical status is P2.

OPERATIVE REPORT

LOCATION: Inpatient, Hospital

PATIENT: Laurence Hooper

ATTENDING PHYSICIAN: Gary Sanchez, MD

SURGEON: Gary Sanchez, MD

PREOPERATIVE DIAGNOSIS: Perforated appendicitis.

POSTOPERATIVE DIAGNOSIS: Same.

ANESTHESIA: General.

ANESTHESIOLOGIST: Janice E. Larson, MD

PROCEDURE: The patient was brought to the operating room, placed under general anesthesia, and prepped and draped sterilely. The patient's advanced age is a concern, since he is 92. A right lower quadrant skin incision was made with a #10 blade, and dissection was carried down through the subcutaneous tissue using electrocautery. The anterior sheath of the rectus fascia was opened. The rectus was retracted medially. The posterior sheath and peritoneum were grasped with curved clamps and sharply incised, allowing entry into the peritoneal cavity. There were a few adhesions, which we took down sharply. We then delivered the appendix up and into the wound. We took down the mesoappendix between Kelly clamps and tied the vascular pedicles with 2–0 silk free ties. The base of the appendix was then crushed. It was tied with 0 Vicryl. It was inverted into the base of the cecum with a 3–0 silk pursestring suture. The abdomen was then irrigated with saline until returns were clear. We closed the posterior sheath and peritoneum with running 0 Vicryl, closed the anterior sheath with interrupted 0 Vicryl, and closed the skin with subcuticular 4–0 undyed Vicryl. Steri-Strips and sterile Band-Aids were applied. All sponge and needle counts were correct. Before the patient left the operating room, the wound was anesthetized with a total of 30 cc of 0.50% Sensorcaine with epinephrine solution.

CPT Code(s): _____

Abstracting Questions

1. What is the main term referenced in the index of the CPT to locate the code?
_____

2. What was the subterm used in the CPT index to locate the anesthesia code?
_____

3. Does the quadrant entered to perform the surgical procedure affect CPT anesthesia code assignment? _____

4. Was the procedure at the abdominal wall or intraperitoneal?
_____

5. Were there any Qualifying Circumstances to report?

_____

6. Who decides what Physical Status Modifier should be reported?

_____

7. Was the anesthesiologist providing service or medically directing cases?

_____

Practice Exercise 3-7: Left Breast Biopsy

Assign anesthesia code(s) only. Do not assign surgery codes. Do not assign diagnosis codes. The patient's physical status is P1.

OPERATIVE REPORT

LOCATION: Outpatient, Hospital

PATIENT: Adrienne Gardener

ATTENDING PHYSICIAN: Gary Sanchez, MD

SURGEON: Gary Sanchez, MD

PREOPERATIVE DIAGNOSIS: Left breast mass.

POSTOPERATIVE DIAGNOSIS: Same.

PROCEDURE PERFORMED: Left breast biopsy.

ANESTHESIA: Local with IV sedation and monitored anesthesia care.

ANESTHESIOLOGIST: Janice E. Larson, MD

PROCEDURE: The patient was brought to the operating room, given IV sedation, and then anesthetized with a total of 30 cc of 1% Sensorcaine with epinephrine solution. Incision was made over the top of the mass with a #15 blade, and dissection was carried down through subcutaneous tissues sharply. We encountered the mass, which appeared to be a fibroadenoma. We excised this sharply. We got the entire lesion. We controlled bleeding with electrocautery. We then closed the skin with subcuticular 4–0 undyed Vicryl. Steri-Strips and sterile Band-Aids were applied. She tolerated this well and was taken to recovery room in stable condition.

Pathology Report Later Indicated: Fibroadenoma.

CPT Code(s): _____

| **Abstracting Questions** |

1. Do you report the sedation with CPT anesthesia codes or medicine codes?

   _____

2. Was the procedure superficial (subcutaneous) or deep (internal structures)?

   _____

Practice Exercise 3-8: Takedown Colostomy and Cholecystectomy

Assign anesthesia code(s) only. Do not assign surgery codes. Do not assign diagnosis codes. The anesthesiologist was supervising two concurrent procedures. The patient's physical status is P2.

OPERATIVE REPORT

LOCATION: Inpatient, Hospital

PATIENT: Simon Sulten

ATTENDING PHYSICIAN: Gary Sanchez, MD

SURGEON: Gary Sanchez, MD

PREOPERATIVE DIAGNOSES
1. Colostomy for obstructing colon cancer.
2. Symptomatic cholelithiasis.

POSTOPERATIVE DIAGNOSES: Same.

PROCEDURE PERFORMED
1. Takedown colostomy with end-to-end colorectostomy.
2. Open cholecystectomy.

ANESTHESIA: General.

ANESTHESIOLOGIST: Janice E. Larson, MD

PROCEDURE: The patient was brought to the operating room, placed under general anesthesia, and prepped and draped sterilely. The previous midline was reopened with the #10 blade, and we excised the old scar. We carried out dissection through subcutaneous tissues using electrocautery. Midline fascia was divided sharply. We entered the peritoneal cavity and entered the midline fascia along the length of the incision. We took down numerous filmy adhesions and ran the small bowel from the terminal ileum to the ligament of Treitz, which appeared normal. First, we placed an Omni retractor and exposed the right upper quadrant. We identified the cystic duct and cystic artery and tied them off with 0 silk ties proximally and distally before transecting them. We then shelled the gallbladder from its fossa using electrocautery. We placed a pack up by the liver bed. We then identified the rectal stump and dissected this free. We then made an elliptical incision around the colostomy opening and carried our dissection down to fascia, freed up the stoma, and fired our TLC 75 stapler across the descending colon. We sent the specimen to pathology for permanent. We mobilized the left colon along the avascular line of Toldt up and around the splenic flexure. Once we had adequate length, we placed a Glassman clamp proximally on the rectum and distally on the descending colon. We then performed a two-layer, hand-sewn, end-to-end anastomosis with an outer layer of 3–0 silk Lembert and inner layer of running 3–0 Vicryl. There was a patent anastomosis, and we could easily milk contents through with no evidence of spilling. We then closed the fascia from the colostomy site with interrupted 0 Vicryl and running 0 PDS. We closed the skin with skin clips. All sponge and needle counts were correct. Patient tolerated this well and was taken to recovery in stable condition.

CPT Code(s): _____

Abstracting Question

1. Was a supervision modifier required? _____

Practice Exercise 3-9: Incision and Drainage of Perirectal Abscess

Assign anesthesia code(s) only. Do not assign surgery codes. Do not assign diagnosis codes. The patient's physical status is P3.

OPERATIVE REPORT

LOCATION: Outpatient, Hospital

PATIENT: Suzy Tarsinski

ATTENDING PHYSICIAN: Gary Sanchez, MD

SURGEON: Gary Sanchez, MD

PREOPERATIVE DIAGNOSIS: Perirectal abscess.

POSTOPERATIVE DIAGNOSIS: Same.

PROCEDURE PERFORMED: Incision and drainage of perirectal abscess.

ANESTHESIA: Spinal.

ANESTHESIOLOGIST: Janice E. Larson, MD

PROCEDURE: The patient was brought back to the operating room, and after a spinal anesthetic had been given, the area of the rectum was cleaned and draped in the usual fashion after the patient had been placed in a jackknife position. An incision was made over the top of this abscess with a #10-blade scalpel. We entered the abscessed cavity, which returned large amounts of purulent material. We broke up the loculations, debrided the necrotic tissue with a #10 blade, and irrigated with a liter of saline. We then were able to pack the cavity with sewed Kerlix. The patient tolerated the procedure well, and all sponges and needles were accounted for at the end of the procedure. Soon she could be transferred to the Post Anesthesia Care Unit in stable condition.

CPT Code(s): _____

Abstracting Question

1. For the purpose of locating an anesthesia code in the CPT manual, what was the location of the I&D? _____

Practice Exercise 3-10: Intracerebral Hematoma

Assign anesthesia code(s) only. Do not assign surgery codes. Do not assign diagnosis codes. The patient is not expected to survive without this procedure.

OPERATIVE PROCEDURE

LOCATION: Inpatient, Hospital

PATIENT: Suzy Kunklemann

ATTENDING PHYSICIAN: Gary Sanchez, MD

SURGEON: Gary Sanchez, MD

PREOPERATIVE DIAGNOSIS: Intracerebral hematoma, right temporal lobe.

POSTOPERATIVE DIAGNOSIS: Intracerebral hematoma, right temporal lobe.

PROCEDURE PERFORMED: Osteoplastic craniotomy, right temporal area; evacuation of intracerebral hematoma.

ANESTHESIA: General.

PROCEDURE: This patient is not expected to survive without this procedure, and at this point we have no other choice but to proceed. Under general anesthesia, the patient's head was placed in the Mayfield pins. The right frontal temporoparietal area was prepped and draped in the usual manner. A linear incision was made extending from the midline of the temporal fossa up to the midportion of the scalp. The skin was incised. The temporalis muscle was separated and divided off the bone. I did a craniotomy here the size of a half dollar coin and made a burr hole. I utilized the craniotome to elevate the bone flap, which was a free bone flap. This was then removed. We placed the Weitlaners into the wound and then incised the dura in a cruciate fashion over the temporal lobe. I then entered the middle temple gyrus, irrigated much of the clot from the temporal and posterior parietal areas, and evacuated the clot from the area. This took copious irrigation. We used cotton balls for hemostasis. I did this numerous times until all the bleeders were coagulated. I then lined the cystic cavity with Gelfoam and coagulated the edges of the raw brain. I closed the dura with 4–0 Vicryl. This was closed in a watertight fashion. I used 2–0 Vicryl to elevate the dura to the bone flap with Wurzburg plates, two of them, using plates and screws. I then closed the scalp in one layer using 0 Vicryl on the temporalis muscle and fascia, and the skin was approximated with 2–0 nylon interrupted mattress sutures. Dressing was applied, and the patient was on the ventilator and discharged to the surgical intensive care unit.

CPT Code(s): _____

Abstracting Question

1. Would a physical status modifier be required? _____

■ CPT/HCPCS LEVEL I MODIFIERS (-22 to -99)

Alters CPT or HCPCS code

Full list, CPT, Appendix A

- Two separate lists
  - One for physician use
  - One for hospital outpatient use

Modifier Functions

Altered (i.e., increased or reduced service)

Bilateral

Multiple

Only portions of service (i.e., professional service only)

More than one surgeon

-22 Increased Procedural Service

Indicates services significantly greater than usual

Accompanied by written report and supportive documentation

-23 Unusual Anesthesia

Use of general anesthesia where local or regional is norm

Example: Highly agitated senile patient

Used only with anesthesia codes

Written report with submission of modifier

-24 Unrelated E/M Services by Same Physician or Other Qualified Health Care Professional During a Postoperative Period

Service not related to surgery

If E/M provided during postoperative global period, no payment considered without -24

-25 Significant, Separately Identifiable E/M Service, by Same Physician or Other Qualified Health Care Professional on the Same Day of the Procedure or Other Service

Documentation must support service

Example: Patient seen for sinus congestion, provider performs H&P, prescribes decongestant, notes and removes lesion on back

Code: Procedure + E/M-25

-26 Professional Component

Professional component (physician, -26)

Technical component (technician + equipment, -TC)

-32 Mandated Service

Mandated by payer, workers' comp, or official body or court of law

Not request of patient, patient's family, or another physician

> **Example:** Workers' Compensation requests examination of person currently receiving disability benefits

-33 Preventive Services

Patient Protection and Affordable Care Act (PPACA)

- Requires coverage without cost to patient of certain preventive services

United States Preventive Services Task Force (USPSTF)

- Grades preventive services
- Example: Grade A: Substantial; Grade B: Moderate

-47 Anesthesia by Surgeon

Surgeon administers regional or general anesthesia

Physician acts as both surgeon and anesthesiologist

Used only with Surgery codes

-50 Bilateral Procedure

Organs that are bilateral

> **Example:** Procedure on kidneys

Caution: Some codes describe bilateral procedures

Typically not used on Integumentary System codes

-51 Multiple Procedure—Three Types

1. Same procedure, different sites
2. Multiple operation(s), same operative session
3. Procedure performed multiple times
   - List most resource-intense procedure first, then descending order of resource intensity
   - Next, other procedure(s) + -51 (unless code is -51 exempt or add-on code)
     Usual procedure payment: 1st 100%, 2nd 50%, 3rd 25%-50%, depending on payer

-52 Reduced Services

Service reduced or not performed to the extent described in code description

There is no other code that accurately reflects the service actually provided

Physician directed reduction

Documentation substantiates reduction

Not to be used for patient unable to pay

Submit regular charge amount, payer will adjust

-53 Discontinued Procedure

Surgical/diagnostic procedures

Procedure started then stopped due to patient's condition

Does not apply to presurgical discontinuance

Submit regular charge, payer will adjust

DO NOT USE -53

- When patient cancels scheduled procedure
- With E/M codes
- With time-based code

-54 Surgical Care Only

Physician provides only procedure (intraoperative); other physician performs preoperative and postoperative service

Documented patient transfer must be in record

Some payers require copy of transfer order

-55 Postoperative Management Only

Physician provides only the care after hospital discharge; report surgical code + modifier -55

If transferred while patient hospitalized, report postoperative management with subsequent hospital codes 99231-99233

Documentation of transfer in medical record

-56 Preoperative Management Only

Physician provided only preoperative care; report surgical code + modifier -56

Not acceptable for Medicare

Usual reimbursement for portions, surgical package

- 10% preoperative
- 70% intraoperative
- 20% postoperative

Each payer determines reimbursement for portions

-57 Decision for Surgery

E/M, 99201-99499

Medicine, 92002, 92004, 92012 and 92014 ophthalmologic services

Medicare: Only for preoperative period of major surgery (day before or day of)

-58 Staged/Related Procedure or Service by Same Physician or Other Qualified Health Care Professional During Postoperative Period

Subsequent procedure planned at time of initial surgery

- During postoperative period of previous surgery in series
  Example: Multiple skin grafts completed in several sessions
- Do not use when code describes total sessions
  Example: 67208 destruction of lesion of retina, one or more sessions
- More extensive than original procedure or
- For therapy following diagnostic procedure (e.g., breast biopsy and subsequent mastectomy)

-59 Distinct Procedural Service

Used to report non-E/M services not normally reported together

- Different session or encounter
- Different procedure
- Different site

Separate incision, excision, lesion, injury

  Example: Physician removes several lesions from patient's leg; also notes a suspicious lesion on torso and biopsies it

- Excision code for lesion removal + biopsy code for torso lesion with -59
- Indicates biopsy as distinct procedure, not part of lesion removal

-62 Two Surgeons

Both function as cosurgeons (equals)

Usually of different specialties

Each reports same code + -62

Each dictates operative/procedure note for their portion

Total reimbursement = 125%; each physician = 62.5%

-63 Procedure Performed on Infants Less Than 4 kg

Kilogram = 2.2 pounds (4 kg = 8.8 lb)

Small size increases complexity

Use with all Surgery section codes except Integumentary System or directed otherwise (see parenthetical guideline following 63702)

-66 Surgical Team

Team: Several physicians with various specialties plus technicians and other support personnel

Very complex procedures

Payers may increase payment up to 50%

- Each physician's service must be documented in the medical record

-76 Repeat Procedure/Service by Same Physician or Other Qualified Health Care Professional

Assigned to indicate necessary service

Example: X-rays before and after fracture repair

-77 Repeat Procedure/Service by Another Physician or Other Qualified Health Care Professional

Performed by one physician, repeated by another physician

Submitted with written report to establish medical necessity and identity of performing physician

• Do not append to E/M codes

-78 Unplanned Return to Operating/Procedure Room by the Same Physician or Other Qualified Health Care Professional Following Initial Procedure for a Related Procedure During Postoperative Period

For complication of first procedure

Example: Patient had outpatient procedure in morning; was returned to operating room in afternoon with severe hemorrhage

Indicates not typographical error

• Medical record must specifically document need for service provided

-79 Unrelated Procedure or Service by Same Physician or Other Qualified Health Care Professional During Postoperative Period

Example: Several days after discharge for procedure, patient returns for unrelated problem

Diagnosis code would also be different

-80 Assistant Surgeon

Reimbursed at 15% to 30%

Payers identify procedures for which they reimburse assistant at surgery

-81 Minimum Assistant Surgeon

Services at a level less than that described in -80

Reimbursed at 10% if services reported with the modifier are recognized by payer

-82 Assistant Surgeon (when qualified resident surgeon not available)

Teaching hospitals

• Have residents who assist as part of education

- Must demonstrate no qualified resident available to use -82
  - Unavailability must be documented in written report

-90 Reference (Outside) Laboratory

Physician has business relationship with outside lab

Physician pays lab

Physician bills payer for lab services

-91 Repeat Clinical Diagnostic Laboratory Test

Repeat same laboratory tests on same day for multiple test results

- e.g., serial troponin levels for acute MI confirmation

Not tests rerun to confirm or negate original test results

Not assigned for malfunction of equipment, loss of specimen, or technician error

-92 Alternative Laboratory Platform Testing

Used to report a laboratory test using portable instrument or kit

Usually single use

86701-86703 HIV testing

-99 Multiple Modifiers

Used when service needs more than one modifier but payer allows for only one modifier with each code

CMS-1500 (Fig. 3-6)

HCPCS Level II Modifiers

Examples of HCPCS Anatomical Modifiers

-LT Left side

-RT Right side

-E1 Upper left, eyelid

-E2 Lower left, eyelid

-E3 Upper right, eyelid

-E4 Lower right, eyelid

	24. A. DATE(S) OF SERVICE From MM	DD	YY	To MM	DD	YY	B. PLACE OF SERVICE	C. EMG	D. PROCEDURES, SERVICES, OR SUPPLIES (Explain Unusual Circumstances) CPT/HCPCS	MODIFIER			
1									19306				

Figure 3-6 CMS-1500 (02/12) allows for multiple placement of modifiers. (Courtesy U.S. Department of Health and Human Services, Centers for Medicare and Medicaid Services.)

-FA   Left hand, thumb

-F1   Left hand, second digit

-F2   Left hand, third digit

-F3   Left hand, fourth digit

-F4   Left hand, fifth digit

-F5   Right hand, thumb

-F6   Right hand, second digit

-F7   Right hand, third digit

-F8   Right hand, fourth digit

-F9   Right hand, fifth digit

-TA   Left foot, great toe

-T1   Left foot, second digit

-T2   Left foot, third digit

-T3   Left foot, fourth digit

-T4   Left foot, fifth digit

-T5   Right foot, great toe

-T6   Right foot, second digit

-T7   Right foot, third digit

-T8   Right foot, fourth digit

-T9   Right foot, fifth digit

-LC   Left circumflex coronary artery

-LD   Left anterior descending coronary artery

-RC   Right coronary artery

Anatomical modifiers are not used with skin procedures

Example: Removal of skin tags, any area

Exception is with codes for procedures on sites including sweat glands, eyelids, and breasts

■ PRACTICE EXERCISES

Practice Exercise 3-11: Massive Debridement

OPERATIVE REPORT

LOCATION: Inpatient, Hospital

PATIENT: Pam Tieg

ATTENDING PHYSICIAN: Leslie Alanda, MD

SURGEON: Gary Sanchez, MD

PREOPERATIVE DIAGNOSES
1. Massive abdominal wound.
2. Status post multiple small-bowel fistula repair.

POSTOPERATIVE DIAGNOSES
1. Massive abdominal wound.
2. Status post multiple small-bowel fistula repair.

SURGICAL FINDINGS: There was a 28 × 50-cm open wound in the abdomen extending predominantly to the right over past the midline on the left with a more inferior extension near the inguinal ligament. The primary areas of concern were pockets that were at least 8 to 10 cm in diameter in their total dimensions that had undermined in the retroperitoneal space behind the bowel. This contained malodorous fat necrosis and other necrotic tissue, and the odor smelled like Gram-negative organisms. We noted that the bowel was anterior in this space and probably came down on the psoas muscle posteriorly on the right side. Also, there were various areas of fat necrosis overlying the superficial aspect of the wound and fat necrosis along the edges of the wound that was quite malodorous. Multiple cultures and sensitivities were obtained, particularly of the area around the ileostomy site, the large area of fat necrosis in the left side of the abdomen, and the two undermined retroperitoneal areas. There was some extrusion of the mesh with the surrounding coagulative necrosis superiorly.

SURGICAL PROCEDURE: Massive debridement of open abdominal wound and status post multiple enterotomy repairs, small bowel.

ANESTHESIA: General, administered through tracheostomy tube.

ESTIMATED BLOOD LOSS: Approximately 50 cc.

ADDENDUM: Dr. White was called to observe the wound at his request and advised us regarding the dissection retroperitoneally in the proximity of the bowel in the area.

PROCEDURE: The abdomen was prepped as well as possible considering the conditions with Betadine scrub and solution and draped in a routine sterile fashion. A major 3-cm area of fat necrosis was initially debrided, and I debrided multiple sites of fat necrosis over the exposed surface of the wound, and then along the marginal surface there were multiple sites that were malodorous. Culture and sensitivity were obtained of the original fat necrosis area, the area around the ileostomy, and the more malodorous areas along the skin edges. We then, on the right side, lifted up the abdominal contents and dissected behind this, encountering foul-smelling, anaerobic-smelling collection of tissue, which probably consisted of old blood clot and fat necrosis. This was gently curetted out without entering the bowel. The bowel was in immediate proximity. We came down on what appeared to be the psoas area, which apparently connected with this pocket on the right side. We packed the right side with metronidazole-soaked Kerlix roll and vaginal packing, then also did the same on the left side. We covered the areas of the wound that were most accessible with fine mesh gauze soaked in metronidazole. ABD pads were then applied. The patient tolerated the procedure well and left the area in good condition.

CPT Code(s): _____

ICD-9-CM Code(s): _____

Abstracting Questions

1. Was debridement superficial, deep, or both? _____

2. Was the skin debridement code selection affected by the infection?

   _____

3. Does the skin debridement code include the retroperitoneal exploration?

   _____

4. Was there a CPT code for re-exploration of a recent abdominal surgery site?

   _____

5. Why would code 11008 not be reported? _____

6. Were there different diagnosis codes required to report the necrotic status of abdominal fat, skin, and retroperitoneum? _____

Practice Exercise 3-12: Nevus Excision

OPERATIVE REPORT

One week prior to this report, Dr. Erickson, plastic surgeon, removed a portion of a nevus from the right arm of Leonardo Zapata. Dr. Erickson believed that a further excision was necessary but wanted another opinion. Mr. Zapata was referred to Dr. Matalo to obtain his opinion on the further excision (staged procedure). Dr. Matalo recommended further excision, and today Dr. Erickson performed the other surgery. The follow-up for the first procedure was 10 days.

LOCATION: Outpatient, Hospital

PATIENT: Leonardo Zapata

PRIMARY CARE PHYSICIAN: Ronald Green, MD

SURGEON: Mark Erickson, MD

INDICATION: This patient had a 1-cm lesion excised from the right arm approximately 1 week ago. There was a question as to whether or not this was a Spitz nevus versus melanoma, and this was referred to Dr. Matalo at the New York Clinic for a second opinion. His opinion was that this was a Spitz nevus, and further conservative excision was recommended if that had not already been done. Since we only took a 5-mm margin, we are going to take about another 1 cm or so off around the previously excised area.

PREOPERATIVE DIAGNOSIS: Spitz nevus, right arm.

POSTOPERATIVE DIAGNOSIS: Spitz nevus, right arm.

SURGICAL FINDINGS: A healed incision of the right arm 2 cm in diameter.

ANESTHESIA: Six cc of 1% Xylocaine with 1:100,000 epinephrine.

PROCEDURE: The arm was prepped with Betadine solution and draped in the routine sterile fashion. The lesion was anesthetized and excised elliptically. Bleeders were electrocoagulated, and the wound was closed with interrupted subcuticular 3–0 Monocryl sutures and two twists of 4–0 Prolene. Half-inch Steri-Strips were applied. The patient tolerated the procedure well and left the area in good condition. He will use the sling that he used with his previous incision.

Pathology Report Later Indicated: Nevus, right arm, re-excision. Skin showing biopsy site with fibrosis, granulation tissue, and suture.

CPT Code(s): _____

ICD-9-CM Code(s): _____

Abstracting Questions

1. Is a modifier required to indicate the patient is in the global period from a previous procedure? _____

2. What modifier reports a more extensive procedure than the initial procedure performed during the global period of a previous procedure?

   _____

3. What was the excised diameter of the initial excision? _____

4. What is the excised diameter for the re-operation? _____

Practice Exercise 3-13: Echocardiogram

Remember to report only the profession portion of the service when the physician is not an employee of the facility in which the service is being provided.

ECHOCARDIOGRAM REPORT

LOCATION: Outpatient, Hospital

PATIENT: Loralee Branigan

ATTENDING/ADMIT PHYSICIAN: James Noonar, MD

RADIOLOGIST: Morton Monson, MD

PERSONAL PHYSICIAN: Ronald Green, MD

INDICATIONS: Valvular heart disease, atrial fibrillation, left ventricular dysfunction.

The M-Mode echo measurements are listed on the accompanying data sheet. They are essentially within normal limits.

The two-dimensional echocardiogram clearly demonstrates some thickening and calcification of the mitral valve leaflets as well as thickening of the aortic valve leaflets. The aortic valve opening is normal, and the mitral valve opening is probably normal as well. Left ventricular contractility is definitely diminished. The ejection fraction is in the range of about 20-25% only.

The Doppler and color Doppler studies do confirm the presence of mild tricuspid insufficiency. The RV systolic pressure is 32 mm Hg, which is consistent with mild pulmonary hypertension.

CONCLUSION: Depression of left ventricular function, as described above, with mild valvular pathology, as described above.

CPT Code(s): _____

ICD-9-CM Code(s): _____

Abstracting Questions

1. What approach was used for the cardiac echocardiogram? _____

2. Is the Doppler study also reported? _____

3. Is the Doppler color flow study reported? _____

4. What modifier is required on the CPT code? _____

Practice Exercise 3-14: Cervical Cerclage Preoperative Examination

LOCATION: Outpatient, Clinic

PATIENT: Chandelle Jackson

ATTENDING PHYSICIAN: Andy Martinez, MD

SURGEON: Andy Martinez, MD

ADMITTING DIAGNOSIS: Decreased cervical length with suspected incompetent cervix.

PROCEDURE PLANNED: Cervical cerclage.

HISTORY OF PRESENT ILLNESS: The patient is a 26-year-old woman, gravida 5, para 2, whose last menstrual period was August 12 of this year, giving her an estimated date of confinement of May 17 of next year. This presently places her at 19 weeks and 3 days gestation. Her due date has been confirmed by pelvic ultrasound, the earliest of which was at 15 weeks gestation. We suspect possible incompetent cervix. The patient does have a history of two preterm deliveries, the first was 3 years ago in March when she delivered at 32 weeks after a 7-hour labor. Her previous obstetrician had therefore discussed with her that perhaps a cervical cerclage would be appropriate. Her history did not seem overly convincing for incompetent cervix. She had had LEEP procedure about 5 years ago. She then had a miscarriage the following year, for which she had a D&C, and then had a therapeutic abortion 2 years later. I have been following cervical length on this pregnancy. On initial scan at 15 weeks' gestation, cervical length was not performed but a week later was found to be 2.7 cm. Follow-up ultrasound done at 17 weeks' gestation showed cervical length to be 3.1 cm. The most recent ultrasound from 19 weeks' gestation showed cervical length decreased to 2.5 cm, and with the patient's questionable history the decision has been made to proceed with cervical cerclage.

OBSTETRIC AND GYNECOLOGIC HISTORY: As noted above.

PAST MEDICAL AND SURGICAL HISTORY: The patient had a tonsillectomy at age 14 and a hallex vagus correction at age 20.

MEDICATIONS: Prenatal vitamins.

PHYSICAL EXAMINATION: Blood pressure: 108/60. Height: 5'6". Weight: 132 lb. Lungs: Clear to auscultation bilaterally. Heart: Sounds normal. Abdomen: Gravid with uterus palpable at the level of the umbilicus. Fetal heart rate is in the 140s. Bimanual examination was carried out, and the cervix is long, soft, and closed.

ASSESSMENT AND PLAN: The patient has had two previous preterm deliveries with history questionable for incompetent cervix, and now has decreased cervical length of 2.5 cm on ultrasound at 19 weeks' gestation. After discussing risks and alternatives, the patient has consented to proceed with cervical cerclage. She is aware of the risks, such as general anesthetic, hemorrhage, infection, ruptured membranes, and ultimately loss of the pregnancy. She does, however, consent to proceed, and the surgery has been scheduled for tomorrow.

CPT Code(s): _____

ICD-9-CM Code(s): _____

Abstracting Questions

1. What section of the CPT would be referenced to locate a code to report the service provided in this report? _____

2. Was the patient admitted to the hospital after the clinic examination?

   _____

Practice Exercise 3-15: Ethmoidectomy, Sphenoidotomy, and Septoplasty

Ready for a challenge? This case will give your coding skills an excellent workout. There will be five service codes and five diagnosis codes. The most extensive procedure is the septoplasty, and that code will be sequenced first.

LOCATION: Outpatient, Hospital

PATIENT: Russell Price

ATTENDING PHYSICIAN: Jeff King, MD

SURGEON: Jeff King, MD

PREOPERATIVE DIAGNOSES
1. Septal deviation.
2. Bilateral sinonasal polyposis.
3. Pansinusitis.
4. Bilateral inferior turbinate hypertrophy.
5. Nasal obstruction.

POSTOPERATIVE DIAGNOSIS: Same as Preoperative.

PROCEDURES PERFORMED
1. Bilateral endoscopic total ethmoidectomy.
2. Bilateral endoscopic maxillary antrostomy with removal of polyps from maxillary sinus.
3. Bilateral endoscopic sphenoidotomy.
4. Septoplasty.
5. Bilateral inferior turbinate overfracture.

ANESTHESIA: Endotracheal.

INDICATIONS: A 43-year-old male with history of nasal trauma that resulted in a septal deviation. He also has a history of bilateral sinonasal polyposis and has undergone prior polypectomy and sinus surgery. The patient now has recurrent disease. This was confirmed on examination and the CT scan. He also has bilateral inferior turbinate hypertrophy. The patient also has a history of severe snoring. He is to undergo correction of his nasal obstruction and sinusitis to see if that will help. If not, further evaluation of his snoring will be done.

PROCEDURE: After consent was obtained, the patient was taken to the operating room and placed on the operating table in supine position. After an adequate level of general endotracheal anesthesia was obtained, the patient was positioned for nasal and sinus surgery. The patient's nose was packed with cotton pledgets soaked with 4% cocaine. After several minutes, 1% Xylocaine with 1:100,000 epinephrine was infiltrated into the nasal portion of the polyps as well as the septum bilaterally and the inferior turbinates. Nasal hairs were trimmed. Attention was first focused on the right side. Using the 5-degree sinuscope and the microdebrider, the nasal portions of the polyps were removed. Polyps were noted both medial and lateral to the middle turbinate. There was also some scarring from the middle turbinate to the lateral nasal wall. This scar tissue was also removed with a microdebrider. Subsequently, polyps in the middle meatus and anterior posterior ethmoid areas were removed with microdebrider.

The maxillary sinus ostia area was cleared of polyps, and then the ostium was widened in a posterior-to-inferior direction. Polyps within the sinus near the ostia were also removed. The area was then packed with cotton pledgets soaked with 1:50,000 units of epinephrine. Attention was then focused on the left side, where a similar procedure was performed. Again, polyps were noted to be both medial and lateral to the middle turbinate remnant. Polyps were obstructing the maxillary sinus drainage area and were also cleared. The left side was packed with a pledget soaked with epinephrine solution. Attention was refocused on the right side, where further polyps were removed from the sphenoid/ethmoid area. Remnant of the superior turbinate was also cleared of polyps. The sphenoid sinus ostium was cleared of polyps. The area was then packed with cotton pledget soaked with epinephrine solution. Similar procedure was then performed on the left side. Attention was then focused on the nasal septum. Utilizing a right hemitransfixion incision, mucoperichondrium and mucoperiosteal flaps were elevated. The cartilaginous septum was noted to be severely attenuated and deviated with several fractured areas. Deviated portions were removed. This does not leave much support for the nasal tip area. If this is a problem in the future, this will need to be reconstructed. The deviated portion of the bony septum and spurs off the maxillary crest were then removed.

Attention was then focused on the inferior turbinates, which were outfractured. The hemitransfixion incision was then closed with an interrupted 4–0 chromic suture. A quilting suture of 4–0 plain gut was then performed. The pledgets in the sinus area were then removed. There was some oozing from the ethmoid as well as the sphenoid sinus areas. As such, these areas were coated with FloSeal and then packed lightly with strips of Surgicel soaked with local solutions. Bacitracin ointment was then applied. Silastic splints were then placed on both sides of the nasal septum and secured with nylon suture. The nose was then packed bilaterally. Packs consisted of a Merocel sponge with a gloved finger coated with Bacitracin ointment. It was inflated with location solution. Nasal dressing was applied.

The patient tolerated the procedure well, and there was no break in technique. The patient was extubated and taken to the postanesthetic care unit in good condition. Fluids administered included 2000 cc RL. Blood loss was less than 150 cc. Preoperative medications included 12 mg Decadron and 1 gram Ancef IV.

CPT Code(s): _____

ICD-9-CM Code(s): _____

Abstracting Questions

1. Maxillary Sinus

   a. Were polyps/tissue removed? _____

   b. What additional work was done to this sinus? _____

2. Sphenoid Sinus

   a. Were polyps/tissue removed? _____

3. Ethmoid Sinus

   a. Were polyps/tissue removed? _____

   b. Was this anterior, posterior, or both? _____

4. Inferior Turbinates

   a. Was there specific work done on this area? _____

5. What modifiers were appended extensively to the majority of CPT codes that reported the services provided in this case? _____

6. What does the diagnosis "pansinusitis" indicate? _____

■ SURGERY SECTION (10021-69990)

Largest CPT Section

Section Format

Divided by subspecialty, e.g., Integumentary, Cardiovascular

Notes and Guidelines

Throughout section

Information varied and extensive

"Must" reading

Subsection notes apply to entire subsection

Subheading notes apply to entire subheading

Category notes apply to entire category

Parenthetical information (Fig. 3-7)

Unlisted Procedure Codes

Used only when more specific code not found in Category I or Category III

Written report accompanies submission

Each unlisted code service paid on case-by-case basis

Separate Procedures

"(Separate procedure)" follows code description

Usually minor surgical procedure

Incidental to more major procedure:

- Breast biopsy before radical mastectomy would not be reported unless results of biopsy resulted in mastectomy, modifier -59 appended to biopsy code

- Appendectomy performed incidentally when other abdominal surgery is performed

Separate procedures reported when

- Only procedure performed

- With another procedure

  - On different site

  - Unrelated to major procedure

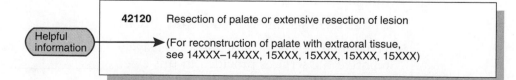

Figure **3-7** Parenthetical information in the CPT manual.

Major Guideline of Surgical Packages

Usually include

- Preoperative (before, preop)

- E/M service subsequent to decision for surgery but prior to surgery date

- Intraoperative (during, intraop)

- Postoperative (after—also known as global period, postop)

  - Post-anesthesia recovery (PAR)

  - Follow-up office visits

- Local/topical anesthesia and digital block

To report these bundled services separately is "unbundling"

Remember to use modifiers during global period for unrelated E/M, return to OR, etc.

Supplies

Supplies that are beyond those typically included in the procedure are reported separately

> *Example:* Report surgical tray with

- 99070 CPT, Medicine section

- A4550 HCPCS

Special Report

Submitting an unlisted service or one that is unusual, variable, or new may require a special report, as listed in Guidelines

Demonstrates medical necessity/appropriateness of service

Contains pertinent information describing service in terms of

- Nature

- Extent

- Need for procedure

- Time

- Effort

- Equipment necessary

May also include complexity of symptoms, final diagnosis, physical findings, procedures, concurrent problems, and follow-up care

GENERAL SUBSECTION (10021, 10022)

Fine needle aspirations with or without (w/wo) imaging guidance

Pathology 88172, 88173, and 88177 are for evaluation of fine needle aspirate

INTEGUMENTARY SYSTEM SUBSECTION (10040-19499)

Often used in all specialties of medicine

Not just surgeons or dermatologists; wide range of physicians

Subheadings of Integumentary Subsection

- Skin, Subcutaneous, and Accessory Structures
- Nails
- Pilonidal Cyst
- Introduction
- Repair (Closure)
- Destruction
- Breast

Skin, Subcutaneous and Accessory Structures (10030-11646)

Introduction and Removal (10030)

Report percutaneous image-guided fluid drainage of a catheter collection from soft tissue

- Example: Abscess, seroma, cyst, hematoma, or lymphocele

Reported once for each individual collection drained

Incision and Drainage (10040-10180)
I&D of abscess, carbuncle, boil, cyst, infection, hematoma, pilonidal cyst

- Lancing (cutting of skin)
- Aspiration (removal by puncturing lesion with a needle and withdrawing fluid)

Gauze or tube may be inserted for continued drainage

Excision—Debridement (11000-11047)
Dead tissue cut away and washed away with sterile saline

11000, 11001 Eczematous or infected skin

11004-11006 Debridement of infected area based on location and depth of necrotizing tissue (subcutaneous tissue, muscle, and fascia)

+11008 Removal of prosthetic material or mesh from abdominal wall

11010-11012 Foreign material with open fracture or dislocation

- Skin, subcutaneous tissue, muscle fascia, muscle, and bone

11042-11044 Subcutaneous tissue, muscle, bone

- Debridement partial thickness based on 20 square centimeters or less

11045, 11046, and 11047 Based on each additional 20 square centimeters

Paring or Cutting (11055-11057)
Removal by scraping or peeling (e.g., removal of corn or callus)

Codes indicate number: 1, 2-4, 4+

Biopsy (11100, 11101)
Skin, subcutaneous tissue, or mucous membrane biopsy

Not all of lesion removed

- All lesion removed = excision

Do not use modifier -51

Codes indicate number: 1 or each additional

Tissue removed during excision, shaving, etc., and submitted to pathology is NOT reported separately as a biopsy

- Rather, it is included in the code for the excision

Skin Tag Removal (11200, 11201)

Benign lesions

Removed with scissors, blade, chemicals, electrosurgery, etc.

Do not use -51

- Codes indicate number: Up to and including 15 lesions and each additional 10 lesions or part thereof

Shaving of Lesions (11300-11313)

Removed by transverse incision or sliced horizontally

Based on

- Size (e.g., 1.1-2.0 cm)
- Location (e.g., arm, hand, nose)

Does not require suture closure

- Report most extensive lesion first with no modifier, then least extensive lesions with modifier -51

Benign/Malignant Lesions (11400-11646)

Codes divided: Benign or malignant

Physician assesses lesion as benign or malignant

Codes include local anesthesia and simple closure

Report each excised lesion separately

Lesion size

- Taken from physician's notes
- Includes greatest diameter plus narrowest margins of two sides (Fig. 3-8)

  Example: A benign lesion measuring 0.5 cm at widest point is removed with 0.5-cm margin at narrowest point (each side, 0.5 + 0.5 = 1.0 cm). Reported as 1.5-cm lesion excision (11402)

  - Do not take size from pathology report—storage solution shrinks tissue
  - Margins (healthy tissue) are also taken for comparison with unhealthy tissue
  - Re-excisions following initial excision of malignant lesion coded as excision of malignant lesion

All excised tissue pathologically examined

Codes 11400-11646 report excision of lesion

Destroyed lesions have no pathology samples

  Example: Laser or chemical

Lesion closure

- Simple or subcutaneous closure included in removal
- Reported separately
  - Layered or intermediate, 12031-12057 (Repair—Intermediate)
  - Complex, 13100-13153 (Repair—Complex)

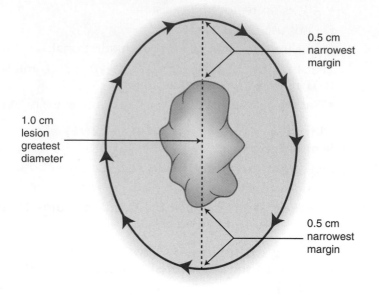

Figure **3-8** Calculating the size of a lesion.

Nails (11719-11765)

Includes toes and fingers

Types of services

• Trimming, debridement, removal, biopsy, repair

Pilonidal Cyst (11770-11772)

Codes divided by

• Simple

• Extensive

• Complicated

Introduction (11900-11983)

Types of services

• Lesion injections (therapeutic or diagnostic), tattooing, tissue expansion, contraceptive insertion/removal, hormone implantation services, and insertion/removal of non-biodegradable drug delivery implant

Repair (Closure) (12001-13160)

Repair Factors in Wound Repair

As types of wounds vary, types of wound repair also vary

Length, complexity (simple, intermediate, complex), and site must be documented

• Length measured in centimeters

• Measured prior to closure

Types of Wound Repair

Simple. Superficial, epidermis, dermis, or subcutaneous tissue

- One-layer closure
- Dermabond closure
- Medicare report Dermabond closure with G0168

Intermediate. Layered closure of deeper layers of subcutaneous tissue and superficial fascia with skin closure

- Single-layer closure can be coded as intermediate if extensive debridement required

Complex. Greater than layered; may include multiple layers of tissue and fascia or extensive debridement

> *Example:* Scar revision, complicated debridement, extensive undermining, stents, extensive retention sutures

Included in Wound Repair Codes
Simple ligation of vessels in an open wound

Simple exploration of nerves, blood vessels, and exposed tendons

Normal debridement

- Additional codes for debridement can be used when
  - Gross contamination requires prolonged cleaning
  - Appreciable amounts of devitalized/contaminated tissue are removed to expose healthy tissue
  - Debridement is provided without immediate primary closure

Grouping of Wound Repair
Add together lengths by

- **Complexity** of Wound
  - Simple, intermediate, complex

- **Location** of Wound
  - e.g., face, ears, eyelids, nose, lips

1 inch = 2.54 cm

> *Example:* **Same complexity, same codes description location:** Intermediate repairs of 2.9-cm laceration of leg and 1.1-cm laceration of buttocks. 2.9 + 1.1 = 4.0 cm (12032)

> *Example:* **Different complexity:** Intermediate repair of 2.9-cm laceration of leg and simple repair of 1.1-cm laceration of buttocks. 2.9-cm intermediate repair (12032) and 1.1-cm simple repair (12001)

> *Example:* **Same complexity, different code description locations:** Intermediate repair of 2.9-cm laceration of leg and intermediate repair of 1.1-cm laceration of nose. 2.9-cm intermediate repair of leg (12032) and 1.1-cm intermediate repair of nose (12051)

Do Not Group Wound Repairs That Are
Different complexities

> *Example:* Simple repair and complex repair

Different locations as stated in the code description

> *Example:* Simple repairs of scalp (12001) and nose (12011)

Adjacent Tissue Transfer, Flaps, and Grafts (14000-15778)

Information Needed to Code Graft

Type of graft—adjacent, free flap, etc.

Donor site (from)

Recipient site (to)

Any repair to donor site

Size of graft

Adjacent Tissue Transfer/Rearrangement (14000-14350)

Includes lesion excision and/or repair (e.g., Z-plasty, W-plasty, V-plasty, Y-plasty, rotation flap, advancement flap)

Codes based on size and location of graft

Primary defect results from excision of lesion

Secondary defect results from formation of flap

To select code, add the size of the primary and secondary defects together

Skin Replacement Surgery (15002-15278)

15002-15005 Site preparation based on size and site

15040-15261 Autografts/Tissue Cultured Autografts

- 15050-15278 Graft codes by type and size
- 15271-15278 Skin substitute grafts

Split-thickness: Epidermis and some dermis (Fig. 3-9)

Full-thickness: Epidermis and all dermis

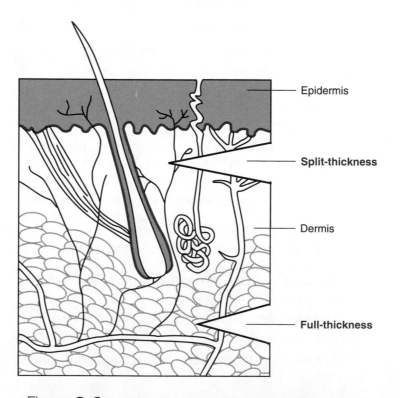

Figure **3-9** Split-thickness and full-thickness skin grafts.

Allograft: Donor graft

Xenograft: Nonhuman donor

Flaps (15570-15777)
Some skin left attached to blood supply

- Keeps flap viable

Donor site may be far from recipient site

Flaps may be in stages

Codes divided by location and size

Formation of flap (15570-15576)

- Based on recipient location: Trunk, scalp, nose, etc.

Transfer of flap (15650): Previously placed flap released from donor site

- Also known as walking or walk up of flap

- 15777 is an add-on code to report soft tissue reinforcement with biological implants

Muscle, Myocutaneous, or Fasciocutaneous Flaps (15732-15738)

- Based on recipient location; head and neck, trunk, upper or lower extremity

- Repairs made with
  - Muscle
  - Muscle and skin
  - Fascia and skin

- Flaps rotated from donor to recipient site

- Includes closure donor site unless skin graft or local flaps are necessary

Other Procedures (15780-15879)
Many cosmetic procedures including:

- Dermabrasion
- Chemical peel
- Blepharoplasty
- Rhytidectomy
- Excessive skin excision

Pressure (Decubitus) Ulcers (15920-15999)
Excision and various closures

- Primary, skin flap, muscle, etc.

Many codes "with ostectomy"

- Bone removal

Locations

- Coccygeal (end of spine)
- Sacral (between hips)

• Ischial (lower hip)

• Trochanteric (outer hip)

Site preparation only: 15936, 15937, 15946, 15956 or 15958

• Defect repair of donor site reported separately

Burns Local Treatment (16000-16036)

Codes for small, medium, and large

Must calculate percentage of body burned using Rule of Nines for adults (Fig. 3-10)

• <5% small

• 5% to 10% medium

• >10% large

Lund-Browder for children (Fig. 3-11)

• Proportions of children differ from adults

• Heads are larger

Often require multiple debridements and redressing

Based on

• Initial treatment of 1st-degree burn (16000)

• Size

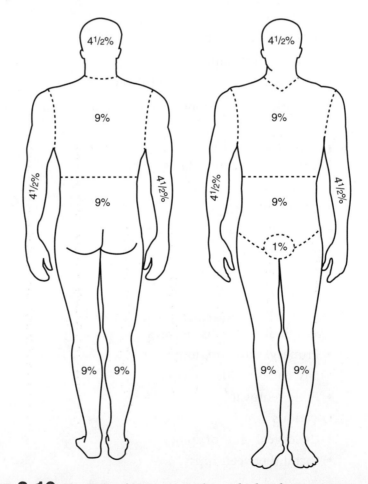

Figure **3-10** The Rule of Nines is used to calculate burn area on an adult.

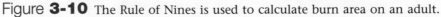

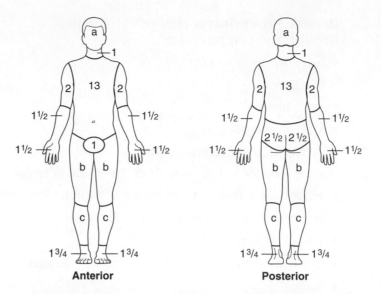

Anterior   **Posterior**

Relative percentage of body surface areas (% BSA) affected by growth

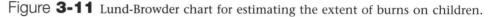

	0 yr	1 yr	5 yr	10 yr	15 yr
a – 1/2 of head	9 1/2	8 1/2	6 1/2	5 1/2	4 1/2
b – 1/2 of 1 thigh	2 3/4	3 1/4	4	4 1/4	4 1/2
c – 1/2 of lower leg	2 1/2	2 1/2	2 3/4	3	3 1/4

Figure **3-11** Lund-Browder chart for estimating the extent of burns on children.

Report percent of burn and depth

Destruction (17000-17286)
Ablation (destruction) of tissue

- Laser, electrosurgery, cryosurgery, chemosurgery, etc.

- Benign/premalignant or malignant tissue

- Malignant tissue is based on location and size of lesion

- Benign/premalignant is based on the number of lesions removed/destroyed or size (sq cm)

Mohs Micrographic Surgery (17311-17315)
Surgeon acts as pathologist and surgeon

Removes one layer of lesion at a time

Continues until no malignant cells remain

Based on stages and number of specimens per stage indicated in medical record

Other Procedures (17340-17999)
Treatment of acne

- Cryotherapy

- Chemical exfoliation

- Electrolysis

- Unlisted procedures

Breast Procedures (19000-19499)
Divided based on procedure

- Incision

- Excision

- Introduction

- Mastectomy Procedures

- Repair and/or Reconstruction

Use excision of lesion codes if entire lesion is removed during incisional biopsy

Use additional code for placement of radiological marker

Mastectomies based on extent of procedure

- Wide excision

- Removal of neoplasm, capsule, and surrounding margins

- Radical

- Wide excision and anatomical structure surrounding neoplasm

    Example: Muscle or fascia

- Conservative partial mastectomy in which lesion is removed with adequate margins (19301)

- Axillary dissection and partial mastectomy, 19302

- Radical and modified radical (19305, 19306, and 19307) based on extent

Confirm whether pectoral muscles, axillary, or internal lymph nodes were removed

19307 most common and includes breast and axillary lymph node removal

Code removal of lymph nodes separately unless included in code description

Bilateral procedures, use -50

Biopsy/Removal of Lesion

Incisional biopsy: Incision made into lesion and small portion of lesion removed

Excisional biopsy: Entire lesion removed

Open incisional biopsy most complex (19101)

Percutaneous needle core biopsy without imaging guidance (19100)

- Same procedure with imaging guidance based on guidance method:
    - 19081, 19082 stereotactic
    - 19083, 19084 ultrasound
    - 19085, 19086 magnetic resonance

Complete, simple removal of a mass is reported with 19120

Lesion may be preoperatively marked with localization devices (clip, metallic pellet, wire, needle, radioactive seed) based on guidance method:

- 19281, 19282, mammographic

- 19283, 19284, stereotactic

- 19285, 19286, ultrasound

- 19287, 19288, magnetic resonance

■ PRACTICE EXERCISES

Practice Exercise 3-16: Excision, Cheek Lesion

OPERATIVE REPORT

LOCATION: Outpatient, Hospital

PATIENT: Mary Carbono

ATTENDING PHYSICIAN: Gary Sanchez, MD

SURGEON: Gary Sanchez, MD

PREOPERATIVE DIAGNOSIS: Right cheek lesion, unspecified behavior.

POSTOPERATIVE DIAGNOSIS: Right cheek lesion, unspecified behavior.

PROCEDURE PERFORMED: Excision of lesion, right cheek.

ANESTHESIA: General anesthetic by inhalational mask technique.

PROCEDURE: Following informed consent from the patient's mother, the patient was taken to the operating room and placed supine on the operating room table. The appropriate monitoring devices were placed on the patient, and general anesthesia was induced. It was maintained by inhalation mask technique. The right cheek was prepped and draped in a sterile fashion. The lesion, which was about 1.6 cm, somewhat raised, and erythematous, was injected at its base with 0.5 cc of 1% Xylocaine with 1 : 100,000 epinephrine. A #15-blade scalpel was used to perform a shave excision. No suture was placed. A sterile bandage was applied. The patient tolerated the procedure well. She was allowed to recover from general anesthesia and was transferred to the recovery room in good condition.

Pathology Report Later Indicated: Benign lesion of cheek.

CPT Code(s): _____

ICD-9-CM Code(s): _____

Abstracting Questions

1. What method was used to excise the lesion? _____

2. Does the pathologic status of the report affect CPT code assignment?
   _____

3. Does the size and location of the lesion affect CPT code assignment?
   _____

4. Does the pathologic status of the lesion affect the diagnosis code?
   _____

Practice Exercise 3-17: Right Breast Wide Excision

OPERATIVE REPORT

LOCATION: Outpatient, Hospital

PATIENT: Jane Doe

ATTENDING PHYSICIAN: Gary Sanchez, MD

SURGEON: Gary Sanchez, MD

PREOPERATIVE DIAGNOSIS: Mass, right breast.

POSTOPERATIVE DIAGNOSIS: Mass, right breast.

OPERATIVE PROCEDURE: Right breast mass excision.

PROCEDURE: With the patient under general anesthesia, the breast and chest were prepped and draped in a sterile manner. An elliptical incision was made about the palpated mass, including the area around the nipple. This was excised all the way down to the fascia of the breast and then submitted for frozen section. Frozen section revealed a carcinoma of the breast with what appeared to be a good margin all the way around it. We then maintained hemostasis with electrocautery and proceeded to close the breast tissue using 2–0 and 3–0 chromic. The skin was closed using 4–0 Vicryl in a subcuticular manner. Steri-Strips were applied. The patient tolerated the procedure well and was discharged from the operating room in stable condition.

Pathology Report Later Indicated: Primary, malignant neoplasm of the right breast nipple.

CPT Code(s): _____

ICD-9-CM Code(s): _____

Abstracting Questions

1. Does the pathologic status of the lesion affect CPT code assignment?

   _____

2. Does the size of the lesion affect CPT code assignment? _____

3. Does the pathologic status of the lesion affect the diagnosis code?

   _____

4. Does the location of the lesion affect the diagnosis code? _____

5. Does the gender of the patient affect either code? _____

Practice Exercise 3-18: Thenar Flap Coverage

OPERATIVE REPORT

Assign an E code to indicate how this injury occurred in addition to the diagnosis and service codes.

LOCATION: Outpatient, Hospital

PATIENT: Leslie May

ATTENDING PHYSICIAN: Gary Sanchez, MD

SURGEON: Gary Sanchez, MD

PREOPERATIVE DIAGNOSIS: Oblique volar amputation tip, right middle finger, while working on machinery.

POSTOPERATIVE DIAGNOSIS: Oblique volar amputation tip, right middle finger, while working on machinery.

PROCEDURE: Thenar flap coverage, tip, right middle finger.

ANESTHESIA: General.

PROCEDURE: The patient was brought to the operating room, and general anesthesia was induced. Right upper extremity was prepped with Betadine and draped in a sterile fashion. The limb was exsanguinated with a tourniquet inflated to 250 mm Hg for 45 minutes. Using 4× magnification loupes, we debrided the fingertip. It was a volar oblique amputation. However, there was loss of distal phalanx down to about half of the sterile nail matrix. We trimmed the nail plate back to the level of the bone, we debrided the wound, and it was quite clean. We then fabricated a thenar flap using a piece of paper glove as a template. We traced this out on the thenar eminence. We then incised this and elevated the flap with fatty tissue. The radialward digital nerve to the index finger was exposed, and we covered this over with muscle with 4–0 Vicryl suture. We next harvested a split-thickness skin graft from the ulnar aspect of the hand using the Davol dermatome. We then placed this graft in place and sutured it over the defect in the palm with 5–0 Vicryl suture. Tegaderm was then placed over the donor site on the ulnar aspect of the hand.

We then placed the finger down in the palm and then attached the flap with interrupted 5–0 nylon sutures. This covered the defect on the finger nicely. We next applied Xeroform over all wounds and applied wet cotton balls over the graft site to hold it in place, then placed as compression a hand bandage with fluffs, Kerlix, Kling, and plaster splints immobilizing the hand in an intrinsic plus position. The tourniquet was released, and good circulation returned to the hand.

The patient tolerated the procedure well. She went to the recovery room in excellent condition. She will be dismissed as an outpatient today with plans for follow-up back in the office in appropriately 2 weeks.

CPT Code(s): _____

ICD-9-CM Code(s): _____

Abstracting Questions

1. Was this an adjacent tissue transfer flap? _____

2. Was the CPT code selection based on the recipient or donor site?

_____

3. Can the split-thickness skin graft for repair of the donor site be reported separately?

   _____

4. What HCPCS modifier would be appropriate to append to the CPT code reported for the formation of the pedicle flap? _____

5. Does the way in which the amputation occurred affect the diagnosis code selection? _____

6. If the type of machinery used during the procedure were specified, what other type of diagnosis code would you have reported? _____

Practice Exercise 3-19: Laceration Repair

OPERATIVE REPORT

Assign an E code to indicate how the injury occurred.

LOCATION: Outpatient, Hospital

PATIENT: Rod Seim

ATTENDING PHYSICIAN: Gary Sanchez, MD

SURGEON: Gary Sanchez, MD

PREOPERATIVE DIAGNOSIS: Multiple simple lacerations, right middle finger due to arrow.

POSTOPERATIVE DIAGNOSIS: Multiple simple lacerations, right middle finger due to arrow.

PROCEDURE PERFORMED: Simple closure of lacerations to right middle finger.

ANESTHESIA: Ring block.

PROCEDURE: Ring block anesthesia was achieved with 1% Xylocaine without epinephrine. Once the ring block was successful, the patient was taken to the scrub sink and the finger gently scrubbed and thoroughly irrigated with water. Once the finger was cleansed, repair was performed. The patient had a small nick (1 cm) in the lateral band. This was tacked together with one 4–0 nylon suture. There was noted to be no dirt on the tendon after irrigating the finger. To minimize the risk for infection, it was elected to just loosely close this. The 5-cm, J-shaped wound was then closed with four 4–0 nylon sutures just to approximate the skin. Some fat at the edge of the volar wound was debrided with scissors, and some abrasion of the epidermis was also debrided with scissors. The volar wound was then closed with two 4–0 nylon sutures. Dressing and a TubeGauz dressing were then applied. The patient tolerated this well.

CPT Code(s): _____

ICD-9-CM Code(s): _____

Abstracting Questions

1. What type of repair was performed (simple, intermediate, complex)?
   _____

2. Does the location on the body of the repair affect the choice of the CPT code assignment? _____

3. Does the size of the repair affect the choice of CPT code? _____

4. Does the repair to the nick in the tendon affect the diagnosis coding?
   _____

Practice Exercise 3-20: Minimal Debridement

OPERATIVE REPORT

The patient is returned to the operating room during the postoperative period of a previous procedure.

LOCATION: Inpatient, Hospital

PATIENT: Pam Tieg

ATTENDING PHYSICIAN: Leslie Alanda, MD

SURGEON: Gary Sanchez, MD

PREOPERATIVE DIAGNOSES
1. Massive abdominal wound with multiple sites of fat necrosis and retroperitoneal tissue necrosis, predominantly fat.
2. Draining sinus, anterior abdominal wall.

POSTOPERATIVE DIAGNOSES
1. Massive abdominal wound with multiple sites of fat necrosis and retroperitoneal tissue necrosis, predominantly fat.
2. Draining sinus, anterior abdominal wall.

SURGICAL FINDINGS: There are about 10 sites of fat necrosis scattered throughout the anterior abdominal wall, but the posterior aspect of the wound (i.e., in the retroperitoneal space that is obliterated by the overhang of bowel) appeared to be clean as far as we could tell, and certainly there was no odor.

SURGICAL PROCEDURE
1. Minimal debridement of anterior abdominal wall wound.
2. Collection of specimen for amylase.

ANESTHESIA: General endotracheal.

PROCEDURE: The patient's abdomen was prepped with Betadine scrub and solution and draped in the routine sterile fashion. Multiple sites of fat necrosis were debrided, and one area of protrusion of the mesh was debrided. There was some clear fluid leaking from a sinus in the anterior abdominal wall, and we collected 2 cc of fluid from this and submitted it for amylase. The wound was then repacked with Kerlix-soaked dressings using 0.5% metronidazole, and fine mesh gauze was applied to the anterior abdominal wound. The patient seemed to tolerate the procedure well and left the area in good condition. We additionally did spray Hemaseel into a pocket in the retroperitoneal area where there was some bleeding that did not respond to cautery, and it was thought that this was more the nature of generalized oozing, and therefore the Hemaseel and packing were used for control.

CPT Code(s): _____

ICD-9-CM Code(s): _____

Abstracting Questions

1. Was the retroperitoneum re-explored? _____

2. Does the return to the operating room require a modifier appended to the surgical procedure code? _____

MUSCULOSKELETAL SYSTEM SUBSECTION (20005-29999)

Subsection divided: Anatomic site, then service (e.g., excision)

Used extensively by orthopedic surgeons

- Many codes commonly used by variety of physicians

Extensive notes

Most common

- Fracture and dislocation treatments
- "General" subheading
- Arthroscopic procedures
- Casting and strapping

Eponyms are "things" named after "people"

> *Example:* Barr procedure is a tendon transfer of the lower leg (27690-27692) and, Mitchell and Chevron or concentric type procedure is a complex metatarsal osteotomy (bunion correction) (28296)

- Procedures are often referred to with eponyms
- Check the index of the CPT manual for directions to eponym codes

Fracture Treatment

Type of treatment depends on type and severity of fracture

Diagnosis codes must support the procedure codes and document the medical necessity

Open: Surgically opened to view or remotely opened to place nail across fracture site

- Open reduction with internal fixation is ORIF

Closed: Not surgically opened

Percutaneous: Insertion of devices through skin or a remote site

- Percutaneous fracture treatment neither open nor closed

Treatment terms should not be confused with **types** of fractures:

- Open fracture: Fractured bone penetrates skin
- Closed fracture: Fractured bone does not penetrate skin

Traction

- Application of force to align bone
- Force applied by internal device (e.g., wire, pin) inserted into bone (skeletal fixation)
- Application of force by means of adhesion to skin (skin traction)

Manipulation

Use of force to return bone back to normal alignment by manual manipulation (reduction) or temporary traction

Codes often divided based on whether manipulation was or was not used

Dislocation

Bone displaced from normal joint position

Treatment: Return bone to normal joint location

Subheading "General"

Begins "Incision" (20005)

Depth: Difference between Integumentary and Musculoskeletal incision codes

Musculoskeletal used when underlying bone or muscle is involved or procedure is deep subcutaneous

Wound Exploration (20100-20103)

Traumatic penetrating wounds

Divided by wound location

Includes

- Enlargement
- Debridement
- Foreign body(ies) removal
- Ligation
- Repair of tissue and muscle

Use additional code for repair of major structures or blood vessels

Not used for integumentary repairs

  - Unless the repair requires extension, enlargement, or exploration

Repair of major structure is reported instead when exploration leads to repair

Excision (20150-20251)

Biopsies for bone and muscle

Divided by

- Type of biopsy (bone/muscle)
- Depth
- Some by method

Can be percutaneous needle or excisional

Does not include tumor excision, which is coded separately

Biopsy with excision: Code only excision

Introduction or Removal (20500-20697)

Codes for

- Injections
- Aspirations
- Insertions
- Applications
- Removals
- Adjustments

Therapeutic sinus tract injection procedures

- Not nasal sinus
- Abscess or cyst with passage (sinus tract) to skin
- Antibiotic injected with use of radiographic guidance

Removal of foreign bodies lodged in muscle or tendon sheath

Integumentary removal codes for removal from skin

Injection into

- Tendon sheath
- Tendon origin
- Ligament
- Ganglion cyst
- Trigger points

Placement of needles or catheters into muscle and/or soft tissue

- For interstitial radioelement application

Arthrocentesis: Injection "and/or" aspiration of a joint

- Both aspiration and injection reported with one code (20600-20610)
- Codes based on joint size: Small, intermediate, major
- Do not unbundle and report aspiration/injection with two codes

External fixation

Device that holds bone in place

- Application, adjustment, removal under anesthesia

Code fracture treatment and external fixation device (EFD)

- Unless treatment and fixation both included in fracture care code description
- Adjustment to (20693) and removal of (20694 [under anesthesia]) EFD are coded separately

Replantation (20802-20838)

Used to report reattachment of amputated limb

Code by body area

Grafts (or Implants) (20900-20938)

Autogenous grafts: Used to report harvesting through separate incision of

- Bone
- Cartilage
- Tendon
- Fascia lata
- Tissue

Fascia lata grafts: From upper lateral thigh where fascia is thickest

Some codes include obtaining grafting material (not coded separately)

Some grafts are add-on codes for spine surgery only (20930-20938)

Other Procedures (20950-20999)

Monitoring interstitial fluid pressure (interstitial for compartment syndrome, etc.)

- Pressure increases due to increased accumulation of fluids, causing blood supply to be compromised

Bone grafts identified by donor site

Free osseocutaneous flaps: Bone grafts

• Taken along with skin and tissue overlying bone

Electrical stimulation

• Used to speed bone healing
• Placement of stimulators externally or internally
• Ultrasound also used externally

Soft Tissue Tumors

Codes identify excision of soft tissue and subfascial (intramuscular) tumors

• Subcutaneous soft tissue tumors: Below skin but above deep fascia
• Fascial or subfascial soft tissue tumors: Within or below deep fascia (not bone)
• Soft tissue tumors: May involve resection from one or more layer (i.e., subcutaneous, subfascial)

Example: 21011-21016 to report subcutaneous, subfascial, and soft tissue tumors

Arthrodesis

Fixation of joint (arthro = joint, desis = fusion)

• Bony structures of joint fused together to form one solid bone
• Fixation with pins, wires, rods, etc. to hold the joint immobile

Often performed with other procedure such as fracture repair

• Arthrodesis of the spine is also called spinal fusion

Subsequent Subheadings

After General subheading, divided by anatomic location

• Anatomic subheadings divided by type procedure

Example: Subheading "Head" divided by procedure

• Incision
• Excision
• Manipulation
• Head Prosthesis
• Introduction or Removal
• Repair, Revision, and/or Reconstruction
• Fracture and/or Dislocation
• Other Procedures
• Fracture and/or Dislocation

Spine and Spinal Instrumentation

Insertion of spinal instrumentation reported in addition to arthrodesis (fusion)

Many add-on codes reported in addition to definitive procedure

Spine (Vertebral Column), 22100-22899, divided by repair location (Fig. 3-12)

• Cervical (C1-C7)

C1 = Atlas

C2 = Axis

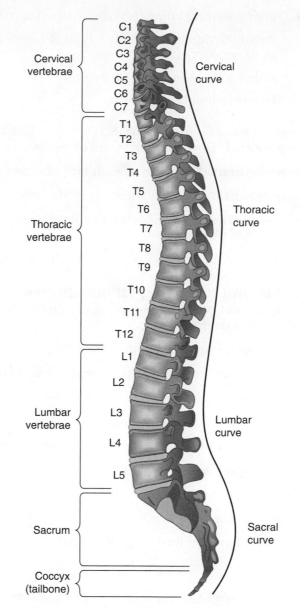

Figure **3-12** The spinal cord is part of the central nervous system (CNS) and extends from the brain to the lower back.

- Thoracic (T1-T12)
- Lumbar (L1-L5)
- Sacral (S1-S5)
- Coccyx (tailbone)

Vertebral segment: Single complete vertebral bone with articular processes and laminae

Vertebral interspace: Non-bony compartment between two vertebral bodies which contains the disc

Single level = two vertebrae and the disc that separates them

Percutaneous vertebroplasty

- Use of polymethylmethacrylate injected into the vertebral space
  - Polymethylmethacrylate is a type of bone cement/glue similar to the texture of silicone
  - Adheres bone fragments together
  - Fills vertebral body defects

Types of spinal instrumentation

Segmental: Devices at each end of repair area + at least one other attachment

Nonsegmental: Devices at each end of defect only

Approach: Pay special attention to the approach used to perform the surgery

- Several different approaches to spine: Most common are anterior (front) and posterior (back)

- Most spinal instrumentation codes divided based on approach

Casts and Strapping (29000-29799)
Replacement procedure or initial placement to stabilize without additional restorative treatment

>   *Example:* Application of wrist splint or cast for wrist sprain

Initial fracture treatment includes placement and removal of first cast

- Subsequent cast applications coded separately

- Payers have strict individual reimbursement policies for subsequent casting

Application not coded when part of surgical procedure

>   *Example:* Application of wrist splint or cast for wrist sprain

Initial fracture treatment includes placement and removal of first cast

Elastic bandage application is not billed separately

Removal bundled into surgical procedure

Supplies reported separately

Endoscopy/Arthroscopy (29800-29999)
Surgical arthroscopy always includes diagnostic arthroscopy

Codes divided by joint

- Subdivided by procedure

Be aware of subterms and bundled procedures within code descriptions

Note: Parenthetical information following codes indicates codes to use if procedure was an open procedure

■ PRACTICE EXERCISES

Practice Exercise 3-21: Arthroplasty and Spur Excision

LOCATION: Outpatient, Hospital

PATIENT: Merry Hoffert

PRIMARY CARE PHYSICIAN: Frank Gaul, MD

SURGEON: Mohomad Almaz, MD

PREOPERATIVE DIAGNOSIS: Arthritis, secondary impingement, right ankle.

POSTOPERATIVE DIAGNOSES
1. Osteoarthritic change, grade 3/4 tibia, medial shoulder of the talus, right ankle.
2. Osteophytic spurring with secondary impingement, both hard and soft tissue anterior talotibial articulation, right ankle.
3. Impinging soft tissue entity, anterolateral aspect of the ankle.

PROCEDURES PERFORMED
1. Abrasion arthroplasty, right ankle.
2. Excision of osteoarthritic spurs of the anterior articular margin, distal tibia.

PROCEDURE: After a satisfactory level of general anesthesia and the patient in a supine position, the extremity was prepped and draped in a routine sterile manner. At this time we proceeded with the establishment of routine arthroscopic portals. We entered from an anteromedial direction with camera, anterolateral direction with camera, and anterolateral direction with in-cutting device. At this setting there was a proud prominence of secondary scar tissue formation. We proceeded with its resection at this time. There were also areas of secondary eburnation change diffusely of grade 2/3 about the lateral aspect of the talus and focally grade 3/4 changes about the medial shoulder of the talus and the tibia as they articulate. There was also the demonstration with dorsiflexion of secondary abutment of soft tissue and proud tibial spurring. At this setting, with use of mechanical in-cutting device, we reamed back the abutment of the diarticular tibia and also at this time proceeded with abrasion chondroplasty and arthroplasty procedures where appropriate of the distal articular tibial plafond and the talus proper.

Medial and lateral recesses were evaluated at this time and were otherwise unremarkable. The posterior confines of the ankle other than the areas of graded arthritic change as noted above were otherwise unremarkable. With completion of this element of the procedure we simply proceeded with closure of portal sites. Both preprocedure and postprocedure arthroscopic photos were obtained for documentation purposes. The patient tolerated the procedure well and was transported to the recovery room in a stable manner.

CPT Code(s): _____

ICD-9-CM Code(s): _____

Abstracting Questions

1. What approach was used for this procedure? _____
2. Was the procedure limited or extensive? _____

Practice Exercise 3-22: Steroid Injection

LOCATION: Outpatient, Clinic

PATIENT: Kim Ortega

PRIMARY CARE PHYSICIAN: Frank Gaul, MD

SURGEON: Mohomad Almaz, MD

PROCEDURE PERFORMED: Steroid injection.

INDICATIONS: Left shoulder subacromial bursitis.

PROCEDURE: This procedure was done in the procedure area in the hospital.

After obtaining consent, area of the left shoulder was prepped in the usual fashion with Betadine; 6 cc of 1% lidocaine with 1 cc of Kenalog was injected in the left subacromial bursa without difficulty. The patient tolerated the procedure well without immediate complications. There was moderate relief of pain afterward.

The patient was advised to call me if she experiences any signs of infection, such as fever, chills, erythema, or swelling. She will call me in 3 days and tell me how she is doing.

CPT Code(s): _____

ICD-9-CM Code(s): _____

Abstracting Questions

1. What is the medical term for inserting a needle into a joint?

   _____

2. Would the joint into which the needle is inserted affect CPT code assignment?

   _____

Practice Exercise 3-23: Fascial Sling Arthroplasty

LOCATION: Outpatient, Hospital

PATIENT: Becky Wellington

PRIMARY CARE PHYSICIAN: Ronald Green, MD

SURGEON: Mohomad Almaz, MD

PREOPERATIVE DIAGNOSIS: Degenerative arthritis carpometacarpal joint, left thumb.

POSTOPERATIVE DIAGNOSIS: Same as Preoperative.

PROCEDURES PERFORMED: Fascial sling arthroplasty, left thumb.

ANESTHESIA: General.

PROCEDURE: The patient was brought to the operating room and a general anesthetic was induced. The left upper extremity was prepped with Betadine and draped in a sterile fashion. The limb was exsanguinated and tourniquet inflated to 250 mm Hg for 40 minutes. With 4× magnification loupes, we made a Chevron incision at the base of the thumb metacarpal. Dissection was carried down to the CMC joints, preserving subcutaneous nerves and vessels. We made a longitudinal arthrotomy incision and exposed the trapezium. We then morselized the trapezium and slowly removed the pieces with the rongeur. We carefully removed the entire trapezium, preserving the underlying FCR tendon. There was eburnated bone at the base of the first metacarpal. We then placed a drill hole through the base of the first metacarpal from its dorsal surface to its volar ulnar base. We opened this up to accept the tendon transfer. We next harvested the flexor carpi radialis tendon through two incisions, a short 1-cm incision over the tendon at the distal wrist flexor crease and an incision parallel to this 10 cm up the forearm at the myotendinous junction, where the FCR was transected at the floor of the thumb. Both volar forearm wounds were then closed with 5–0 nylon suture.

We next transferred the FCR tendon through the hole at the base of the first metacarpal, which effectively slung the first metacarpal up to the second metacarpal. We then pinned this to the second metacarpal with a 0.045 Kirchner wire bent and cut off outside the skin. We next sutured the tendon to the hole in the first metacarpal with 4–0 Vicryl sutures and packed bone graft into the hole to secure this. We then placed a 4–0 Vicryl suture in the floor of the wound, placed two Bunnell needles over the limbs of this, and then threaded the tendon onto this in an accordion fashion. We tied this Vicryl, pulled the tendon down into the defect, where the trapezium was excised, and filled this nicely. We then proceeded with capsular closure, imbrication of the capsule, and closed this with 4–0 Vicryl sutures. The appearance was excellent. We irrigated the wound with sterile saline and closed the skin with interrupted 5–0 nylon sutures. Next, we applied Xeroform, and a thumb spica compression hand bandage was then applied with plaster splints immobilizing the thumb. The tourniquet was released, and good circulation returned to the hand.

The patient tolerated the procedure well and went to the recovery room in excellent condition. She will be dismissed as an outpatient today with plans for follow-up back in the office in approximately 2 weeks.

DISCHARGE MEDICATION: Lorcet, 30 tablets.

Pathology Report: No specimen was sent.

CPT Code(s): _____

ICD-9-CM Code(s): _____

Abstracting Questions

1. On what area of the body was the arthroplasty performed? _____

2. Was the tendon transfer bundled into the arthroplasty? _____

3. Are modifiers reported with these procedures? _____

Practice Exercise 3-24: Excision Bone Tumor

LOCATION: Outpatient, Hospital

PATIENT: Tyron Banks

PRIMARY CARE PHYSICIAN: Leslie Alanda, MD

SURGEON: Mohomad Almaz, MD

PREOPERATIVE DIAGNOSIS: Bone tumor, distal lateral right femur.

POSTOPERATIVE DIAGNOSIS: Same as Preoperative.

PROCEDURES PERFORMED: Excision bone tumor, distal right femur.

ANESTHESIA: General.

PROCEDURE: The patient was brought to the operating room and a general anesthetic was induced. Right lower extremity was prepped with Betadine and draped in a sterile fashion. The limb was exsanguinated, and tourniquet was inflated to 300 mm Hg for 25 minutes. Ioban drape was applied. A standard 4-inch longitudinal anterolateral incision was made beginning at the lateral patellar region and extending proximally. Dissection was carried down through the lateral parapatellar region and lateral parapatellar arthrotomy was performed. We entered down to the lateral femur where the tumor was palpable. This appeared to represent a chondroma on the lateral femur. We elevated the soft tissue and periosteum off of this and then used osteotomes to sharply excise this and gradually take this down to its base. It appeared to be bleeding normal bone, and at that point we did put bone wax on the bone. We then closed the periosteum with a running 0 Vicryl suture, then closed the fascia and joint with a running 0 Vicryl suture, and then closed the skin with a subcuticular 2–0 Vicryl suture and a running 4–0 Monocryl suture. Steri-Strips were applied with gauze dressing, Kling, ABD, Kerlix, and a Coban. The tourniquet was released, and good circulation returned to the leg.

The patient tolerated the procedure well. He will be dismissed as an outpatient today with plans for follow-up in the office in approximately 2 weeks.

DISCHARGE MEDICATIONS: Tylenol #3, 30 tablets.

Pathology Report Later Indicated: Benign neoplasm.

CPT Code(s): _____

ICD-9-CM Code(s): _____

Abstracting Questions

1. From what body part was the bone tumor excised? _____

2. Was a graft required to repair the defect? _____

3. Was any fixation required? _____

4. What report is required to correctly assign a diagnosis to the excision?

_____

Practice Exercise 3-25: Excision of Mass, Bursa

LOCATION: Outpatient, Hospital

PATIENT: Brittany Lionel

PRIMARY CARE PHYSICIAN: Ronald Green, MD

SURGEON: Mohomad Almaz, MD

PREOPERATIVE DIAGNOSIS: Mass, left prepatellar bursa.

POSTOPERATIVE DIAGNOSIS: Same as Preoperative.

PROCEDURES PERFORMED: Excision of mass, left prepatellar bursa.

ANESTHESIA: Local infiltration with 1% Xylocaine, supplemented with IV sedation.

PROCEDURE: The patient was placed in the supine position on the operating room table. She pointed out the mass on the anterior aspect of her left knee, which was a very small mass, perhaps 2 or 3 mm in diameter. This bothers her when she kneels on her left knee, and she wanted it removed. We therefore marked it with a marking pen since it was not a large mass but was still nevertheless fairly easily palpable.

We then prepped her left knee with Betadine and draped it in a sterile fashion. She was given IV sedation. We then infiltrated the area around the mass with 1% Xylocaine. Once adequate anesthesia had been achieved, we exsanguinated the left leg with Esmarch bandage and inflated a tourniquet to 225 mm Hg. The total tourniquet time was about 6 minutes.

We created an incision in a longitudinal fashion directly over this mass and carried it down through the subcutaneous tissue. We very quickly found this mass, which was perhaps half the size of a pea (0.5 cm). It was fairly firm, and we sent it to pathology. It appears to be part of the left prepatellar bursa. We then excised some of the adjacent bursal tissue. We found this was located directly over the left patella and the patella was very visible underneath this mass. We then probed the area, looking for any other masses. We then thoroughly irrigated the area and closed the subcutaneous tissue with 2–0 Vicryl and the skin with 3–0 nylon suture. Pressure was applied to this area, and the tourniquet was released after 6 minutes of tourniquet time. We then applied a 4 × 4 dressing and an Ace wrap over this. She was then awakened and taken from the operating room in good condition, breathing spontaneously. The final sponge and needle counts were correct. She tolerated this procedure very well.

Pathology Report Later Indicated: Benign mass of left prepatellar bursa.

CPT Code(s): _____

ICD-9-CM Code(s): _____

Abstracting Questions

1. What was the body location of the tumor? _____

2. What was the size of the mass? _____

RESPIRATORY SYSTEM SUBSECTION (30000-32999)

Anatomic site arrangement, such as:

- Nose

- Larynx

Further subdivided by procedure, such as:

- Incision

- Excision

Endoscopy

Endoscopy in all subheadings except Nose

Each preceded by "Notes"

Endoscopy Rule One
Code full extent of endoscopic procedure performed

> *Example:* Procedure begins at mouth and ends at bronchial tube

- Bronchial tube = full extent

Endoscopy Rule Two
Code correct approach

> *Example:* For removal:

- Interior lung lesion via endoscope inserted through mouth

- Exterior lung lesion via endoscope inserted through skin into chest

Incorrect approach = incorrect code = incorrect or no reimbursement

Endoscopy Rule Three
Diagnostic endoscopy always included in surgical endoscopy

> *Examples:*

- Diagnostic bronchial endoscopy begins

- Identified foreign body

- Removed foreign body (surgical endoscopy)

- Only surgical endoscopy reported

Multiple Procedures

Frequent in respiratory coding

- **Watch for bundled services**

Sequence primary procedure first, no modifier

Sequence secondary procedures next, with -51

Bilateral procedures often performed, use -50

Format for reporting chosen by payer

> *Example:* Nasal lavage

- 31000×2

- 31000 and 31000-50

- 31000-50
- 31000-RT and 31000-LT

Nose (30000-30999)

Used extensively by otorhinolaryngologists (ear, nose, and throat [ENT] specialists)

Also used by wide variety of physicians in other specialties

Approach to nose

- External approach, use Integumentary System
- Internal approach, use Respiratory System

Incision (30000-30020)

Bundled into Incision codes are drain or gauze insertion and removal

Supplies reported separately

Excision (30100-30160)

Contains intranasal biopsy codes

Polyp excision, coded by complexity

- Excision includes any method of destruction, even laser
- Use -50 (bilateral) for both sides

Turbinate excision and resection

- Three turbinates: Superior, middle, inferior
- Excision of inferior turbinate, 30130
- Excision of superior or middle turbinate, 30999
- Submucous resection of inferior turbinate, 30140
- Submucous resection of superior or middle turbinate, 30999

Introduction (30200-30220)

Common procedures

> *Example:* Injections to shrink nasal tissue or displacement therapy (saline flushes) to remove mucus

- Displacement therapy performed through nose

Removal of Foreign Body (30300-30320)

Distinguished by the site of removal, whether at office or hospital (requires general anesthesia)

Repair (30400-30630)

Many plastic procedures

- Rhinoplasty (reshaping nose internal and/or external)
- Septoplasty (rearrangement or repair of nasal septum)

Destruction (30801-30802)

Use of ablation (removing by cutting)

Used for removal of excess nasal mucosa or to reduce turbinate inflammation

Based on intramural or superficial extent of destruction

- **Intramural:** Deeper mucosa
- **Superficial:** Outer layer of mucosa

Other Procedures (30901-30999)

Control of nasal hemorrhage

- Packing
- Ligation
- Cauterization
- The packing may be anterior or posterior

Accessory Sinuses (31000-31299)

Subheadings include:

Incision (31000-31090)

Excision (31200-31230)

Endoscopy (31231-31297)

Other Procedures (31299)

Codes for lavage (washing) of sinuses

- Cannula (hollow tube) placed into sinus
- Sterile saline solution flushed through

Procedures may involve multiple codes when multiple locations are accessed

Example: 31020, Sinusotomy, maxillary, can be coded with 31050 sinusotomy, sphenoid, and 31070 sinusotomy, frontal

Use -50 (bilateral) for both sides

Maxillary sinusotomy may use an external and intranasal approach to creating passage between sinus and nose

- Used to clear blocked or infected sinus
- Intranasal sinusotomy, 31020
- External sinusotomy, radical (such as Caldwell-Luc)

  Access through mouth

  Incision above eyetooth

  Sinus is cleaned

  New opening created or existing opening enlarged

Repair of fractures occurring during procedure may be coded separately if not included in code description

Larynx (31300-31599)

Excision (31300-31420)

Laryngotomy: Open surgical procedure to expose larynx

- For removal procedure (e.g., tumor)

May be confused with Trachea/Bronchi codes for tracheostomy used to establish airflow

Introduction (31500-31502)
Used to establish, maintain, and protect air flow

Endotracheal intubation, establishment of airway

Based on planned (ventilation support) or emergency procedure

Endoscopy (31505-31579)
Uses terms *indirect* and *direct*

- **Indirect:** Tongue depressor with mirror used to view larynx

- **Direct:** Endoscopy passed into larynx; physician directly views vocal cords

Repair (31580-31590)
Several plastic procedures and fracture repairs

Laryngoplasty procedures based on purpose

Fracture code is open reduction code

Trachea and Bronchi (31600-31899)

Incision (31600-31614)
Most codes: Tracheostomy divided by

- Planned (ventilation support), based on age

- Emergency

Divided by type

- Transtracheal or cricothyroid (location of incision)

Endoscopy (31615-31661)
Bronchoscope may be inserted into nose or mouth

Rigid endoscopy performed under general anesthesia

Flexible endoscopy usually performed under local or moderate (conscious) sedation

Bronchial Thermoplasty (31660-31661)

- Treatment for severe asthma in which radiofrequency is utilized to produce heat in the airways that results in the reduction of the airway smooth muscles

Introduction (31717-31730)
Catheterization

Instillation

Aspiration

Tracheal tube placement

Excision, Repair (31750-31830)
Repairs of trachea and bronchi

Lungs and Pleura (32035-32999)

Incision (32035-32225)
Thoracotomy. Surgical opening of chest to expose to view.

Used for

- Biopsy

- Cyst
- Foreign body removal
- Cardiac massage, etc.

Excision/Removal (32310-32540)
Biopsy codes in both Excision and Incision categories

- Excisional biopsy with percutaneous needle
- Incisional biopsy with chest open

Also services of pleurectomy, pneumocentesis, and lung removal

- **Segmentectomy:** 1 segment
- **Lobectomy:** 1 lobe
- **Bilobectomy:** 2 lobes
- **Total Pneumonectomy:** 1 lung

Thoracentesis. Needle inserted into pleural space for aspiration (withdrawal) of fluid and/or air (32554, 32555)

Introduction and Removal (32550-32557)
- Insertion of indwelling tunneled pleural catheter (removal 32552)
- Tube thoracostomy
- Placement of interstitial device(s) for radiation therapy guidance
- Thoracentesis and percutaneous pleural drainage

Destruction (32560-32562)
- Chemical pleurodesis
- Fibrinolysis, initial day, subsequent day

CARDIOVASCULAR SYSTEM SUBSECTION (33010-37799)

CV coding may require codes from
- **Radiology:** Diagnostic studies
- **Medicine:** Nonsurgical and percutaneous
- **Surgery:** Open and percutaneous

Both Medicine and Surgery sections contain invasive procedures

Cardiology Coding Terminology

Invasive: Enters body
- Incision

    Example: Opening chest for removal (e.g., tumor on heart)
- Percutaneous
    - Placement of catheter into artery or vein through the skin by means of wire threaded through needle and catheter slid over wire

    Example: PTCA (percutaneous transluminal coronary angioplasty) procedure

Percutaneous—wire threaded through needle placed through skin into vessel and catheter placed over wire

- Cut down—small nick made into vessel under direct vision and catheter inserted

    Example: Catheter inserted into femoral or brachial artery

Common catheters are:

- Broviac
- Hickman
- HydroCath
- Arrow multi-lumen
- Groshong
- Dual-lumen
- Triple-lumen

Noninvasive: Procedures that do not break skin

> *Example:* Electrocardiogram

Electrophysiology (EP): Study of electrical system of heart

> *Example:* Study of irregular heartbeat (arrhythmia)

- EP studies are in Medicine section, 93600-93662
- Electrophysiologic Operative Procedures are in Surgery section, 33250-33266

Nuclear Cardiology: Diagnostic and treatment specialty; uses radioactive substances to diagnose cardiac conditions

> *Example:* Myocardial perfusion and cardiac blood pooling imaging studies

■ Cardiovascular in Surgery Section

Codes for Procedures

Heart/Pericardium (33010-33999)

- Pacemakers, valve disorders

Arteries/Veins (34001-37799)

Heart/Pericardium (33010-33999)

Both percutaneous and open surgical

- Cardiologists often use percutaneous intervention; cardiovascular or thoracic surgeons often use open surgical procedures

Extensive notes throughout

Frequent changes with medical advances

Examples of categories of Heart/Pericardium subheading

- Pericardium
- Cardiac Tumor
- Pacemaker or Pacing Cardioverter-Defibrillator

Examples of services

- Pericardiocentesis: Percutaneous withdrawal of fluid from pericardial space (pericarditis) (33010-33011)
- Cardiac Tumor: Open surgical procedure for removal of tumor on heart (33130)

Pacemakers or Pacing Cardioverter-Defibrillators (33202-33249)

Devices that assist heart in electrical function

- Differentiate between temporary and permanent devices
- Differentiate between one-chamber (one lead) and dual-chamber (two leads) devices

Divided by where pacer placed, approach, and type of service

Patient record indicates revision or replacement

- Pacemaker pulse generator is also called a battery
- Pacemaker leads are also called electrodes

Usual follow-up 90 days (global period)

Placed

Atrium (single chamber)

- Pulse generator and one or more electrodes in atrium (single-chamber pacemaker)

Ventricle (single chamber)

- Pulse generator and one or more electrodes in ventricle (single-chamber pacemaker)

Both (dual chamber)

- Pulse generator and one electrode in right ventricle and one electrode in right atrium

Biventricular, right ventricle, right atrium, and coronary sinus

- Pulse generator and one electrode in right ventricle, one electrode(s) may be placed in right atrium, and one electrode in the coronary sinus over the left ventricle

Approach

Epicardial: Open procedure to place electrodes on heart

Transvenous: Through vein to place in heart (endoscopic)

Type of service

Initial placement or replacement of all or part of device

Number of leads placed is important in code selection

Electrophysiologic Operative Procedures (33250-33266)

Surgeon repairs defect causing abnormal rhythm

Chest opened to full view

- Cardiopulmonary (CP) bypass usually used

Endoscopy procedure

- Without cardiopulmonary bypass

Codes based on reason for procedure and if CP bypass used

Patient-Activated Event Recorder (33282-33284)

Also known as cardiac event recorder or loop recorder

Internal surgical implantation required

Divided based on whether device is being implanted or removed

Cardiac Valves (33361-33478)

Divided by valve

- Aortic, mitral, tricuspid, pulmonary

Subdivided by whether replacement, repair, resection and use of bypass machine

33361-33369 report transcatheter aortic valve replacement and implant

Coronary Artery Bypass Graft (CABG)
CABG performed for bypassing coronary arteries severely obstructed as in atherosclerosis or arteriosclerosis

Determine what was used in repair

- Vein (33510-33516)
- Artery (33533-33536)
- Both artery and vein (33517-33523 and 33533-33536)

Based on number of bypass grafts performed and if combined venous and arterial grafts are used

> *Example:* Three venous grafts

Venous Grafting Only for Coronary Artery Bypass (33510-33516)

Based on number of grafts being replaced

Combined Arterial-Venous Grafting (33517-33530)

Divided based on number of grafts and if initial procedure or reoperation

Procuring saphenous vein included, unless performed endoscopically

These codes are never used alone

- Arterial-Venous codes (33517-33523) report only **venous** graft portion of procedure
- Always used with Arterial Grafting codes (33533-33536)

> *Example:* 3 vein grafts and 2 arterial grafts = 33519 and 33534

Open procurement of saphenous vein is included in procedure (not coded separately)

Code harvesting of saphenous vein graft separately when endoscopic video-assisted procurement is performed (33508)

Code harvesting separately for upper extremity or femoral vein

Arterial Grafting for Coronary Artery Bypass (33533-33548)

Divided based on number of grafts

Obtaining artery for grafting included in codes, except

- Procuring upper-extremity artery (e.g., radial artery), coded separately (35600)

Several codes (33542-33548) for myocardial resection, repair of ventricular septal defect (VSD), and ventricular restoration

Endovascular Repair of Descending Thoracic Aorta (33880-33891)

Placement of an endovascular aortic prosthesis for repair of descending thoracic aorta

- Less invasive than traditional approach of chest or abdominal incision

Synthetic aortic prosthesis placed via catheter

- Report fluoroscopic guidance separately 75956-75959

> Fluoroscopic guidance codes include diagnostic imaging prior to placement and intraprocedurally

Stent-graft (endoprosthesis) is deployed to reinforce weakened area

Arteries and Veins Subheading (34001-37799)

Only for noncoronary vessels

- Divided based on whether artery or vein involved

  Example: Different codes for embolectomy, depending on artery or vein

Catheters placed into vessels for monitoring, removal, repair

Nonselective or selective catheter placement

- Nonselective: Direct placement without further manipulation

- Selective: Place and then manipulate into further order(s)

Catheter placement example

- Nonselective: 36000 Introduction of needle into vein

- Selective: 36012 Placement of catheter into second-order venous system

Vascular Families Are Like a Tree

First-order (main) branch (tree trunk)

Second-order branch (tree limb)

Third-order branch (tree branch)

Brachiocephalic vascular family (Fig. 3-13)

- Report farthest extent of catheter placement in a vascular family; labor intensity is increased with the extent of catheter placement

Embolectomy and Thrombectomy (34001-34490)

Embolus: Dislodged thrombus

Thrombus: Mass of material in vessel located in place of formation

- May be removed by dissection or balloon

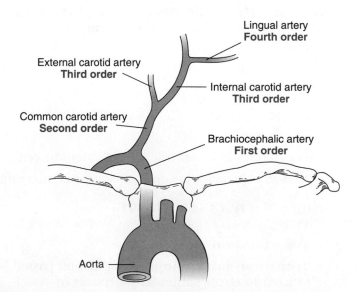

Figure **3-13** Brachiocephalic vascular family with first-, second-, third-, and fourth-order vessels.

Balloon: Threaded into vessel, inflated under mass, pulled out with mass

- Codes are divided by site of incision and whether artery or vein

Venous Reconstruction (34501-34530)
Types of repairs
- Valve of the femoral vein

- Vena cava

- Saphenopopliteal vein anastomosis

Aneurysm
Aneurysm: Weakened arterial wall causing a bulge or ballooning

Repair by removal, bypass, or coil placement

Endovascular repair (34800-34900) from inside vessel

Direct (35001-35152) from outside vessel

Endovascular Repair of Abdominal Aortic Aneurysm (34800-34834)
Fluoroscopic guidance: Use Radiology 75952 or 75953

Includes access, catheter manipulation, balloon angioplasty, stent placement, site closure

Reported separately: Introduction of guideline and catheters

Other procedures performed at same time coded separately

Endovascular Repair of Iliac Aneurysm (34900)
Extensive notes preceding codes—"must" reading

Uses fluoroscopic guidance, report Radiology 75954

Includes introduction, positioning, and deployment of graft, stent and balloon angioplasty

Reported separately: Introduction of guidewire and catheters

Repair Arteriovenous Fistula (35180-35190)
Abnormal passage from artery or vein

Divided based on fistula type
- Congenital

- Acquired/traumatic

- By site

Repair methods
- Autogenous graft—fistula created artery to vein

- Non-auto fistula—biocompatible tube connecting artery to vein

Angioplasty (35450-35476)
Divided as open or percutaneous and by vessel
- **Transluminal:** By way of vessel

- **Transluminal Angioplasty:** Catheter passed into vessel and a balloon is inflated to crush/flatten fatty deposits in vessel

  - Placement of eluding or noneluding stents coded in addition to catheter placement

Noncoronary Bypass Grafts (35500-35671)
Divided by
- Vein
- In-Situ Vein (veins repaired in their original place)
- Other Than Vein

Code by type of graft and vessels being used to bypass

Example: 35506 Bypass graft, with vein; carotid-subclavian
- Graft attached to carotid and to subclavian, bypassing defect of subclavian

Procurement of saphenous vein graft is included and not reported separately

Harvesting of upper-extremity vein (35500) or femoropopliteal vein (35572) is reported separately

Vascular Injection Procedures (36000-36598)
Divided into
- Intravenous
- Intra-arterial—Intra-aortic
- Venous
- Central venous access procedures

Used for many procedures, including
- Local anesthesia
- Introduction of needle
- Injection of contrast material
- Preinjection and postinjection care related to injection procedure

Example: Injection of opaque substance for venography (radiography of vein)

Central Venous Access (CVA) Procedures
Long term use for medication/chemotherapy administration and short-term use for monitoring

Approach
- Central: jugular, subclavian, or femoral vein
- Peripheral: basilic or cephalic vein

Categories
1. Insertion
2. Repair
3. Replacement, partial or complete
4. Removal
5. Other central venous access procedure
6. Guidance for vascular access

Insertion (36555-36571)
Insertion of newly established venous access
- Tunneled under skin (e.g., Hickman, Broviac, Groshong)
- Nontunneled (e.g., Hohn catheter, triple lumen, PICC)
- Central (e.g., subclavian, internal jugular, femoral, inferior vena cava)
- Peripheral (basilic or cephalic vein)

Codes divided by tunneled/non-tunneled, with/without port, central/peripheral, and age

Repair (36575-36576)

Repair of malfunction without replacement with or without subcutaneous port or pump

Repair of central venous access device

No differentiation between age of patient or central/peripheral insertion

Replacement (Partial or Complete) (36578-36585)

Partial (36578) is replacement of catheter only

Complete (36580-36585) is replacement through same venous access site

Differentiated by tunneled/non-tunneled, central/peripheral, and with or without subcutaneous port or pump

Removal (36589, 36590)

To be used for tunneled catheter

Removal of non-tunneled catheter is not reported separately

Other Central Venous Access Procedures (36591-36598)

Collection of blood specimen

Declotting of catheter or access device by thrombolytic agent

Mechanical removal of obstructive material from around catheter or within lumen

Guidance for Vascular Access

77001, Fluoroscopic guidance for central venous access device placement, replacement, or removal

- Reported in addition to primary procedure

76937, Ultrasound guidance for vascular access

- Reported in addition to primary procedure

Transcatheter Procedures (37184-37217)

Arterial mechanical thrombectomy (37184-37186)

- Removal of thrombus by means of mechanical device

  From artery or arterial bypass graft

Venous mechanical thrombectomy (37187-37188)

- Removal of a thrombus by means of a mechanical device

  From vein

Arterial and venous mechanical thrombectomy may be performed as primary procedure or add-on

- Includes

  Introduction of device into thrombus

  Thrombus removal

  Injection of thrombolytic drug(s), if used

  Fluoroscopic and contrast guidance

  Follow-up angiography

- Report separately

  Diagnostic angiography

  Catheter placement(s)

Diagnostic studies

Pharmacologic thrombolytic infusion before or after (37211-37214, 75896, 75898)

Other interventions

Other Procedures (37191-37217)

- Used to report a variety of transcatheter procedures

   Example: Transcatheter biopsy, therapy, infusion for thrombolysis or antispasmotic treatment of a vessel, retrieval of foreign object, occlusion or embolization, and intravascular stents

Endovascular Revascularization (Open or Percutaneous, Transcatheter) (37220-37235)

■ Cardiovascular in Medicine Section

Services can be

- Invasive or noninvasive
- Diagnostic or therapeutic

Subheadings

- Therapeutic Services and Procedures
- Cardiography
- Cardiovascular Monitoring Services
- Implantable and Wearable Cardiac Device Evaluations
- Echocardiography
- Cardiac Catheterization
- Intracardiac Electrophysiologic Procedures/Studies
- Peripheral Arterial Disease Rehabilitation
- Noninvasive Physiologic Studies and Procedures
- Other Procedures

Therapeutic Services and Procedures (92920-92998)

Types of services

- Cardioversion
- Infusions
- Thrombolysis
- Catheter placement

Codes divided by

- Method (e.g., balloon, blade)
- Location (e.g., aortic or mitral valve)
- Number (e.g., single or multiple vessels)

Intracoronary Brachytherapy (92974)

Uses radioactive substances to destroy re-stenosis of coronary vessel

Patients have had stent placed in coronary vessel

Stent "re-stenosis" (re-formation of plaque)

Add-on code

Includes moderate sedation

Cardiologist: Places guidewire and catheter

Radiation oncologist: Places radioactive elements

Cardiography (93000-93042)

Types of services

- Stress tests
- Holter monitor
- Electrocardiogram

Separate codes for components of study, such as

- 93000 global
- 93005 tracing only
- 93010 interpretation and report only

Codes report professional and/or technical components, so do not append -26 or -TC

Cardiovascular Monitoring Services (93224-93278)

Diagnostic procedures in-person or by means of remote technology to assess cardiovascular rhythm via ECG

- Holter monitors, 93224-93227
- Mobile telemetry, 93228, 93229
- Event monitors, 93268-93272
    - Patient depresses a button on portable monitor when feeling a sensation (event), such as a flutter or dizziness

Codes divided based on type of monitoring and time

Implantable and Wearable Cardiac Device Evaluations (93279-93299)

Diagnostic medical procedures for cardiac rhythm devices

- Devices are internal or external
- In-person or remote assessments

Codes divided by

- Type of Service
    Implantation
    Interrogation
    Programming
- Devices, such as:
    Implantable cardioverter-defibrillator
    Implantable loop recorder
- Number of leads or chambers
- Monitoring period must exceed 10 days

Implantation procedures (93279-93291)

- Reported once per procedure

Interrogation device evaluation of implantable cardioverter-defibrillator (ICD) or pacemaker (93293-93296)

- ICDs may act as defibrillator or pacemaker
- Report interrogation or monitoring once per 90-day period

Interrogation device evaluation implantable cardiovascular monitor system (93297-93299)

- Report interrogation or monitoring once per 30-day period

Echocardiography (93303-93352)

Noninvasive diagnostic procedure
Ultrasound detects presence of cardiac or vascular disease

Codes divided by

- Approach
- Extent of study (e.g., limited, complete)
- Service provided (e.g., probe only, interpretation and report)

Cardiac Catheterization (93451-93572)

Used to identify valve disorders, abnormal blood flow

Many bundled services in catheterization codes

Examples:

- Introduction
- Positioning/Repositioning of catheter
- Pressure readings inside heart or vessels
- Blood samples
- Rest/Exercise studies
- Final evaluation and report
- Many codes are -51 exempt
- Many codes include moderate (conscious) sedation

Three components of coding cardiac catheterization

1. Placement of catheter
2. Injection
3. Imaging supervision, interpretation, and report

Most codes have all three components in the code

- Example: 93456 includes catheterization, injection, imaging

Some codes require multiple codes

- Example: 93531 reports catheterization for congenital cardiac anomalies, injection code (93563/93564) must be added

Intracardiac Electrophysiologic Procedures/Studies (93600-93662)

Services to diagnose and treat conditions of electrical system of heart

- Arrhythmic induction
- Mapping
- Ablation

EP system of heart

Electrical conduction system

Electrical recording codes divided based on location of recording device

Example: Bundle of His or right ventricle

Pacing: Temporary pacing to stabilize beating of heart

Example: Intraventricular or intra-arterial pacing

Peripheral Arterial Disease (PAD) Rehabilitation (93668)

Rehabilitation sessions: 45-60 minutes

Use of motorized treadmill/track/bicycle to build patient's CV function

Supervised by exercise physiologist or nurse

If E/M is provided by physician, service is reported separately

Noninvasive Physiologic Studies and Procedures (93701-93790)

Category contains codes for services such as

- **Plethysmography:** Recordings of changes in size of body part when blood passes through it
- **Electronic Analysis:** Checks electronic function of devices, such as pacemakers

- **Ambulatory Blood Pressure Monitoring:** Outpatient basis over 24-hour period
- **Thermograms:** Visual recordings of body temperature

Other Procedures (93797-93799)

Codes 93797 and 93798 report professional outpatient cardiac rehabilitation services, per session

- With or without ECG monitoring

■ Cardiovascular in Radiology Section

Radiology section, Heart (75557-75574) and Aorta/Arteries (75600-75791) subsections

Prior to 1992, Radiology section contained codes for entire CV procedures

Major revision to CV radiology codes 1992

Divided complete procedures into two components: technical and professional

> *Example:* Angiography

- Technical component angiography—remains in Radiology section
- Professional component injection—moved to Surgery section

Complete angiography requires radiology code and surgery code

Reflects common practice of cardiologist's performing injection and radiologist's performing angiography

Contrast Material

Often radiologic procedures use contrast material to improve image

Many codes have contrast material bundled into service

- "with contrast" or "with or without contrast"

Only injected contrast qualifies as "with contrast"

Contrast not included in description but used in procedure: Code contrast material and injection separately

- Specify site where service is received to differentiate between global (total), technical, and professional components of the procedure

Non-hospital-based (not employed by hospital) physician usually performs procedure in hospital outpatient department: Use -26 to report only professional component

---

A COMPONENT CODING EXAMPLE

Two physicians (cardiologist and radiologist from same facility) perform angiography of third-order brachio-cephalic artery with contrast

- Cardiologist places catheter (36217), Surgery section
- Radiologist performs angiography (75658), Radiology section
- Supply of contrast material (99070), Medicine section

HEMIC AND LYMPHATIC SYSTEM SUBSECTION (38100-38999)

Divisions

- Spleen
- General
- Lymph Nodes and Lymphatic Channels

Spleen Subheading (38100-38200)

Spleen easily ruptured, causing massive and potentially lethal hemorrhage

Excision:

- Splenectomy: Total or partial/open or laparoscopic

Often done as part of more major procedure

- Bundled into major procedure
- Repair
- Laparoscopy

General (38204-38243)

Bone Marrow
Codes divided based on

- Preservation
- Preparation
- Purification
- Aspiration
- Biopsy
- Harvesting
- Transplantation

Hematopoietic Progenitor Cell (HPC)

- Obtained from bone marrow, peripheral blood apheresis, umbilical cord blood

Types of cells
Allogenic: Same species (38240)
Autologous: Patient's own (38241)

Lymph Nodes and Lymphatic Channels Subheading (38300-38999)

Two types of lymphadenectomies:

1. **Limited:** Pelvic and para-aortic lymph nodes only for neoplasm staging
2. **Radical:** Aortic and/or splenic lymph nodes and surrounding tissue for neoplasm staging

Often bundled into more major procedure (e.g., prostatectomy)

Do not unbundle and report lymphadenectomy separately

MEDIASTINUM AND DIAPHRAGM SUBSECTION (39000-39499)

Incision codes for foreign body removal, biopsy, or drainage

Excision codes for removal of cyst or tumor

Diaphragm (39501-39599)

Only two categories: Repair and Other Procedures

Includes hernia and laceration repairs

■ PRACTICE EXERCISES

Practice Exercise 3-26: Angiogram

Assign the codes for the catheterizations only.

RADIOLOGY REPORT

LOCATION: Inpatient, Hospital

PATIENT: Joy Gigel

ORDERING PHYSICIAN: John Hodgson, MD

ATTENDING/ADMIT PHYSICIAN: Frank Gaul, MD

RADIOLOGIST: Morton Monson, MD

PERSONAL PHYSICIAN: Frank Gaul, MD

EXAMINATION: Carotid/cerebral angiogram.

CLINICAL SYMPTOMS: Intracranial bleed.

CAROTID/CEREBRAL ANGIOGRAM: The patient is a 54-year-old female who was found to have an intracranial bleed. Carotid/cerebral angiogram was requested by Dr. Hodgson, neurosurgery.

APPROACH: Right common femoral artery.

VESSELS INJECTED
1. Proximal thoracic aorta.
2. Right common carotid artery.
3. Right internal carotid artery.
4. Left common carotid artery.
5. Left vertebral artery.

FOLLOW-UP: Dr. Hodgson.

Prior to the start of the study, the procedure was explained to the patient's husband by Dr. Hodgson, including risks, complications, and alternatives. The patient's husband understood and consented to the exam. This study was performed on an emergency basis.

The patient was prepped and draped in the usual sterile fashion. Utilizing single wall technique following administration of local anesthesia (1% lidocaine), a #5 French flush catheter was introduced into the right common femoral artery through a vascular sheath, and the tip was advanced into the proximal thoracic aorta. Contrast was injected, and sequential digital subtraction angiography films were obtained.

The flush catheter was then exchanged for a #4 French Osborne catheter for select evaluation of both common carotid arteries, as well as the right internal carotid artery and the left vertebral artery. Again, contrast was injected, and multiple views of the carotid bifurcations and cerebral vessels were obtained.

On arch injection, there is no significant stenosis at the origin of the great vessels. There is an antegrade flow in both vertebral arteries. Please note that the right vertebral artery is somewhat smaller when compared to the left.

On evaluation of the carotid bifurcations, there is no evidence of narrowing or irregularity.

On evaluation of cerebral vessels, there is no evidence of aneurysm, extravasation, or arteriovenous malformation. Please note that there is marked medial and superior displacement of the vessels in the right middle cerebral artery distribution. There is also midline shift of all the cerebral structures of the left as well as midline shift to the left of the anterior cerebral arteries. These findings are consistent with the patient's intraparenchymal bleed predominantly in the right temporal lobe seen on CT study from an outside institution.

The patient tolerated the procedure well. The puncture site was closed with sutures utilizing the Perclose device. There was no evidence of bleeding, hematoma, or change in peripheral pulses at the termination of the study.

IMPRESSION: Carotid/cerebral angiogram with multiple findings as described above.

Dr. Hodgson was present during this examination.

CPT Code(s): _____

ICD-9-CM Code(s): _____

Abstracting Questions

1. What CPT Appendix could you reference to understand how to code the procedure performed in the report? _____

2. What vessels were evaluated? _____

3. Are right and left HCPCS modifiers appended to the catheter insertion codes? _____

4. Are both the right common carotid and right internal carotid reported? _____

5. Is the left common carotid reported? _____

6. Is the left vertebral artery reported? _____

7. Why does the proximal thoracic aorta not get reported? _____

Practice Exercise 3-27: Dialysis Catheter Replacement

LOCATION: Outpatient, Hospital

PATIENT: Sally Perez

ATTENDING PHYSICIAN: George Orbitz, MD

SURGEON: George Orbitz, MD

PREOPERATIVE DIAGNOSIS: ESRD.

POSTOPERATIVE DIAGNOSIS: ESRD.

PROCEDURE PERFORMED: Dialysis catheter replacement.

ANESTHESIA: Local.

DESCRIPTION OF PROCEDURE: After obtaining consent, the 46-year-old patient was put in the Trendelenburg position. The area of the right IJ vein where the catheter was placed was prepped in the usual fashion. A guidewire was advanced without difficulty. The old dialysis catheter was taken out. Tip was sent for culture. A new 11.5 French 13.5-cm temporary dialysis catheter was advanced through the right IJ vein over the guidewire using the Seldinger technique without difficulty. Both ports had good blood return. Both ports were flushed with saline and heparin. The catheter was secured to the skin. The patient tolerated the procedure well without immediate complications.

CPT Code(s): _____

ICD-9-CM Code(s): _____

Abstracting Questions

1. Was the catheter placement venous or arterial? _____

2. Was this an open or percutaneous insertion? _____

3. Was the catheter a central or peripheral insertion? _____

4. Was this reported as an insertion or a replacement? _____

5. What was the principal reason for the encounter? _____

Practice Exercise 3-28: Catheter Placement

Report the services, diagnosis(es), and any sedation provided to this patient by the interventional radiologist.

LOCATION: Outpatient, Hospital

PATIENT: John Cane

PRIMARY CARE PHYSICIAN: Rapheal White, MD

INTERVENTIONAL RADIOLOGIST: Edward Riddle, MD

EXAMINATION: Right IVJ Port-a-Cath placement.

CLINICAL SYMPTOMS: Primary lung cancer. Access required for chemotherapy.

PORT-A-CATH PLACEMENT: Informed consent was obtained from this 26-year-old patient. The right neck and infraclavicular region were prepped and draped in the usual sterile fashion. Skin and subcutaneous tissues were infiltrated with 1% lidocaine with epinephrine. Under ultrasound guidance, access was obtained into the right jugular vein, and over a 0.035 J-tip guidewire the needle was exchanged for a 10 French peel-away sheath. A subcutaneous pocket was created in the right infraclavicular region using blunt dissection. A 9.6 French Bard single-lumen Port-a-Cath was placed into the pocket and a subcutaneous tunnel created from the pocket to the right IJV puncture site. The 9.6 French catheter was advanced through the tunnel and placed through the peel-away sheath. The sheath was removed. Under fluoroscopic observation the distal tip of the catheter was positioned in the right atrium. The pocket was closed using subcutaneous interrupted sutures with 4–0 Vicryl and a subcuticular stitch with 4–0 Vicryl. The right neck incision site was closed using vertical mattress suture technique with 3–0 Ethilon.

Patient received conscious sedation for 45 minutes. The patient's pulse oximeter and vital signs were monitored throughout the exam. There were no complications. The patient tolerated the procedure well and left the radiology department in stable condition.

A single digital spot radiograph obtained demonstrates the single-lumen port placed via a right IJV approach with the distal tip of the catheter in the right atrium.

CPT Code(s): _____

ICD-9-CM Code(s): _____

Abstracting Questions

1. Was the catheter inserted by the radiologist? _____

2. Was the catheter inserted into the venous or arterial system?

   _____

3. Was the catheter inserted centrally or peripherally? _____

4. Was the catheter tunneled? _____

5. Was a subcutaneous port/pump inserted? _____

6. Does the age of the patient affect code assignment? _____

7. What were the two types of guidance used? _____

8. The catheter inserted was used for access for what purpose? _____

Practice Exercise 3-29: Aortogram

LOCATION: Outpatient, Hospital

PATIENT: Theodore Lambert

PRIMARY CARE PHYSICIAN: Ronald Green, MD

INTERVENTIONAL RADIOLOGIST: Edward Riddle, MD

EXAMINATION: Arch aortogram with bilateral carotid and cerebral arteriograms.

CLINICAL SYMPTOMS: Previous stroke; carotid artery stenosis.

AORTOGRAPHIC TECHNIQUE: Informed consent was obtained. The right groin was prepped and draped in the usual sterile fashion. Skin and subcutaneous tissues were infiltrated with 1% lidocaine. Access was obtained of the right common femoral artery, and over a 0.035 Bentson guidewire the needle was exchanged for a 5 French sheath. Over the guidewire a 5 French Pigtail catheter was threaded to the aortic arch and angiography was performed in the LAO projection during mechanical injection of contrast through the catheter. The catheter was exchanged for a 5 French H1H catheter. The right vertebral artery was selectively catheterized using the H1H and a 0.035 angled Glidewire. Posterior fossa arteriogram was performed during hand injection of contrast through the catheter. This was performed in AP and lateral projections.

The right common carotid artery was selectively catheterized using the Glidewire and H1H catheter. Right carotid arteriogram was performed in three projections during mechanical injection of contrast through the catheter. AP and lateral cerebral arteriography on the right was performed during mechanical injection of contrast through the catheter.

The left common carotid artery was selectively catheterized using the Glidewire and H1H. Left carotid arteriogram was performed during hand injection of contrast through the catheter. Cerebral arteriogram was performed on the left during hand injection of contrast through the catheter.

Catheter and sheath were removed. Hemostasis was obtained using a 6 French AngioSeal device. The patient received conscious sedation. His pulse oximeter and vital signs were monitored throughout the exam. There were no complications. He tolerated the procedure well and left the radiology department in stable condition.

ARCH AORTOGRAM: The arch is unremarkable. Origins of the great vessels are normal in caliber with no stenosis seen. Subclavian arteries are patent. Bilateral vertebral arteries are patent. Left common carotid artery is small in caliber and indicates that the left internal carotid artery is completely occluded.

POSTERIOR FOSSA ARTERIOGRAM: Visualized distal right vertebral artery is patent. Basilar artery is unremarkable, as are the bilateral posterior cerebral arteries. No aneurysm is seen. No anterior cerebral arterial circulation is noted on this posterior fossa injection.

RIGHT CAROTID ARTERIOGRAM: Calcified atheromatous disease of the carotid bulb and proximal internal carotid artery is noted. There is approximately 30-40% diameter narrowing of the carotid bulb, with no significant stenosis seen involving the proximal internal carotid artery. There is a 90-95% diameter narrowing of the proximal external carotid artery.

LEFT CAROTID ARTERIOGRAM: The common carotid artery is small in caliber, with the distal common carotid artery demonstrating a high-grade stenosis with a "string sign." The internal carotid artery is completely occluded.

RIGHT CEREBRAL ARTERIOGRAM: The distal internal carotid artery and the intracranial internal carotid artery are widely patent. The right anterior and middle cerebral artery and their distribution are unremarkable, with no stenosis seen. No hypervascular or hypovascular mass is present. No aneurysm is seen. The left anterior and middle cerebral arterial supply is provided via a patent anterior communicating artery. No abnormalities are seen on the left anterior or middle cerebral arterial supply.

LEFT CEREBRAL ARTERIOGRAM: As discussed above, the left cerebral anterior circulation is provided from the right cerebral anterior circulation. There is no intracranial supply on the left seen via external carotid branches. No reconstitution of the left internal carotid artery is seen.

IMPRESSION
1. Negative arch aortogram with a small-caliber left common carotid artery.
2. Negative posterior fossa arteriogram.
3. 30-40% diameter narrowing of the carotid bulb on the right, with no significant stenosis of the right internal carotid artery seen.
4. Complete occlusion of the left internal carotid artery.
5. The left anterior and middle cerebral arteries receive their supply via patent anterior communicating artery from the right anterior arterial circulation.

CPT Code(s): _____

ICD-9-CM Code(s): _____

Abstracting Questions

1. What does LAO stand for? _____

2. In the Left Carotid Arteriogram section of the report, the radiologist refers to a "string sign." What is a string sign? _____

Practice Exercise 3-30: Extremity Angiogram

LOCATION: Outpatient, Hospital

PATIENT: George Ball

PRIMARY CARE PHYSICIAN: Ronald Green, MD

SURGEON: Gary Sanchez, MD

INTERVENTIONAL RADIOLOGIST: Edward Riddle, MD

EXAMINATION: Right lower extremity angiogram and thrombolysis.

CLINICAL SYMPTOMS: Cold right foot.

RIGHT LOWER EXTREMITY ANGIOGRAM AND THROMBOLYSIS: This 62-year-old male presented a month ago with ischemic changes below the knee of the right lower extremity. Some years earlier, the patient had a femoral-popliteal Gore-Tex graft placed. At the time of the angiogram a month ago, there was clot of virtually all the arteries commencing in the distal external iliac artery. We saw very few collateralizations extending into the right lower extremity. Subsequent lytic procedure cleared the Gore-Tex graft and the popliteal artery, but there was then very hard material in the distal popliteal artery that was resistant to the tPA lysis. Subsequently, the patient was taken to the operating room by Dr. Sanchez, where he placed a vein graft from the proximal third of the Gore-Tex graft and inserted it into the posterior tibial artery. The patient then did very well. He now presents acutely with ischemic changes of the right foot.

The patient is on heparin and had been taking Plavix and aspirin as an outpatient. The present procedure was performed via the left femoral artery with single-wall micropuncture entry and placement of a 5 French sheath. A 5 French Omni Flush catheter was then positioned into the right external iliac artery for examination of the right lower extremity.

There is a patency of the right external iliac artery to the junction with the common femoral artery. The common femoral artery is virtually occluded. One or two proximal branches are arising from the artery. The superficial femoral artery and the Gore-Tex graft are occluded. There was also no visualization of the saphenous vein graft. Some collaterals from the deep femoral artery can be visualized at the level of the knee. Although these are scant, they are certainly more than we appreciated when the patient initially arrived here last month.

Utilizing a long Glidewire, I obtained access into the Gore-Tex graft. While traversing the Gore-Text graft, I kept the curve of the wire pointed anteromedially, hoping that we might enter the vein graft. I was able to extend the Glidewire all the way to the knee. Subsequently, a Mewissen catheter with 15 cm of holes was placed proximally with the most proximal hole in the beginning of the clot in the common femoral artery. Coaxially, a Katzen wire with 12 cm of holes was positioned into the graft. tPA was then commenced through both catheters. The patient was medicated with intravenous Versed and fentanyl. He will return to the angiographic suite in the morning.

IMPRESSION: Complete occlusion of the patient's superficial femoral artery, Gore-Tex femoral-popliteal graft, and saphenous graft that extends from the Gore-Tex graft to the posterior tibial artery. Coaxial system has been appropriately placed and tPA lysis started.

CPT Code(s): _____

ICD-9-CM Code(s): _____

Abstracting Question

1. The furthest extent of this selective catheterization was to what vessel
_____ _____ artery and to this order? _____

DIGESTIVE SYSTEM SUBSECTION (40490-49999)

Divided by anatomic site from mouth to anus + organs that aid digestive process

Example: Liver and gallbladder

Many bundled procedures

Endoscopy

Diagnostic procedure always bundled into surgical endoscopic

Code to furthest extent of procedure

Endoscopy Terminology

Notes define specific terminology

Code descriptions are specific regarding

- Technique and depth of scope

    Esophagoscopy: Esophagus only

    Esophagogastroscopy: Esophagus and past diaphragm

    Esophagogastroduodenoscopy: Esophagus and beyond pyloric channel

- Proctosigmoidoscopy: Rectum and sigmoid colon (6-25 cm)

- Sigmoidoscopy: Entire rectum, sigmoid colon, and may include part of descending colon (26-60 cm)

- Colonoscopy: Entire colon, rectum to cecum, and may include terminal ileum (greater than 60 cm)

Laparoscopy and Endoscopy

Some subheadings have both laparoscopy (outside) and endoscopy (inside) procedures

Example: Subheading Esophagus

- Endoscopy views inside

- Laparoscopy—scope inserted through umbilicus; views from outside

Hemorrhoidectomy and Fistulectomy Codes (46200-46320)

Divided by

- Location
  - Internal
  - External
- Complexity
  - Simple: No repair procedure involved
  - Complex: Includes repair procedure and fissurectomy
- Anatomy
  - Subcutaneous: No muscle involvement
  - Submuscular: sphincter muscle
- Complex fistulectomy involves excision/incision of multiple fistulas

Hernia Codes (49491-49659)

Divided by

- Type of hernia

  Example: Inguinal, femoral

- Initial or subsequent repair
- Age of patient determines code choice
- Clinical presentation

  - **Strangulated:** Blood supply cut off
  - **Incarcerated:** Cannot be returned to cavity (not reducible)

Additional code is used for implantation of mesh or prosthesis for incisional or ventral hernias only

- Open or laparoscopic surgical approaches

■ PRACTICE EXERCISES

Practice Exercise 3-31: Orogastric Tube Placement

OPERATIVE REPORT

The intraoperative KUB was provided by the radiologist, and you are only reporting the services of Dr. Friendly.

LOCATION: Outpatient, Hospital

PATIENT: Otto Garth

ATTENDING/ADMIT PHYSICIAN: Alma Naraquist, MD

SURGEON: Larry P. Friendly, MD

INDICATION: Feeding, patient with gastroparesis.

PROCEDURE: The patient was placed in the sitting position and then tilted to the right with a wedge. CORFLO was placed at the level of 19 cm without any complications. KUB was then done demonstrating the tip of the CORFLO in the third portion of the duodenum. After confirmation of postpyloric position of the CORFLO, the patient was started on UltraCal at 10 cc/hour.

CPT Code(s): _____

ICD-9-CM Code(s): _____

Abstracting Questions

1. What does KUB stand for? _____

2. What type of tube is a CORFLO? _____

Practice Exercise 3-32: Gastrojejunostomy Placement

Because this is an interventional radiologist performing the procedure, report both the procedure and the radiology services.

RADIOLOGY REPORT

LOCATION: Outpatient, Hospital

PATIENT: Betty Frye

ORDERING PHYSICIAN: Ronald Green, MD

ATTENDING/ADMIT PHYSICIAN: Ronald Green, MD

INTERVENTIONAL RADIOLOGIST: Monica Hamilton, MD

EXAMINATION: Gastrojejunostomy placement.

CLINICAL SYMPTOMS: Malnutrition needing nutritional support.

INDICATION: The patient is a 69-year-old female requiring tube feeding. Placement of a #14 French Shetty gastrojejunostomy catheter was requested by Dr. Green for nutritional support.

Prior to the start of the study, the procedure was explained to the patient, including the risks, complications, and alternatives. The patient understood and consented to the procedure.

PERCUTANEOUS GASTROJEJUNOSTOMY PLACEMENT: The patient was prepped and draped in the usual sterile fashion. Using ultrasound guidance, we localized the edge of the liver. Through a previously placed nasogastric tube, the stomach was distended with air.

Using fluoroscopic guidance following administration of local anesthesia (1% lidocaine), we performed gastropexy utilizing four Medi-Tech T-tacks at the mid to distal aspect of the stomach.

Using multiple wires and catheters, an extra-stiff guidewire was ultimately placed with the tip in the proximal jejunum. Following multiple dilatations, a #14 French Shetty gastrojejunostomy catheter was placed with the tip in the proximal jejunum. A small amount of contrast was administered, which revealed adequate placement. There is no evidence of extravasation or other significant abnormalities.

The patient tolerated the procedure well. There was no evidence of bleeding at the termination of the study.

IMPRESSION: Placement of a #14 French Shetty gastrojejunostomy catheter with the tip in the proximal jejunum, as described above.

CPT Code(s): _____

ICD-9-CM Code(s): _____

Abstracting Questions

1. What was the approach for insertion of the gastrostomy tube?

   _____

2. Was the ultrasonic guidance separately reported? _____

3. Was the radiology service to check placement separately reported?

   _____

Practice Exercise 3-33: Cystotomy

OPERATIVE REPORT

Dr. Martinez operated on this patient yesterday. The patient presents to the emergency department with an acute abdomen. You are to report only Dr. Martinez's services.

LOCATION: Inpatient, Hospital

PATIENT: Patti Bryan

ATTENDING PHYSICIAN: Gary Sanchez, MD

SURGEONS: Paula Smithson, MD, and Andy Martinez, MD

PREOPERATIVE DIAGNOSES
1. Acute abdomen.
2. Hematuria with suspected bladder injury.

POSTOPERATIVE DIAGNOSES
1. Iatrogenic cystotomy with urine extravasation into the peritoneal cavity.
2. Peritonitis.
3. Extensive intestinal adhesions.

PROCEDURES PERFORMED
1. Exploratory laparotomy.
2. Closure of cystotomy.
3. Extensive intestinal adhesiolysis.

SURGICAL INDICATIONS: This patient is a 32-year-old female who had undergone a Hasson laparoscopy that I performed yesterday. She presented to the emergency department last night with abdominal pain and findings of an acute abdomen. She also had a leukopenia. She was not running a fever. She was noted on insertion of the catheter into the bladder to have some grossly bloody urine.

OPERATIVE FINDINGS: There was less than 1-cm laceration in the dome of the bladder that was extravasating through the bladder. There was a large amount of urine in the peritoneal cavity and some slightly foul-smelling purulent fluid as well. This looked relatively murky and was just not plain urine. There were multiple intestinal adhesions, mostly involving the small bowel. No perforation of the bowel could be detected. The appendix was normal.

OPERATIVE DESCRIPTION: After induction of general anesthesia with patient in the supine position, the abdomen was prepped and draped. The abdomen was opened through a midline hypogastric incision excising her old scar on the way in. The above findings were noted initially, and Dr. Smithson was able to isolate the small bladder dome laceration. This was smaller than one would expect if a 5-mm laparoscopic trocar had gone through the bladder. I believe that the edge of the bladder probably was nicked. Dr. Smithson will dictate her note concerning the cystotomy repair. We then ran the bowel in its entirety from the ligament of Treitz on down to the ileocecal junction. There were multiple interloop adhesions, which were lysed by Dr. Smithson. She will dictate her note separately. Some omental adhesions were also lysed. After copious irrigation of the abdominal cavity, we then irrigated with heparinized lactated Ringer's and left some of the Ringer's in the abdomen. The peritoneum was closed with a running 2–0 Vicryl. The fascia was closed with interrupted figure-of-eight 0 Vicryl, and the skin closed with staples. Blood loss estimation was 100 cc. The patient received 3000 cc of lactated Ringer's during the case.

Specimens to pathology were cultures of the peritoneal fluid. A Foley catheter was changed at the end of the case. The patient was returned to the recovery room in stable condition.

CPT Code(s): _____

ICD-9-CM Code(s): _____

Abstracting Questions

1. What procedures were performed during this operative session?
   _____

2. Which of the procedures did Dr. Martinez perform? _____

3. Were any modifiers required for the two surgeons involved in the same session and if so, which modifier? _____

Practice Exercise 3-34: Small-Bowel Anastomosis

OPERATIVE REPORT

LOCATION: Inpatient, Hospital

PATIENT: Dona Kelly

ATTENDING PHYSICIAN: Ronald Green, MD

SURGEON: Daniel G. Olanka, MD

PREOPERATIVE DIAGNOSIS: Multiple intestinal fistulas.

POSTOPERATIVE DIAGNOSIS: Multiple intestinal fistulas.

PROCEDURE PERFORMED: Excision of abdominal wall and small bowel with primary anastomosis of small bow.

PRELIMINARY NOTE: This patient is well known to us. She has had multiple abdominal procedures to try to repair a very large abdominal wall hernia. She is outside the postoperative period of the hernia repair. She basically has no abdominal cavity left, and all her intestine resides outside the abdomen. There is such a drag on her abdominal wall that she has developed fistulas at the base of where the bowel rests against the mesh, and these have become unmanageable in the home setting. On this basis, we take this very high-risk patient to the operating room, with appropriate counseling for the family about the dire consequences.

OPERATIVE NOTE: With the patient under general anesthesia, the abdomen was prepped and draped in a sterile manner. A long incision was made above the area of the fistulas, and we began to work our way down onto the mesh. Unfortunately, we entered the bowel at multiple points and had multiple enterotomies into the small bowel *(small intestine)* and colon *(large intestine)*. Finally we got everything freed up and were able to resect some of the abdominal wall that had adherent small bowel to it *(this indicates that part of the small intestine was removed)*. We were able to repair all of the enterostomies and a right colotomy using two layers of suture, an inner layer of Vicryl, and an outer layer of silk. We then copiously irrigated the abdominal field and used some large retention-type sutures to bring the wound together for partial closure. It is our hope that the bowel that remains is viable *(this indicates that part of the bowel was removed)*. This procedure took substantially greater time than typically would be required. *(This statement indicates -22 may be assigned.)* We measured it at approximately 200 cm of length of her small bowel, and we are hopeful that this will be enough for her to nourish adequately.

CPT Code(s): _____

ICD-9-CM Code(s): _____

Abstracting Questions

1. Was a portion of the large or small intestine removed?_____

2. What statement indicates that modifier -22 would be appended to the CPT code?_____

Practice Exercise 3-35: Pyloroplasty

OPERATIVE REPORT

Report only Dr. White's surgical services. Note in this case that the surgeon began the procedure as a percutaneous liver biopsy, but because the patient could not hold his breath long enough for the biopsy to be obtained, Dr. White decided to discontinue the percutaneous biopsy and take the patient directly to the operating room for an open procedure. Two surgeons (co-surgeons) are performing this case. Dr. Sanchez, in his operative report, states that the patient was turned to a lateral position, prepped, and draped and the chest was opened to expose the esophagus. The distal esophagus was mobilized under direct vision and divided above the diseased segment. The distal esophagus and the attached proximal stomach were removed. The remaining stomach was pulled into the chest and connected to the stump of the proximal esophagus. Drains were placed and a chest tube inserted and the incision was closed.

LOCATION: Inpatient, Hospital

PATIENT: Ted Boyd

ATTENDING PHYSICIAN: Larry Friendly, MD

PRIMARY CARE PHYSICIAN: Ronald Green, MD

SURGEONS: Loren White, MD, and Gary Sanchez, MD

PREOPERATIVE DIAGNOSIS: Barrett's esophagus with severe dysplasia, possible carcinoma.

POSTOPERATIVE DIAGNOSIS: Barrett's esophagus with severe dysplasia, possible carcinoma, hemangioma liver.

PROCEDURES PERFORMED
1. Exploratory laparotomy.
2. Biopsy of liver lesion.
3. Immobilization of stomach with pyloroplasty.
4. Placement of feeding tube.

PRELIMINARY NOTE: This patient is a 63-year-old man who has been referred by Dr. Green for a bleeding esophageal lesion. This was seen and scoped, and the patient was markedly anemic. Biopsies showed it to be severe dysplasia with possible cancer present. He has had a rather extensive workup including complete cardiac workup. CT of the abdomen showed some lesions within the liver, which we tried to have biopsied percutaneously, but the patient could not hold his breath well enough and the lesions were too close to the diaphragm, so we do not have a tissue diagnosis on these. After all this workup we are taking the patient to the operating room for exploration. Assuming that he does not have disease metastatic to the liver, we will proceed with an esophagogastrectomy in the Ivor-Lewis technique. The abdominal portion of the procedure, which I am dictating, will be done by myself, and then Dr. Sanchez will do the chest portion of the procedure.

OPERATIVE NOTE: With the patient under general anesthesia, the abdomen was prepped and draped in a sterile manner. Midline incision was made from the xiphoid to below the pubis. Sharp dissection was carried down into the peritoneal cavity, and hemostasis was maintained with electrocautery. We began by exploring the abdominal cavity. The liver was carefully palpated. The area that had been identified on CT was at the very apex of the right lobe of the liver, we could feel this area; it did not have a thickened feel to it but was more consistent with an area of hemangioma. There was a small secondary lesion on the undersurface of the right lobe. A **wedge biopsy** of this was taken and it did return a diagnosis of hemangioma. The rest of the liver appeared normal, and I thought that we did not need to proceed with anything further. We thus began with mobilization of the stomach, taking down the greater curvature vessels, preserving the gastroepiploica. We carried our dissection all the way up into the hiatal hernia, preserving the blood supply to the spleen and not injuring it. We were then able to detach the left gastric artery such that the stomach was tethered on its other vasculature but appeared completely viable. All these vessels were taken down with clamps and ligatures of 2–0 silk. We then circumferentially went around the esophagus and carried our dissection all the way back toward the pylorus. We then had the entire stomach freed up from pylorus all the way up to the diaphragm. *(The esophagus has been mobilized where it passes through the diaphragm and the stomach has been totally freed up so that when the chest is opened Dr. Sanchez will perform the remaining part of the surgery.)* The stomach appeared viable with reasonable circulation. A Heineke-Mikulicz **pyloroplasty** was then performed opening the pylorus in one direction and closing it in another using interrupted 3–0 silk sutures to complete the pyloroplasty. With this accomplished, we then picked up the **jejunum** approximated 40 or 50 cm beyond the ligament of Treitz and placed a red rubber **feeding tube** using a Witzel technique; this was a number 18-2. This was attached to the skin and brought out through a separate stab incision. The abdominal cavity was then checked for hemostasis and everything appeared to be intact. We then closed the incision using running 0–loop nylon. We closed the skin with staples. A sterile dressing was applied. With all this completed, the patient remained in the operating room and will be positioned by Dr. Sanchez for the thoracic portion of the procedure.

Pathology Report Later Indicated: Hemangioma.

CPT Code(s): _____

ICD-9-CM Code(s): _____

Abstracting Questions

1. Can the discontinued percutaneous liver biopsy be reported?

   _____

2. If reporting the percutaneous liver biopsy, what modifier(s) is/are required?

   _____

3. Was the wedge biopsy reported? _____

4. Dr. White performed an immobilization and what other procedure?

   _____

5. Was the Barrett's and hemangioma reported separately? _____

URINARY SYSTEM SUBSECTION (50010-53899)

Anatomic division

- Kidney
- Ureter
- Bladder
- Urethra

Further divided by procedure, such as:

- Incision
- Excision
- Introduction
- Repair
- Laparoscopy
- Endoscopy

Kidney Subheading (50010-50593)

Endoscopy codes are for procedure performed through previously established stoma or incision

Caution: Codes may be unilateral or bilateral

Introduction Category (50382-50398)

Codes divided by renal pelvis catheter procedures or other introduction procedures

Renal pelvis catheters further divided; internally dwelling or externally accessible

Catheters for drainage and injections and for radiography

Aspirations

Insertion of guidewires

Tube changes

Usually reported with radiology component

Ureter Subheading (50600-50980)

Caution: Codes may be unilateral or bilateral

Divided by type of procedure

- Incision
- Excision
- Introduction
- Repair
- Laparoscopy
- Endoscopy

Bladder Subheading (51020-52700)

Includes codes for

- Incision
- Removal
- Excision
- Introduction
- Urodynamics
- Repair
- Laparoscopy
- Endoscopy
- Cystoscopy
- Urethroscopy
- Cystourethroscopy
- Transurethral surgery
- Vesical Neck and Prostate

Many bundled codes

> ***Example:*** Urethral dilation is included with insertion of cystoscope

Urodynamics (51725-51798)

Procedures relate to motion and flow of urine

Used to diagnose urine flow obstructions

Bundled: All instruments, equipment, fluids, gases, probes, catheters, technician's fees, medications, gloves, trays, tubing, and other sterile supplies

Vesical Neck and Prostate (52400-52700)

Contains codes for transurethral resection of the prostate (TURP)

> ***Example:*** 52601 reports a complete transurethral electrosurgical resection of the prostate and includes vasectomy, meatotomy, cystourethroscopy, urethral calibration and/or dilation, internal urethrotomy, and control of any postoperative bleeding

Other approaches are reported with 55801-55845

> ***Example:*** 55801 reports a removal of the prostate gland (prostatectomy) through an incision in the perineum and includes vasectomy, meatotomy, urethral calibration and/or dilation, internal urethrotomy, and control of any postoperative bleeding

MALE GENITAL SYSTEM SUBSECTION (54000-55899)

Penis

Testis

Epididymis

Tunica Vaginalis

Scrotum

Vas Deferens

Spermatic Cord

Seminal Vesicles

Prostate

Biopsy Codes

Located in anatomical subheading to which the codes refer

> *Example:* Biopsy codes in subheadings

- Epididymis (Excision)

  > *Example:* 54800, needle biopsy of epididymis

- Testis (Excision)

  > *Example:* 54500, needle biopsy of testis

Penis (54000-54450)

Incision codes (54000-54015) differ from Integumentary System codes

- Penis incision codes assigned for deeper structures

Destruction (54050-54065)
Codes divided by

- Extent: Simple or extensive

- Method of destruction, e.g., chemical, cryosurgery

Extensive destruction can be by any method

Excision (54100-54164)
Commonly used codes are biopsy and circumcision

Introduction (54200-54250)
Many procedures for corpora cavernosa (spongy bodies of penis)

- Injection procedures for Peyronie disease (toughening of corpora cavernosa)

- Treatments for erectile dysfunction (ED)

Repair (54300-54440)
Many plastic repairs

Some repairs are staged (more than one procedure)

- Stage indicated in code description

REPRODUCTIVE SYSTEM PROCEDURES (55920)

Code 55920 reports the placement of catheters/needles into pelvic organs/genitalia

- For subsequent interstitial radioelement application

INTERSEX SURGERY SUBSECTION (55970-55980)

Only 2 codes within subsection

1. Male to female

2. Female to male

Complicated procedures completed over extended period of time

Performed by multiple physicians with extensive specialized training

FEMALE GENITAL SYSTEM SUBSECTION (56405-58999)

Anatomic division: From vulva to ovaries

• Many bundled services

Vulva, Perineum, and Introitus (56405-56821)

Skene's gland reported with Urinary System, Incision or Excision codes

• Group of small mucous glands, lower end of urethra

  • Paraurethral duct

Incision (56405-56442)

I&D of abscess of vulva, perineal area, or Bartholin's gland

Marsupialization (56440)

Cyst incised

Drained

Edges sutured to sides to keep cyst open, creating a pouchlike repair

Destruction (56501, 56515)

Lesions destroyed by variety of methods

• Destruction = Eradication (not to be confused with excision; excision is removal)

Divided by simple or extensive destruction

• Complexity based on physician's judgment

• Stated in medical record

Destruction has no pathology report

Excision (56605-56740)

Biopsy includes

• Local anesthetic

• Biopsy

• Simple closure

Code based on number of lesions biopsied

Vulvectomy. Surgical removal of portion of vulva (56620-56640)

Based on extent and size of area removed

Extent

• Simple: Skin and superficial subcutaneous tissues

• Radical: Skin and deep subcutaneous tissues

Size

- Partial: <80% vulvar area

- Complete: >80% vulvar area

Extent and size indicated in operative report

Repair (56800-56810)

Includes plastic repair

Read notes following category

- If repair procedure for wound of genitalia, use Integumentary System code

Endoscopy (56820-56821)

By means of a colposcope with or without biopsy(s)

Vagina (57000-57426)

Codes divided based on service, e.g., incision, excision

Introduction (57150-57180)

Includes vaginal irrigation, insertion of devices, diaphragm, cervical caps

Report device inserted separately

- 99070 or HCPCS National Level II codes, such as A4261 (cervical cap)

Repair (57200-57335)

For nonobstetric repairs

- Obstetric repairs, report Maternity Care and Delivery codes

Manipulation (57400-57415)

Dilation: Speculum inserted into vagina, which is enlarged by dilator

Endoscopy/Laparoscopy (57420-57426)

Colposcopy codes based on purpose

- e.g., biopsy, diagnostic

Includes code for laparoscopic approach for repair of paravaginal defect

Cervix Uteri (57452-57800)

Cervix uteri, narrow lower end of uterus

Services include endoscopy, excision, repair, manipulation

Excision (57500-57558)

Conization codes

Conization: Removal of cone of tissue from cervix

LEEP (loop electrocautery excision procedure) technology may be used for conizations or loop electrode biopsies

Corpus Uteri (58100-58579)

Many complex procedures

- Often very similar wording in code descriptions

- Requires careful reading and specific documentation in the medical record

Excision (58100-58294)

Dilation and curettage (D&C, 58120) of nonobstetric uterus

- After dilation, curette used to scrape uterus

- Coded according to circumstances: Obstetrical or nonobstetrical

Do not report postpartum hemorrhage service with 58120

- Report 59160—Maternity and Delivery code

Many hysterectomy codes

- Based on approach (vaginal, abdominal), extent (uterus, fallopian tubes, etc.), and weight of uterus

Often secondary procedures performed with hysterectomy

Do not report secondary, related minor procedures separately

Introduction (58300-58356)

Common procedures

- e.g., insertion of an IUD

Report supply of device separately

Specialized services

- e.g., artificial insemination procedures

Used to report physician component of service

Component coding

- Necessary with catheter procedures for hysterosonography

- Notes following codes indicate radiology guidance component codes

Laparoscopy/Hysteroscopy (58541-58579)

Laparoscopic approach for:

- Removal of myomas

- Radical hysterectomy

- Supracervical and laparoscopic vaginal hysterectomies

Codes divided by tissue removed and weight of uterus

- Hysteroscopy codes divided on procedure performed (e.g., lysis of uterine adhesions, endometrial ablation)

Oviduct/Ovary (58600-58770)

Oviduct. Fallopian tube
Incision category contains tubal ligations

- When during same hospitalization (but not at same session as delivery), is reported separately

Laparoscopy (58660-58679)
Through abdominal wall

Codes in the laparoscopy and hysteroscopy section are divided by procedure performed (e.g., lysis of adhesions, removal adnexal structures)

Caution: If only diagnostic laparoscopy

- Do not report Female Genital System codes
- Report 49320, Digestive System

Many codes can be reported separately with appropriate modifiers

> ***Example:*** 58660 Laparoscopy, surgical, with lysis of adhesions, can be reported with any of the indented codes that follow 58660 (58661-58673)

Ovary (58800-58960)

Two categories only: Incision and Excision

Incision: Primarily for drainage of cysts and abscesses

- Divided by surgical approach

Excision: Biopsy, wedge resection, and oophorectomy

In Vitro Fertilization (58970-58976)

Specialized codes used by physicians trained in fertilization procedures

- Codes divided by type of procedure and method used

MATERNITY CARE AND DELIVERY SUBSECTION (59000-59899)

Divided by service, such as:

- Antepartum and Fetal Invasive Services

  Amniocentesis

  Fetal non-stress test

  Fetal monitoring during labor
- Type of delivery

  Vaginal delivery

  C-section

  Delivery after previous C-section
- Abortion

Gestation

Fetal gestation: Approximately 266 days (40 weeks)

EDD: Estimated Date of Delivery

- 280 days from last menstrual period (LMP)

Trimesters
First, LMP to week 12

Second, weeks 13-27

Third, week 28 to EDD

Global Package and Delivery

Uncomplicated maternity care includes

- Antepartum care = Before delivery

- Delivery

- Postpartum care = After delivery

Antepartum Care Includes

Initial and subsequent H&P (history and physical)

Blood pressures

Weight

Routine chemical urinalysis

Fetal heart tones

Monthly visits to 28 weeks

Twice-a-month visits, weeks 29 to 36

Weekly visits from week 37 to delivery

Listed in notes preceding 59000

- Services not related to antepartum care are reported separately

    Example: Pregnant female with complaint of suspicious mole on left shoulder

    - Visits OB/GYN physician, who provides antepartum care

    - Service regarding mole, not antepartum care, requires good documentation in the maternity record and a specific diagnosis relative to the treatment provided

Delivery Includes

Admission to hospital with admitting H&P

Management of uncomplicated labor

Vaginal or cesarean section delivery

- Complications coded separately

- Listed in notes preceding 59000

Postpartum Care Includes

Normal follow-up care for 6 weeks after delivery

- Hospital visits, office visits

- Listed in notes preceding 59000

Antepartum and Fetal Invasive Services (59000-59076)

Amniocentesis: Insertion of needle into pregnant uterus, withdrawal of fluid (59000, 59001)

- Ultrasound guidance with 59000 (76946)

- Ultrasound guidance included with 59001

- Component coding often part of services in subheading

Fetal services: Include stress tests, blood sampling, monitoring, and therapeutic procedures

Excision (59100-59160)
Postpartum curettage: Removes remaining pieces of placenta or clotted blood (59160)

Nonobstetric curettage: 58120 (Corpus Uteri, Excision)

Introduction (59200)
Insertion of cervical dilator: Used to prepare and soften the cervix for an abortive procedure or delivery (for abortive procedure, see 59855)

Cervical ripening agents may be introduced to prepare cervix

• Separate procedure and not reported when part of more major procedure

Repair (59300-59350)
Only for repairs during pregnancy

Repairs done as a result of delivery or during pregnancy

Episiotomy or vaginal repair by other than attending physician

Suture closure (cerclage) of cervix or repair of uterus (hysterorrhaphy)

Routine Global Obstetric Care
Includes antepartum, delivery, and postpartum care

59400, Vaginal delivery

59510, Cesarean delivery

59610, Vaginal delivery after previous cesarean delivery (VBAC)

59618, Cesarean delivery following attempted vaginal delivery after previous cesarean delivery

Note: Take care when assigning diagnosis codes for normal versus complicated delivery. ICD-9-CM states specific guidelines for a normal delivery.

Episiotomies and Use of Forceps
Included in delivery

Not reported separately

Physician Provides Only Portion of Global Routine Care, Delivery
59409, Vaginal delivery only

59514, Cesarean delivery only

59612, Vaginal delivery only, after previous cesarean delivery

59620, Cesarean delivery only, following attempted vaginal delivery after previous cesarean delivery

Delivery of Twins
Payers differ on reporting format

• -22 (Unusual Procedural Services)

• -51 (Multiple Procedures)

Abortion Services (59812-59857)

Spontaneous: Happens naturally (for a complete spontaneous abortion, report with a code from the E/M section [99201-99233])

Incomplete: Requires medical intervention

Induced: Intentional termination of pregnancy

Missed: Fetus dies naturally but does not abort during first 22 weeks of gestation

Septic: Abortion with infection

Medical intervention

• Dilation and curettage or evacuation (suction removal)

• Intra-amniotic injections (saline or urea)

• Vaginal suppositories (prostaglandin)

■ PRACTICE EXERCISES

Practice Exercise 3-36: Renal Tumor Excision

LOCATION: Inpatient, Hospital

PATIENT: Brian Eberhoft

ATTENDING PHYSICIAN: Leslie Alanda, MD

SURGEON: Ira Avila, MD

PREOPERATIVE DIAGNOSIS: Right renal tumor.

POSTOPERATIVE DIAGNOSIS: Complex right renal cyst (acquired).

PROCEDURE PERFORMED: Right renal exploration; de-roofing of right renal cyst.

ANESTHESIA: General.

CLINICAL NOTE: Mr. Eberhoft is a 78-year-old gentleman found to have an enlarging right complex renal mass. This does not enhance but has irregular boundaries and has increased in size over the past year. It is located on the medial posterior part of the right kidney adjacent to the renal hilum. Options were discussed with the patient, and he elected to proceed with exploration and possible partial nephrectomy or radical nephrectomy depending on findings.

PROCEDURE: The patient was given a general endotracheal anesthetic as well as an epidural for intraoperative and postoperative analgesia. An incision was made over the tip of the 10th rib and the tip of the 10th rib excised. A small hole in the pleura was created, which was closed at the end of the case.

The patient has very poor fascial structures and very poor superficial muscle development. The peritoneal space was entered and the kidney identified. The Omni retractor was used for exposure. The ascending color was reflected off of Gerota's fascia. The duodenum had made a large turn over top of the renal hilum, and the duodenum was kocherized carefully. The renal vein and renal artery were identified, isolated, and surrounded with vessel loops.

The kidney was mobilized. The adrenal was quite superficial within Gerota's fascia, and the fascia was accidentally torn during the mobilization of the kidney. This was controlled with hemoclips. There was a large perinephric fat pad that was mobilized with the kidney initially, and then Gerota's fascia opened posteriorly. The area in question was identified. The patient had some reaction around the area, but this was not significant. There was a lot of fat adherent to the kidney that was dissected off the posterior region around the renal hilum to identify the mass. The mass appeared to be cystic in origin. A total of 3 cc of cyst fluid was aspirated from this and sent for cytology.

The cyst room was then opened. There was only a very small part of the cyst visible at the renal surface. Inspection of the cyst wall showed it to be smooth without masses. A small vessel was seen coursing inferiorly. This was cauterized. The renal pelvis was identified and Jelco catheter placed, and 5 cc of methylene blue–stained saline was injected through this to ensure that there was no communication with the cyst cavity and the renal pelvis. There was none.

The entire cyst wall was then cauterized. It was packed with Surgicel. Surgicel was also placed over the adrenal gland to help ensure hemostasis. Hemostasis was ensured. Vessel loops were removed. The kidney was then returned to renal fossa. A 10-mm Jackson-Pratt drain was left through a left lower quadrant stab wound and was placed adjacent to the de-roofed renal cyst.

The peritoneum was inspected, and there was no other abnormality identified on laparotomy.

The abdominal wall was then closed with three layers of 1 Vicryl. The skin was closed with surgical clips. A dressing was applied. Abdominal binder was applied. Prior to beginning closure of the abdominal wall, the rent in the pleura was closed with 3–0 Vicryl. Air was removed using a red rubber catheter in the usual fashion.

Sponge and needle counter were reported correct. The patient had a Foley catheter placed intraoperatively, and he had good urine output throughout the case. Estimated blood loss was 300 cc. He was transferred to the recovery room in good condition.

CPT Code(s): _____

ICD-9-CM Code(s): _____

Abstracting Questions

1. Was this procedure reported as an excision, even though the cyst was drained and the cyst wall retained? _____

2. Was de-roofing of renal cyst the same as an excision? _____

3. Did the accidental tear of the fascia require a separate, reportable repair? _____

4. Was a modifier reported? _____

5. Was the diagnosis for an acquired or congenital renal cyst? _____

Practice Exercise 3-37: Renal Mass

LOCATION: Inpatient, Hospital

PATIENT: Myra Grossman

ATTENDING PHYSICIAN: Ronald Green, MD

SURGEON: Ira Avila, MD

PREOPERATIVE DIAGNOSIS: Right renal mass.

POSTOPERATIVE DIAGNOSIS: Right renal cyst (acquired).

PROCEDURE PERFORMED: Laparoscopic exploration of kidneys, de-roofing, and biopsy of right renal mass.

ANESTHESIA: General.

SURGICAL INDICATIONS: This is a 20-year-old female who has a complex right renal cyst. She has been evaluated and worked up by Dr. Green. Options have been discussed, and she has elected to proceed with the exploration.

PROCEDURE: The patient was prepped and draped in the right flank position. A Foley catheter was placed. An incision was made. A retroperitoneal laparoscopic approach was used to approach the kidney, the cyst isolated, vessels identified and surrounded with vessel loops. The cyst was then aspirated and contents sent for cytology. The roof was ablated free and the base biopsied. There was some bleeding from the bases, which was controlled with 3–0 Chromic suture ligature. 3–0 Chromic sutures were used to close the cyst defect. A 10-mm flat Jackson-Pratt drain was left through a separate stab wound and sutured to the skin. The wound was closed with Vicryl and skin with clips. The patient tolerated the procedure well and was transferred to the recovery room in good condition. Estimated blood loss was 100 cc.

Pathology Report Later Indicated: Both pathology and cytology reports demonstrating benign cyst.

CPT Code(s): _____

ICD-9-CM Code(s): _____

Abstracting Question

1. What surgical approach was used for this procedure? _____

Practice Exercise 3-38: Abdominal Hysterectomy

OPERATIVE REPORT

LOCATION: Inpatient, Hospital

PATIENT: Maggie Brock

ATTENDING PHYSICIAN: Andy Martinez, MD

SURGEON: Andy Martinez, MD

PREOPERATIVE DIAGNOSES

1. Chronic menorrhagia.

2. Uterine fibroids.

POSTOPERATIVE DIAGNOSES

1. Chronic menorrhagia.

2. Uterine fibroids.

PROCEDURE PERFORMED: Total abdominal hysterectomy and bilateral salpingo-oophorectomy.

ANESTHESIA: General endotracheal.

SURGICAL INDICATION: This patient is a 48-year-old multiparous female who had had problems with chronic menorrhagia, unsuccessfully treated with hormone manipulation. She had known fibroids as well. Endometrial biopsy pre-operatively was benign.

OPERATIVE FINDINGS: The uterus was about 10- to 12-week size with multiple leiomyomas. There was a functional-appearing cyst on the left ovary that contained some clear fluid. The right ovary was normal. The appendix was retrocecal but otherwise unremarkable.

OPERATIVE DESCRIPTION: After induction of general anesthesia, the patient was in the supine position. The abdomen and vagina were prepped, and Foley catheter placed; the patient was then draped. The abdomen was opened through a midline hypogastric incision, excising the old skin scar on the way in. Bowel was then packed out of the pelvis and a self-retaining Balfour retractor was placed. The uterus was elevated with clamps at the cornual areas. The left round ligament was clamped, divided, suture ligated with 0 Vicryl. All sutures were 0 Vicryl unless otherwise indicated. The peritoneal lateral to the left infundibulopelvic ligament was opened with Metzenbaum scissors, isolated in the left ovarian vasculature. This pedicle was isolated, clamped, divided, and doubly ligated. An identical procedure was carried out in the structures on the right side. The anterior and posterior leaves of the broad ligament were taken down with Metzenbaum scissors. There was some abnormal scarring and retraction of the bladder flap on the left side due to her prior cesarean sections. We then skeletonized the uterine artery pedicles on either side. The uterine artery pedicles were clamped with curved Rogers clamps, cut, and suture ligated. The cardinal ligaments and paracervical tissue were taken with two bites of straight Heaney-Ballantine clamps and suture ligated. The vaginal angle was then clamped with curved Rogers clamps, cut and held. The anterior vagina was opened with scalpel; then the upper vagina was incised circumferentially with right-angled scissors. The uterus was then removed and handed off. The vaginal angles were sutured with 0 Vicryl, and the vaginal cuff was closed with a series of inter-rupted figure-of-eight 0 Vicryl sutures. There was a small bleeding area on one of the cardinal ligament pedicles on the left side. This was isolated with an Allis clamp and secured with a suture ligature. Sponges were then removed. Sponge and needle counts were correct. The abdominal fascia was closed with interrupted 0 Ethibond sutures and the skin with staples. Blood loss estimation by anesthesia was 250 cc. Specimen to pathology: Uterus, tubes, and ovaries. Final sponge and needle counts were correct.

CPT Code(s): _____

ICD-9-CM Code(s): _____

Abstracting Questions

1. What factors affect CPT code assignment for the abdominal hysterectomy?
   _____

2. What factors affect the diagnosis code selection for the uterine leiomyoma?
   _____

3. What is another name for leiomyoma? _____

Practice Exercise 3-39: Cesarean Section

OPERATIVE REPORT

The physician who performs the cesarean section will also provide the postpartum care in this case.

LOCATION: Inpatient, Hospital

PATIENT: Joan Tisdale

ATTENDING PHYSICIAN: Andy Martinez, MD

SURGEON: Andy Martinez, MD

PREOPERATIVE DIAGNOSES

1. Intrauterine pregnancy at 31 weeks and 6 days.

2. Abruptio placentae.

POSTOPERATIVE DIAGNOSES

1. Intrauterine pregnancy at 31 weeks and 6 days.

2. Abruptio placentae.

PROCEDURE PERFORMED: Primary low transverse cervical cesarean section.

ANESTHESIA: General endotracheal.

SURGICAL INDICATIONS: The patient is a 31-year-old woman, gravida 4, para 3, at 31 weeks 6 days by menstrual dates, who was transferred on an emergency basis because of uterine bleeding. She had an apparent abruption on ultrasound, and the vagina was filled with blood clot. For these reasons, she was taken to surgery for an emergency cesarean section.

OPERATIVE FINDINGS: The infant is female, born at 2007 hours, weighing 2125 grams (4 lb 10 ounces), with Apgar scores of 8 at 1 minute and 9 at 5 minutes. There was a lot of blood in the uterine cavity and some adherent clot to the placenta, estimated to be less than 10% abruption. The tubes and ovaries were normal.

PROCEDURE: The abdomen was prepped and draped. A Foley catheter was in. The patient was then given a general endotracheal anesthetic, and the abdomen was opened through a Pfannenstiel incision. Bladder flap was opened transversely with scissors, and bladder was dissected downward bluntly with a hand. A small incision was made in the myometrium of the lower uterine segment, and then entry into the uterus was accomplished bluntly with a Kelly clamp. Low transverse incision was made with bandage scissors. The infant was delivered without undue difficulty. The infant's mouth and nose were suctioned with a bulb syringe, the cord was clamped and cut, and the infant was handed to Dr. Ortez and the ICN staff. A segment of the cord was taken for cord blood gases, and the placenta was then delivered manually. Inspection of the uterine incision revealed there was a brisk bleeder near the left corner of the incision, and this was oversewn initially and the first layer was a running locked 0 Vicryl. The second layer was a running horizontal Lembert 0 Vicryl. The pelvis was irrigated with saline. The uterine incision was inspected, and there was a small amount of oozing from the incision, which was controlled with a single figure-of-eight 0 Vicryl suture. When hemostasis was adequate and lap sponges were correct, attention was directed toward closure. The peritoneum was loosely approximated in the midline with a couple of mattress sutures of 2–0 Vicryl. A medium Hemovac drain was placed subfascially to exit below the right side of the incision. The fascia was closed with running 0 Vicryl using two strands, one from either side to the middle and tied independently. The skin was closed with staples and the drain sutured to the skin with silk. Estimated blood loss was 1200-1500 cc.

Specimen to pathology was placenta. Final sponge and needle counts were correct.

CPT Code(s): _____

ICD-9-CM Code(s): _____

Abstracting Questions

1. What factor in this case determines the appropriate C-section code?
   _____

2. In addition to the placental abruption, what other two diagnoses must be reported? _____ and _____

Practice Exercise 3-40: Labial Excision

OPERATIVE REPORT

LOCATION: Inpatient, Hospital

PATIENT: Mary Brown

ATTENDING PHYSICIAN: Andy Martinez, MD

SURGEON: Andy Martinez, MD

PREOPERATIVE DIAGNOSIS: Vulvar intraepithelial neoplasia III of the right labia.

POSTOPERATIVE DIAGNOSIS: Vulvar intraepithelial neoplasia III of the right labia.

PROCEDURE PERFORMED: Radical excision, right labia.

PREAMBLE: The patient is a 47-year-old woman who presented with a right labial lesion. This was biopsied and reported as being VIN-III; invasion cannot be ruled out. The decision was therefore made to proceed with radical excision of the right vulva.

PROCEDURE: The patient was taken to the operating room and general anesthetic was administered. The patient was then prepped and draped in the usual manner in lithotomy position, and the bladder was emptied with a straight catheter. The vulva was then inspected. On the right labia majora at approximately the 11-o'clock position, there was a multifocal lesion present. A marking pen was then used to mark out an elliptical incision leaving a 1-cm border on all sides. The skin ellipse was then excised using the knife. Bleeders were cauterized with electrocautery. A running locked suture of 2–0 Vicryl was then placed in the deeper tissues. The skin was finally reapproximated with 4–0 Vicryl in an interrupted fashion. Good hemostasis was thereby achieved. The patient tolerated this procedure well. There were no complications. Estimated blood loss was 75 cc.

Pathology Report Later Indicated: Neoplasia III, carcinoma in situ.

CPT Code(s): _____

ICD-9-CM Code(s): _____

Abstracting Questions

1. In what area of the female genital anatomy is the labia located?

   _____

2. CPT code assignment was affected by the extent (partial/complete) and what other factor? _____

3. Define "in situ." _____

ENDOCRINE SYSTEM SUBSECTION (60000-60699)

Nine glands in endocrine system; only four included in subsection

1. Thyroid
2. Parathyroid
3. Thymus
4. Adrenal

Pituitary and Pineal. *See* Nervous System subsection

Pancreas. Digestive System

Ovaries and Testes. Respective genital systems

Divided into two subheadings

• Thyroid Gland

• Parathyroid, Thymus, Adrenal Glands, Pancreas, and Carotid Body

Carotid Body. Refers to area adjacent to the bifurcation of the carotid artery

Can be site of tumors

Thyroid Gland, Excision Category (60100-60281)

• **Lobectomy:** Partial or subtotal (something less than total)

• **Thyroidectomy:** Total (all)

Thyroid, 1 gland with 2 lobes

NERVOUS SYSTEM SUBSECTION (61000-64999)

Divided anatomically

• Skull, Meninges, and Brain

• Spine and Spinal Cord

• Extracranial Nerves, Peripheral Nerves, and Autonomic Nervous System

Skull, Meninges, and Brain (61000-62258)

Category Examples
Injection, Drainage, or Aspiration

Twist Drills, Burr Hole(s), or Trephine

Conditions that Require Openings Into Brain to
Relieve pressure

Insert monitoring devices

Place tubing

Inject contrast material

Craniectomy or Craniotomy (61304-61576)
Craniectomy involves removal of portion of skull, at operative site, performed emergently to prevent herniation of brain into the brainstem

Craniotomy—bone flap is replaced after surgery

Codes divided by site and condition for which procedure is performed

Surgery of Skull Base (61580-61619)
Skull base: Area at base of cranium

• Lesion removal from this area very complex

Surgery of Skull Base Terminology
Approach procedure used to gain exposure of lesion

Definitive procedure is what is done to lesion

Repair/reconstruction procedure reported separately only if extensive repair

Approach procedure and definitive procedure coded separately

   Example: Removal of an intradural lesion using middle cranial fossa approach

• 61590 approach procedure, middle cranial fossa and

• 61608 definitive procedure of intradural resection of lesion

Cerebrospinal Fluid (CSF) Shunt Category (62180-62258)
Performed to drain fluid

Codes describe, e.g.,

• Placement of devices

• Reprogramming

• Replacement

• Removal of shunting devices

Spine and Spinal Cord (62263-63746)

Codes divided by condition and approach

Often used are

• Unilateral or bilateral procedures (-50)

• Multiple procedures (-51)

• Radiologic supervision and fluoroscopic guidance reported separately

Includes codes for

• Spinal or steroid anesthetic injections 62310-62319

• Intrathecal or epidural catheter placement/implantation 62350-62355

Extracranial Nerves, Peripheral Nerves, and Autonomic Nervous System (64400-64999)

Introduction/Injection of Anesthetic Agent (Nerve Block), Diagnostic or Therapeutic Category (64400-64530)
Includes codes for

• Nerve blocks

   • Bundled when used as anesthesia for procedure

• Paravertebral facet joint injections 64490-64495, diagnostic or therapeutic

Epidural injections 64479-64484

- Used to provide pain relief
- As compared with an epidural catheter placement used for anesthetic purposes

EYE AND OCULAR ADNEXA SUBSECTION (65091-68899)

Terminology extremely important

- Code descriptions often vary only slightly

Understanding of eye anatomy is necessary for proper coding in this subsection

Codes divided anatomically, e.g.,

- Eyeball
- Anterior segment
- Posterior segment
- Ocular adnexa
- Conjunctiva

Some codes specifically for previous surgery

    Example: Insertion of ocular implant, secondary (65130)

Much bundling

    Example: Subheading Posterior Segment, Prophylaxis category notes indicate:

- "The following descriptors (67141, 67145) are intended to include all sessions in a defined treatment period."

Cataracts

Method used depends on type of cataract and surgeon preference

    Nuclear cataract: Most common, center of lens (nucleus), due to aging process

    Cortical cataract: Forms in cortex of lens and extends outward; frequent in diabetics

    Subcapsular cataract: Forms at back of lens, increased rate in diabetics, those who take steroid medications, certain genetic factors, and eye trauma

Lens removal (66830-66986)

- Extracapsular cataract extraction (ECCE)

    Patient retains posterior outer shell of the lens

    Soft cortex and rest of shell is removed in multiple pieces

    Posterior shell helps prevent vitreous prolapse

- Intracapsular cataract extraction (ICCE) is total removal

    Removes lens and capsule in one piece

- Phacoemulsification

    Small incision into eye and introduction of probe

    High-frequency waves fragment cataract (extracapsular); then suctioned out

    Lens placed through same small incision

Eyelids (67700-67999)

Blepharotomy (67700)

- Incision into eyelid for drainage of abscess

Blepharoplasty

- Repair of eyelid
- Codes in Integumentary System (15820-15823) report removal of excess skin
- Codes in Eye and Ocular Adnexa report muscle repairs and slings

  Selection of code depends on technique used to repair eyelid

- Blepharoplasty codes with specific techniques, 67901-67908

AUDITORY SYSTEM SUBSECTION (69000-69979)

Codes divided by

- External Ear (69000-69399)
- Middle Ear (69400-69799)
- Inner Ear (69801-69949)
- Temporal Bone, Middle Fossa Approach (69950-69979)

Understanding of ear anatomy is necessary for proper coding in this subsection

External, middle, and inner ear further divided by procedure

- Incision
- Excision
- Removal
- Repair

Myringotomy and tympanostomy

- Eustachian tube connects middle ear to back of throat for drainage
- Fluid collects in middle ear when tube does not function properly
- Prevents air from entering middle ear and pressure builds
- Surgical intervention

  Myringotomy (incision into tympanic membrane)

  Tympanostomy (placement of PE [pressure equalization] tube)

OPERATING MICROSCOPE SUBSECTION (+69990)

Employed with procedures using microsurgical techniques

Code in addition to primary procedure performed

Do not report separately when primary procedure description includes microsurgical techniques

  Example: 15758 Free fascial flap with microvascular anastomosis

Note that following 15758 is the statement:

- "(Do not report code 69990 in addition to code 15758)" indicating to the coder not to report the use of the operating microscope separately

Do not report 69990 when magnifying loupes are used

■ PRACTICE EXERCISES

Practice Exercise 3-41: Intracerebral Hematoma

OPERATIVE PROCEDURE

LOCATION: Inpatient, Hospital

PATIENT: Suzy Kunklemann

ATTENDING PHYSICIAN: Gary Sanchez, MD

SURGEON: Gary Sanchez, MD

PREOPERATIVE DIAGNOSIS: Intracerebral hematoma (nontraumatic), right temporal lobe.

POSTOPERATIVE DIAGNOSIS: Intracerebral hematoma (nontraumatic), right temporal lobe.

PROCEDURE PERFORMED: Osteoplastic craniotomy, right temporal area; evacuation of intracerebral hematoma.

ANESTHESIA: General.

PROCEDURE: Under general anesthesia, the patient's head was placed in the Mayfield pins. The right frontal temporoparietal area was prepped and draped in the usual manner. A linear incision was made extending from the midline of the temporal fossa up to the midportion of the scalp. The skin was incised. The temporalis muscle was separated and divided off the bone. I did a craniotomy here the size of a half-dollar and made a burr hole. I utilized the craniotome to elevate the bone flap, and this was a free bone flap. This was then removed. We placed the Weitlaners into the wound and then incised the dura in a cruciate fashion over the temporal lobe. I then entered the middle temple gyrus and irrigated much of the clot from the temporal and posterior parietal areas, and evacuated the clot from the area. This took copious irrigation. We used cotton balls for hemostasis. I did this numerous times until all the bleeders were coagulated. I then lined the cystic cavity with Gelfoam and coagulated the edges of the raw brain. I closed the dura with 4–0 Vicryl. This was closed in a watertight fashion. I used 2–0 Vicryl to elevate the dura to the bone flap with Wurzburg plates, two of them, utilizing plates and screws. I then closed the scalp in one layer using 0 Vicryl on the temporalis muscle and fascia, and the skin was approximated with 2–0 nylon interrupted mattress sutures. Dressing was applied, and the patient was on the ventilator and discharged to the surgical intensive care unit.

CPT Code(s): _____

ICD-9-CM Code(s): _____

Abstracting Questions

1. Was the procedure performed a surgical craniotomy? _____

2. Does the area of the skull being opened affect the code? _____

3. What was the purpose of the procedure? _____

4. Does the purpose of the procedure affect the CPT code? _____

Practice Exercise 3-42: Parietal Burr Holes

OPERATIVE PROCEDURE

LOCATION: Inpatient, Hospital

PATIENT: Reed Scaleni

ATTENDING PHYSICIAN: Gary Sanchez, MD

SURGEON: Gary Sanchez, MD

PREOPERATIVE DIAGNOSIS: Subacute subdural hematoma (nontraumatic), right side.

POSTOPERATIVE DIAGNOSIS: Subacute subdural hematoma (nontraumatic), right side.

PROCEDURE PERFORMED: Burr hole times two, right frontal and right posterior parietal.

ANESTHESIA: General.

PROCEDURE: Under general anesthesia, the patient's head was prepped and draped in the usual manner. The incision was made. Straight line linear incisions over the frontal and posterior parietal areas were made on the right side. Retractors were placed. Burr holes remained. The dura was visualized. The bony edges were waxed with beeswax. The dura was incised, both the frontal and the parietal holes. Serosanguineous fluid and clouded blood exuded. I cleaned it out until the supernatant was clear. The brain was found to be pulsating beneath. We then placed two medium-size Penrose drains and closed the galea with 2–0 Vicryl. The skin was approximated with surgical staples, and the Penrose drains were anchored with sutures. A dressing was applied. The patient was discharged to the PAR.

CPT Code(s): _____

ICD-9-CM Code(s): _____

Abstracting Questions

1. What determines the code assignment for burr holes of the skull?

   _____

2. Does the location of the hematoma being drained/aspirated make a difference in the CPT code assignment? _____

3. Was this CPT code reported twice for the two burr holes? _____

4. Was a modifier reported to indicate which side of the skull was drilled?

   _____

Practice Exercise 3-43: Carpal Tunnel

OPERATIVE PROCEDURE

LOCATION: Outpatient, Hospital

PATIENT: Judy Burns

ATTENDING PHYSICIAN: Gary Sanchez, MD

SURGEON: Gary Sanchez, MD

PREOPERATIVE DIAGNOSIS: Left carpal tunnel syndrome.

POSTOPERATIVE DIAGNOSIS: Left carpal tunnel syndrome.

PROCEDURE PERFORMED: Carpal tunnel released, left wrist.

ANESTHESIA: Regional.

PROCEDURE: After a satisfactory level of regional anesthesia, the extremity was addressed once it had been sterilely prepped and draped. Throughout the procedure the patient needed some focal augmentation for sharp pain characteristics at the level of the skin most distally about the skin wound. Sharp dissection was conducted down to the palmaris fascia. We identified the deep transverse ligament. In a blunt manner, we undermined this, and with use of a Freer interposing between deep transverse carpal ligament and the medial nerve, sharply dissected over the Freer, releasing the impinging structures about the carpal canal. The probe palpation, the tendinous structures, and the floor of the carpal canal were otherwise unremarkable. She has at this time an exiting thenar motor branch, which was not obscured. There is an hourglass deformity of the median nerve as noted. At completion of this the wound was irrigated, followed by closure of the dermal planes and application of a splint. The patient tolerated the procedure well and was transported to the recovery room in a stable manner.

CPT Code(s): _____

ICD-9-CM Code(s): _____

Abstracting Question

1. Release of the carpal tunnel has what effect on the median nerve?

_____

Practice Exercise 3-44: Repair of Pseudomeningocele

OPERATIVE PROCEDURE

This patient is returned to the operating room during the postoperative period for a decompression laminectomy performed by the same physician who now performs the pseudomeningocele repair.

LOCATION: Inpatient, Hospital

PATIENT: Debbie Smith

ATTENDING PHYSICIAN: Gary Sanchez, MD

SURGEON: Gary Sanchez, MD

PREOPERATIVE DIAGNOSIS: Pseudomeningocele.

POSTOPERATIVE DIAGNOSIS: Pseudomeningocele.

PROCEDURE PERFORMED: Repair of pseudomeningocele at the L4-5 level just to the left of the midline.

PROCEDURE: The patient was taken to the operating room and underwent placement of a spinal drain by the anesthesiologist. She then underwent induction of a general endotracheal anesthesia. She was flipped to the prone position and was thoroughly prepped and draped. The previous incision was reopened and was extended approximately 1 inch both superiorly and inferiorly. A large amount of spinal fluid came forth. There was a well-epithelialized membrane underneath the subcutaneous tissue extending deep to the muscle. This was excised as much as possible. I first dissected the paraspinal muscles laterally on each side along the L2 vertebra. I identified epithelial lining consistent with a pseudomeningocele. I saw a small leak and thought that I saw spinal fluid coming from the small defect. I gave a Valsalva maneuver, but it was not crystal clear whether this was spinal fluid or merely epidural blood. Anyway, I packed this off with Surgicel, placed a small fat graft, and secured it with a 4–0 Nurolon. I then used the FloSeal and Duragen to seal off the defect. I began reapproximating the muscle when I then noticed that there was spinal fluid again coming from the inferior portion of the incision. I exposed the lamina of L5 bilaterally and placed a retractor. I then noticed that there was a dural defect just to the left of the midline between the L4 and L5 laminae. I did a partial hemilaminectomy of L5 on the left side and was able to place three separate 4–0 Nurolon sutures through the dural defect. Care was taken to depress the nerve within the dural sac with a #4 Penfield. I then directly repaired the dura and did not see any further spinal fluid leakage with a Valsalva maneuver. I then used some FloSeal and strategically placed pieces of Surgicel to cover the defect. I then placed a small piece of Duragen on top of this as well. I irrigated with copious amounts of saline. I then closed the muscle in the deep fascia with interrupted 2–0 Vicryls, which were very closely approximated. I then used interrupted 2–0 Vicryl to close the subcutaneous tissue. The skin was closed with a running 4–0 nylon interlocking stitch. A sterile dressing was placed.

The patient tolerated the procedure well without apparent complications. The spinal drain was sutured in by me at the end of the procedure. She was taken to the recovery room in stable condition. Sponge, instrument, and needle counts were correct times two.

CPT Code(s): _____

ICD-9-CM Code(s): _____

Abstracting Questions

1. Repair of the pseudomeningocele is repair of what? _____

2. What procedure was performed to clear the approach for the repair of the dura tear? _____

3. Does the pseudomeningocele make a difference in the CPT code assignment? _____

4. What modifiers are required? _____

Practice Exercise 3-45: Laminectomy with Foraminotomy

OPERATIVE PROCEDURE

LOCATION: Inpatient, Hospital

PATIENT: Karen Origami

ATTENDING PHYSICIAN: Gary Sanchez, MD

SURGEON: Gary Sanchez, MD

PREOPERATIVE DIAGNOSIS: Severe spinal stenosis from L3 through L5.

POSTOPERATIVE DIAGNOSIS: Severe spinal stenosis from L3 through L5 without neurogenic claudications.

PROCEDURES PERFORMED
1. Bilateral L3 laminectomy with foraminotomy.
2. Bilateral L4 laminectomy with foraminotomy.
3. Bilateral L5 laminectomy with foraminotomy.

INDICATION: This patient is a 79-year-old female who presented with severe neurogenic claudication, left greater than right. Workup included an MRI scan, which showed severe spinal stenosis from L3 through L5. After discussion of the options, she elected to undergo surgery. She was informed that this was an elective surgery and was not life or limb threatening. The risks of the procedure were thoroughly discussed, and the patient consented to proceed.

PROCEDURE: The patient was taken to the operating room and underwent induction after general endotracheal anesthesia in the supine position. She was then flipped to the prone position on the operating room table and the knees were flexed. The lower lumbar spine was thoroughly prepped and draped, and a vertical midline skin incision was made from the L3 to the S1 spinous processes. The skin was infiltrated with local anesthetic prior to making the incision. Using the monopolar cautery, I identified the spinous processes of L2 through S1 bilaterally. Then using the periosteal elevator, I retracted the paraspinal muscles laterally bilaterally. Deep retractors were placed. At this point, I used the handheld rongeur and removed the spinous processes of L4 and L3. An intraoperative x-ray was done to verify the location. At this, the L5 spinous process was then removed. I then alternated between the rongeurs and the high-speed burr, and drilled down the medial facets and the lamina of L5, L4, and L3. I then began using the Kerrison and removed the inferior lamina of L5 and proceeded from a caudal to cephalad direction. I alternated between the high-speed drill and the Kerrison rongeurs and eventually removed the lamina and the medial facets bilaterally of L3 through L5. There was noted to be very severe compression of the thecal sac at the L4-5 level as there was a grade 1 spondylolisthesis at that level. There was also noted to be severe spinal stenosis at the L3-4 level. After an adequate decompression, I made sure that the decompression extended laterally out to the exiting nerve roots on each side bilaterally. The nerve roots were particularly tight at the L4-5 level, where the spondylolisthesis was located. At no time was there a dural tear or spinal fluid leak. I irrigated with copious amounts of saline. Bleeding bone edges were waxed. The gutters were lined with Surgicel, and a piece of Gelfoam was placed over the exposed dura. I irrigated again. I closed the wound in layers with interrupted 0 and 2–0 Vicryl. Skin was closed with a running 3–0 Vicryl subcuticular stitch. Benzoin and one-half-inch Steri-Strips and a sterile dressing were placed.

The patient tolerated the procedure well without apparent complication. She will go to the recovery room after the surgery. Sponge, instrument, and needle counts were correct.

CPT Code(s): _____

ICD-9-CM Code(s): _____

Abstracting Questions

1. In addition to the laminectomy with foraminotomy, what other procedure was performed? _____

2. Which vertebrae were addressed? _____

3. How many codes are necessary to report all three vertebrae?
   _____

4. What modifiers are required? _____

■ RADIOLOGY SECTION (70010-79999)

Radiology: Branch of medicine that uses radiant energy to diagnose and treat patients

Specialist in radiology: Radiologist (doctor of medicine)

Radiology Subsections

1. Diagnostic Radiology
2. Diagnostic Ultrasound
3. Radiologic Guidance
4. Breast/Mammography
5. Bone/Joint Studies
6. Radiation Oncology
7. Nuclear Medicine

Procedures

Fluoroscopy views inside of body, projects onto television screen

Live images by which physician can view function, structure, and defects or anomalies within an organ

> ***Example:*** 71034 chest x-ray with fluoroscopy

Magnetic Resonance Imaging (MRI)

> ***Example:*** 72148 MRI of spinal canal

Tomography or Computed Axial Tomography (CAT or CT Scan)

> ***Example:*** 70450 tomographic scan of head or brain

Planes of Body (Fig. 3-14)

Position and Projection

Position = method of positioning patients for examination

Projection path = pathway traveled by x-ray beam

Component Coding

Three component terms

1. Professional
2. Technical
3. Global

Professional Component

Physician portion of service, includes

- Supervision of technician
- Interpretation of results, including written report

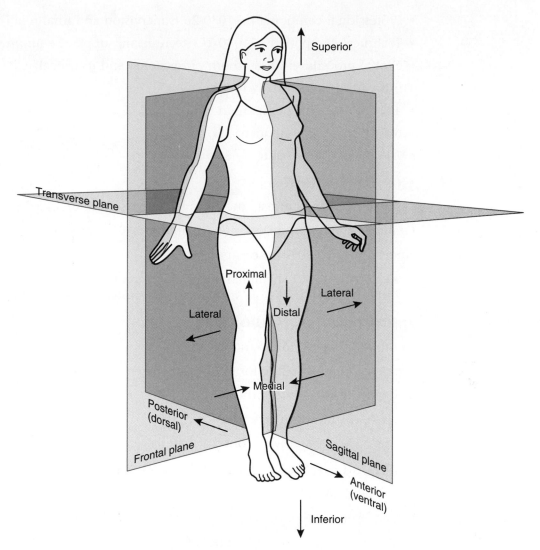

Figure **3-14** Planes of the body.

Technical Component
- Technologist's services
- Equipment, film, and supplies

Global Procedure
Both professional and technical portions of radiology service

Component Modifiers
If only professional component of radiology service provided: add -26

If only technical component provided: add -TC

- -TC HCPCS modifier used with CPT and HCPCS codes

If both professional and technical components of radiology service are provided by physician who owns equipment and facility, pays technician and supplies (global), no modifier is needed

> **Example:** Chest x-ray

- Professional component: 71030-26 (supervision and final report)
- Technical component: 71030-TC (technician, supplies, equipment)
- Global procedure: 71030 (both professional and technical)

Third-party payers usually reimburse

- 40% professional component
- 60% technical component
- 100% global procedure

Contrast Material

Statement "with contrast" indicates injection service included in code

Oral or rectal contrast does not qualify for "with contrast"

Notes indicate codes for components

> *Example:* 75801, Lymphangiography, parenthetical note above code indicates: "For injection procedure for lymphatic system, use 38790"

Interventional Radiologist

Combination radiologist and surgeon

Provides total procedure for cystography with contrast

- Report 74430, x-ray portion
- 51600 for injection procedure
- Plus code for supply of contrast material (e.g., 99070)

DIAGNOSTIC RADIOLOGY SUBSECTION (70010-76499)

Most standard radiographic procedures

Codes often divided by whether contrast material used

Codes further divided by number of views

> *Example:* 71030, Chest x-ray, complete, minimum of 4 views

Used to:

- Diagnose disease
- Monitor disease process—progression or remission
- Therapeutic procedures (guidance)

Diagnostic Procedures Include

X-ray

Computerized axial tomography (CAT or CT scan)

Magnetic resonance imaging (MRI)

Angiography

Fluoroscopy

3D rendering

Computed Axial Tomography (CAT or CT)

X-ray image taken in sections

Computer reconstructs and enhances image

Magnetic Resonance Imaging (MRI)
Uses magnetic fields to produce an image displayed on computer screen

Codes of same area (e.g., spine) divided by whether or not contrast material used

Angiography
Used to view vessel obstructions

Dye injected into vessel

Radiologist uses angiography to diagnose vascular conditions

Example:

- Malformation

- Stroke (cerebrovascular accident, CVA)

- Myocardial infarction (MI)

Remember
- If fewer than total number of views specified in code provided: Report -52, Reduced Service

---

DIAGNOSTIC ULTRASOUND SUBSECTION (76506-76999)
Uses high-frequency sound waves to image anatomic structures

Nine subheadings of Diagnostic Ultrasound

Primarily based on anatomy

A-mode (A = Amplitude)
Technique used to map structure outline in one-dimensional image

M-mode (M = Motion)
Technique used to display one-dimensional movement of structure

B-scan (B = Brightness)
Technique used to display two-dimensional movement of tissues and organs

Known as gray scale ultrasound

Real-Time Scan
Technique used to display both structure and motion with time of organ and tissues in a two-dimensional image

Extent of Study
Codes often divided on extent of study

Example: Extent of scan as follows

- **Complete:** Scans entire body or body region

- **Limited:** Scans part of body, e.g., one organ

- **Follow-up/repeat:** Limited study of part of body that was scanned previously

Three Locations for Ultrasound Services

76506-76999: Radiology codes for diagnostic ultrasound services

93880-93990: Medicine codes for non-invasive vascular studies

93303-93352: Medicine codes for echocardiography

RADIOLOGIC GUIDANCE SUBSECTION (77001-77022)

Guidance

- Fluoroscopic
- Computed tomography
- Magnetic resonance
- Other

BREAST MAMMOGRAPHY SUBSECTION (77051-77059)

Example: Computer-aided detection and screening

Some codes specified unilateral/bilateral

BONE/JOINT STUDIES SUBSECTION (77071-77084)

Example: Bone density, bone mineral density, and joint survey

RADIATION ONCOLOGY SUBSECTION (77261-77799)

Therapeutic use of radiation

Codes both professional and technical services

Subheadings divided based on treatment

Initial consultation, prior to decision to treat, reported with E/M consultation code

- **Outpatient:** 99241-99245
- **Inpatient:** 99251-99255

No reimbursement through CMS for consultation codes

Clinical Treatment Planning—Professional Component (77261-77299)

Includes

- Interpretation of special testing
- Tumor localization
- Determination of treatment volume
- Choice of treatment method
- Determination of number of treatment ports
- Selection of treatment devices
- Other necessary procedures

Clinical Treatment Planning consists of

- Planning
- Simulation

Three Levels of Planning (77261-77263)

1. **Simple:** One treatment area, one port, or one set of parallel ports
2. **Intermediate:** Three or more ports, two separate treatment areas, multiple blocking
3. **Complex:** Complex blocking, custom shielding blocks, tangential ports, special wedges, 3+ treatment areas, special beams

Simulation (77280-77293)

Determining placement of treatment areas/ports for radiation treatment

Does not include administration of radiation

Definitions of Simulation

1. **Simple:** 1 treatment area with 1 port or pair of ports
2. **Intermediate:** 3+ ports, 2 separate treatment areas, multiple blocking
3. **Complex:** Tangential ports, 3+ treatment areas, complex blocking
4. **Computer-generated 3-D:** reconstruction of volume of tumor and critical structures

Medical Radiation, Physics, Dosimetry, Treatment Devices, and Special Services (77295, 77300-77370)

Decision making services of physicians

- Treatment types
- Dose calculation and placement (dosimetry)
- Development of treatment device

Stereotactic Radiation Treatment Delivery (77371-77373)

Delivers large radiation dose to specific tumor sites

- Computer(s) map location
- Radiation delivered to one or more sites

Radiation and Neutron Beam Treatment Delivery (77401-77525)

Technical component of actual delivery of radiation

Information Needed to Code Radiation Treatment Delivery
Amount of radiation delivered

Type of radiation—electron (most common), neutron, or proton

Number of

- Areas treated (single, two, three or more)
- Ports involved (single, three or more, tangential)
- Blocks used (none, multiple, custom)

Reporting Radiation Treatment Management (77427-77499)

Professional (physician) portion of services, including

- Review port films
- Review dosimetry, dose delivery, treatment parameters
- Treatment set-up
- Patient examination for medical E/M

Report in units of five fractions, unless last 3-4 fractions are at the end of the treatment; then you can count the last 3-4 as an additional fraction

Hyperthermia (77600-77615)

Use of heat by means of ultrasound, probes, microwave, etc.

Treatment delivered at three levels:

- External (superficial and deep)
- Interstitial
- Intracavitary

Used in addition to radiation therapy or chemotherapy

Includes three months follow-up after procedure

Clinical Brachytherapy (77750-77799)

Placement of radioactive material into or around site of tumor

- Intracavitary (within body cavity)
- Interstitial (within tissues)

Source
Radioactive element delivers radiation dose over time

> *Example:* Seeds, ribbons, or capsules

- **Ribbons:** Seeds embedded on tape and inserted into tissue
- Tape is cut to desired length, thereby controlling amount of radiation

Clinical Brachytherapy Codes Divided Based on
Number of sources applied

- Simple 1-4
- Intermediate 5-10
- Complex 11+

NUCLEAR MEDICINE SUBSECTION (78012-79999)

Placement of radioactive material into body and measurement of emissions

Used for both diagnosis and treatment

Codes divided primarily on organ system

- Except "Therapeutic," which is for radiopharmaceutical therapies

■ PRACTICE EXERCISES

Practice Exercise 3-46: Cranial CT

RADIOLOGY REPORT

LOCATION: Inpatient, Hospital

PATIENT: Bill Arnold

ORDERING PHYSICIAN: Timothy L. Pleasant, MD

ATTENDING/ADMIT PHYSICIAN: Timothy L. Pleasant, MD

RADIOLOGIST: Morton Monson, MD

PERSONAL PHYSICIAN: Ronald Green, MD

EXAMINATION: Cranial CT.

CLINICAL SYMPTOMS: Altered mental status.

TECHNIQUE: Axial noncontrast CT scan of the head.

INTERPRETATION: There is diffuse mild enlargement of the sulci and ventricles. Periventricular diminished density is present bilaterally and is prominent near the trigones of the lateral ventricles. There is a 1-mm high-density area seen on image 10 in the left posterior temporal occipital region.

In the posterior fossa the fourth ventricle is normal in position. Mildly prominent cerebellar folia are present.

No abnormalities of the orbits, paranasal sinuses, or temporal bone can be seen.

There is a small amount of calcification in the paraclinoid and carotid arteries.

CONCLUSIONS
1. Mild diffuse cerebral atrophy.
2. Periventricular changes consistent with age-related ischemic change.
3. Tiny calcification in the left posterior temporal occipital region. Finding is nonspecific and could reflect previous granulomatous calcification, intraluminal calcification, Pantopaque, or calcification in a lesion. Recommend clinical correlation and cranial MRI if appropriate.
4. Vascular calcifications are present.

CPT Code(s): _____

ICD-9-CM Code(s): _____

Abstracting Questions

1. What was the clinical symptom that prompted this CT? _____

2. Sulci were referred to in the Interpretation section. What are sulci?

_____

Practice Exercise 3-47: Gallbladder Ultrasound

RADIOLOGY REPORT

LOCATION: Outpatient, Hospital

PATIENT: Dan Diel

ORDERING PHYSICIAN: Daniel G. Olanka, MD

ATTENDING/ADMIT PHYSICIAN: Daniel G. Olanka, MD

RADIOLOGIST: Morton Monson, MD

PERSONAL PHYSICIAN: Ronald Green, MD

EXAMINATION: Gallbladder ultrasound.

CLINICAL SYMPTOMS: Increased bilirubin.

GALLBLADDER ULTRASOUND: Examination was technically difficult with some limitations due to overlying leads. Large right pleural effusion identified. Gallbladder is visualized. No obvious gallstones or gallbladder wall thickening. Only short portions of the common hepatic duct and common bile duct are visualized. Common hepatic duct measures 3.6 mm, and common bile duct measures 5.2 mm. These values are within normal limits. There is limited assessment of the liver, which is grossly unremarkable.

IMPRESSION: Gallbladder ultrasound with limitations as discussed above. Grossly unremarkable sonographic appearance of the gallbladder. No obvious dilatation of the common duct. Large right pleural effusion identified.

CPT Code(s): _____

ICD-9-CM Code(s): _____

Abstracting Questions

1. What subcategory within Radiology in the CPT was referenced for assignment of a code for this case? _____

2. What body area was evaluated? _____

3. What code range in the CPT was reviewed to select the ultrasound code?
   _____

4. What modifier was appended to the CPT code? _____

Practice Exercise 3-48: Stress Test

RADIOLOGY REPORT

LOCATION: Outpatient, Hospital

PATIENT: Harry Stein

ORDERING PHYSICIAN: James Noonar, MD

ATTENDING/ADMIT PHYSICIAN: James Noonar, MD

RADIOLOGIST: Morton Monson, MD

PERSONAL PHYSICIAN: Ronald Green, MD

EXAMINATION: Adenosine stress test and resting Myoview, left ventricle, with estimate of left ventricular ejection fraction.

CLINICAL SYMPTOMS: Chest pain.

ADENOSINE STRESS AND RESTING MYOVIEW EVALUATION, LEFT VENTRICLE, WITH ESTIMATE OF LEFT VENTRICULAR EJECTION FRACTION: Clinical information states chest pain. This is a patient with known coronary artery disease. The patient has had prior replacement of aortic and mitral valve 3 to 4 years ago by history. The patient has a previous Cardiolite scan from December 24 two years ago that showed "fixed posterior/inferior wall perfusion defect extending into the cardiac apex." On September 12 of this year, the patient was given adenosine challenge under the supervision of Dr. Dawson, who will report on that portion of the evaluation. On September 12, the patient was injected with 27.2 mCi of technetium-99m–tagged tetrofosmin. Views of the left ventricle were then acquired with a SPECT nuclear medicine camera and reformatted into the standard projections. On September 13, the patient was returned to the nuclear medicine department for resting or redistribution scan and injected with 26.2 mCi of technetium-99m–tagged tetrofosmin. Again, views of the left ventricle were acquired with the SPECT nuclear medicine camera and reformatted into standard projections. Comparison of the stress and resting images shows no area to suggest perfusion defect. Nothing to suggest ischemia or infarct is seen. All segments of the left ventricle are perfused.

IMPRESSION
1. Adenosine challenge as the stress. That will be reported by Dr. Dawson.
2. Normal adenosine stress and resting Myoview evaluation, left ventricle. No region suggesting ischemia or infarct.

ADDENDUM: Previously described fixed perfusion defect involving posterior/inferior wall and apex is no longer seen.

Left ventricular ejection fraction estimated at 66%. This is normal. Normal is 50% or greater.

CPT Code(s): _____

ICD-9-CM Code(s): _____

Abstracting Questions

1. Does use of the SPECT camera affect code assignment? _____

2. Were the left ventricular perfusion and ejection fractions reported separately?

_____

Practice Exercise 3-49: Head Ultrasound

LOCATION: Inpatient, Hospital

PATIENT: Jason Whittle

ATTENDING PHYSICIAN: Rolando Ortez, MD

CLINICAL SYMPTOMS: Premature, weight 1800 grams.

HEAD ULTRASOUND: Sonographic evaluation of the newborn brain was performed through the anterior fontanel. The study was performed in the coronal and sagittal planes. There is a hyperechoic area seen within the right subependymal region. This measures $0.6 \times 0.4 \times 0.5$ cm. I suspect this is a subependymal hemorrhage. There is also an area within the left intraparenchymal region measuring $0.9 \times 1.0 \times 1.4$ cm. This is a hyperechoic area, which may represent an intraparenchymal hemorrhage on the left parietal/occipital region. There is also question of a small septum cavum pellucidum. This is difficult to state for certain, however.

CONCLUSION
1. What appears to be a right subependymal hemorrhage, as discussed above.
2. Hyperechoic area within the left intraparenchymal region. It may also represent a focal area of hemorrhage measuring 1 cm in greatest diameter.
3. Question of small septum cavum pellucidum as a congenital variation. This is very questionable and difficult to assess for the patient's age. The ventricles themselves do not appear to be grossly dilated.

CPT Code(s): _____

ICD-9-CM Code(s): _____

Abstracting Questions

1. In what CPT section was the code to report this service located?

_____

2. In what CPT category of codes was the code to report this service located?

_____

Practice Exercise 3-50: Neonatal Cystourethrogram

LOCATION: Inpatient, Hospital

PATIENT: Crystal Morgan

ATTENDING PHYSICIAN: Rolando Ortez, MD

RADIOLOGIST: Morton Monson, MD

CLINICAL SYMPTOMS: Congenital hydronephrosis.

VOIDING URETHROCYSTOGRAPHY: The study is technically limited due to the infant's inability to cooperate. The urinary bladder was filled to presumed capacity before spontaneous voiding. The bladder capacity is estimated at 25 cc. No immediate, delayed, or voiding reflux is demonstrated.

IMPRESSION: No definite vesicoureteral reflux demonstrated.

CPT Code(s): _____

ICD-9-CM Code(s): _____

Abstracting Questions

1. Was this an acquired or congenital condition? _____

2. What type of evaluation was performed? _____

■ PATHOLOGY AND LABORATORY SECTION (80047-89398)

- Organ or Disease-Oriented Panels
- Drug Testing
- Therapeutic Drug Assays
- Evocative/Suppression Testing
- Consultations (Clinical Pathology)
- Urinalysis
- Molecular Pathology
- Multianalyte Assays with Algorithmic Analyses
- Chemistry
- Hematology and Coagulation
- Immunology
- Transfusion Medicine
- Microbiology
- Anatomic Pathology
- Cytopathology
- Cytogenetic Studies
- Surgical Pathology
- In Vivo (Transcutaneous) Laboratory Procedures
- Other Procedures
- Reproductive Medicine Procedures

Pathology and Laboratory

Codes for laboratory test only

Specimen collection coded separately

Example: Venous blood draw reported with 36415 (Surgery section)

Facility Indicators

Allow additional tests without physician written order

Example: Urinalysis positive for bacteria, built-in indicator for culture

Pathology/Laboratory Caution

Report second or subsequent tests without -51, multiple procedures

Organ or Disease Oriented Panels (80047-80076)

Groups of tests often ordered together

Examples:
- Basic Metabolic Panel
- General Health Panel
- Electrolyte Panel

Rules of Panels

All tests must have been conducted

Do not use -52, Reduced Service

Additional tests, over those in panel, reported separately

If all tests in panel not done

- List each test separately
- Do not use panel code

Drug Testing (80100-80104)

Identifies presence or absence of drug—qualitative analysis

Confirmation conducted to double-check results of positive drug test (80102)

Chromatography procedure in which multiple drugs identified (80100)

- Some machines identify all drugs present in 1 procedure
- Others require 2+ procedures to identify 2+ drugs

Code the number of procedures, not number of drugs tested for

> *Example:*
>
> - 2 procedures to identify 3 drugs = 80100×2
> - 1 procedure to identify 3 drugs = 80100

Does not identify amount of drug present

- Only presence or absence

Other than chromatographic method, each procedure, 80104

Therapeutic Drug Assays (80150-80299)

Reports the presence and amount (quantitative)

Material examined can be from any source

Drugs listed by generic names

> *Example:* Amitriptyline, generic name for brand name Elavil

Evocative/Suppression Testing (80400-80440)

Measures stimulating (evocative) or suppressing agents

Codes report only technical component of service

Additional services reported

- Supplies and/or drugs used in testing (99070 or HCPCS code)

E/M code reported for physician monitoring of test

Consultations (Clinical Pathology) (80500, 80502)

At request of physician

Additional information about specimen

Consultant prepares written report

Levels

Limited without review of medical record

Comprehensive with review of medical record

More Consultation Codes (88321-88334)

Surgical Pathology

Used when pathologist either

- Reviews slides, material, or reports
- Provides consultation during surgery

Reported by number of specimens

Urinalysis (81000-81099)

Tests on Urine

Method of test

- e.g., tablet, reagent, or dipstick

Reason for test

- e.g., pregnancy

Constituents being tested for

- e.g., bilirubin, glucose

Equipment Used

Automated or nonautomated

With or without microscope

Molecular Pathology (81161, 81200-81479)

- 81161, 81200-81383 are Tier 1 procedures that report molecular assay
  - More common gene specific procedures
  - Example, breast cancer gene—81211 (BRCA1 or BRCA2)
- 81400-81479 are Tier 2 procedures to report less commonly performed analyses

Multianalyte Assays with Algorithmic Analyses (81500-81599)

Analyses that use the results of various measures and patient information to predict probabilites in a numeric form

CPT notes and Appendix O provide further detail

Chemistry (82000-84999)

Specific tests on any bodily substances

- Urine
- Blood
- Breath
- Feces
- Sputum

Most are for quantitative (amount of) screenings only

Few report qualitative (presence of) screenings

Samples from different sources reported separately, e.g., blood, feces

Samples taken different times of day reported separately

Hematology and Coagulation (85002-85999)

Laboratory procedures on blood

Example:

- Complete blood count (CBC)
- White blood cell count (WBC)

Codes divided based on method of

- Blood draw
- Test being conducted

Immunology (86000-86849)

Identifying immune system conditions caused by antibodies and antigens

Example: Hepatitis C antibody screening

Tissue Typing (86805-86849)
Compatibility test on tissue

- Match donor to recipient
- Measure/monitor cytotoxic reactions

Transfusion Medicine (86850-86999)

Blood bank codes

Tests performed on blood or blood products

Identifies

- Collection
- Processing
- Typing

Microbiology (87001-87999)

Study of Microorganisms
Identification of organism

Sensitivities of organism to antibiotics

Microbiology Caution: Many code descriptions are similar to those in Immunology (86000-86849), with the only difference being **technique** used

---

Anatomic Pathology (88000-88099)

Postmortem examinations

- Autopsies

Reports only physician service

Codes divided on extent of exam and type of examination—gross versus gross and microscopic

Example: Gross examination without central nervous system (88000)

Cytopathology (88104-88199)

Identifies cellular changes

Common laboratory procedures, e.g., Pap smear

Codes divided by

- Type of procedure
- Technique used

Cytogenetic Studies (88230-88299)

Branch of genetics concerned with cellular abnormalities and pathologic conditions

> *Example:* Chromosomes

Surgical Pathology (88300-88399)

Pathology Terminology

Specimen sample of tissue of suspect area

- Basis of reporting determined by number of labeled specimens

Block: Frozen piece of specimen

Section is a slice of frozen block

Evaluation of Specimens to Determine Disease Pathology

Tissue removed during procedures undergoes pathology evaluation

Operative report usually coded after pathology report received

Pathology reports usually coded with operative report

Unit of measure (88300-88309), specimen

- 2 separately identifiable anus tags, each examined, 88304 × 2
- 1 anus tag examined in 2 different areas of tag, 88304

Types of Pathologic Examination

Microscopic: With microscope

Gross: Without microscope

- 88300, only gross exam code
- Other codes are gross and microscopic

Six Levels of Surgical Pathology

Based on specimen examined (e.g., breast, prostate, lung) and reason for evaluation (e.g., radical procedure for suspected carcinoma)

Levels divided on complexity of examination

> *Example:*
>
> 88305, Colon, Biopsy
>
> 88307, Colon, Segmental Resection, Other than for Tumor
>
> 88309, Colon, Total Resection

Level I

- Specimen can be accurately diagnosed without microscopic examination

Level II
- Gross and microscopic examination is performed on the specimen

Levels III, IV, V, and VI
- Include gross and microscopic examination and additional ascending levels of physician work (increasing difficulty)

Based upon method of or need for removal

Same anatomical site can be listed in each level

Additional service codes 88311-88399 are not included in codes 88300-88309

> **Example:** Special stains (88312)

■ PRACTICE EXERCISES

*Do **not** report the professional modifier -26 for the following reports.*

Practice Exercise 3-51: L3-4 Disc

LOCATION: Outpatient, Hospital

PATIENT: Corrine Wilson

ATTENDING PHYSICIAN: Timothy Pleasant, MD

SURGEON: Timothy Pleasant, MD

PATHOLOGIST: Grey Lonewolf, MD

CLINICAL HISTORY: Lumbar disc L3-4 herniation.

SPECIMEN RECEIVED: L3-4 disc.

GROSS DESCRIPTION: The specimen is labeled with the patient's name and "lumbar disc L3-4" and consists of fibrillary pink-tan tissue fragments. Representative section in one cassette.

MICROSCOPIC DIAGNOSIS: Fragments of fibrocartilage, consistent with herniated disc L3-4.

CPT Code(s): _____

ICD-9-CM Code(s): _____

Abstracting Questions

1. How would the code for this service be referenced in the CPT index?

    _____

2. Was the examination gross, microscopic, or both? _____

3. What was the level of surgical pathology? _____

4. Does the pathologic status of the tissue affect the diagnosis code?

    _____

Practice Exercise 3-52: Uterus, Bilateral Tubes, and Ovaries

LOCATION: Outpatient, Hospital

PATIENT: Tina Highdorn

ATTENDING PHYSICIAN: Ira Avila, MD

SURGEON: Ira Avila, MD

PATHOLOGIST: Grey Lonewolf, MD

CLINICAL HISTORY: Menorrhagia.

SPECIMEN RECEIVED: Uterus, bilateral tubes, and ovaries.

GROSS DESCRIPTION: The specimen is labeled with the patient's name and "uterus, bilateral tubes, and ovaries" and consists of 370 gm; this includes the complete uterus with tubes and ovaries. The uterus measures 14 cm in length × 10 cm in fundal diameter. The specimen is distorted by several bulging areas on the surface. The cervix is transverse. The endometrium is up to 0.3 cm thick and composed of pale tan color. Cut section of the myometrium reveals multiple whirling masses, up to 3 cm in diameter, consisting of white whirling tissue. The fallopian tubes have been surgically divided. The left ovary measures 5 × 4 cm and contains a central cystic structure with smooth lining. A section of the left tube and ovary is placed in cassette labeled 7. The right ovary measures 3 × 2 × 1.5 cm and is composed of wrinkled tan tissue. A section of the right tube and ovary is placed in cassette labeled 8.

MICROSCOPIC DIAGNOSIS: Sections of cervix show squamous metaplasia. Sections of endometrium show tubular glands lined by pseudostratified columnar epithelium. Small nests of endometrial glands and stroma are noted in the superficial myometrium. Sections of myometrium show masses, consisting of interdigitating bands of smooth muscle. Section of left fallopian tube is unremarkable. Section of left ovary shows a follicle cyst. Sections of right fallopian tube are unremarkable. Section of right ovary shows physiologic structures.

DIAGNOSIS
Complete uterus, tubes, and ovaries showing:
1. Squamous metaplasia, cervix.
2. Proliferating endometrium.
3. Adenomyosis, uterus.
4. Multiple intramural leiomyomata.
5. Status post surgical division of fallopian tubes.
6. Follicle cyst, left ovary.

CPT Code(s): _____

ICD-9-CM Code(s): _____

Abstracting Questions

1. When "Metaplasia, cervix" is referenced in the Index of ICD-9-CM you are directed to "omit code." What does this mean? _____

2. The clinical history was menorrhagia. What is menorrhagia?
   _____

3. Why was it not correct to report menorrhagia as the diagnosis?
   _____

Practice Exercise 3-53: Placenta

LOCATION: Inpatient, Hospital

PATIENT: Cindy Kretchenhoff

ATTENDING PHYSICIAN: Ira Avila, MD

SURGEON: Ira Avila, MD

PATHOLOGIST: Grey Lonewolf, MD

CLINICAL HISTORY: 31 weeks, 6 days' gestation, possible placental abruption.

SPECIMEN RECEIVED: Placenta.

GROSS DESCRIPTION: Submitted in formalin, labeled with the patient's name, and "placenta" is 600 gm. Discoid placenta measuring 18 × 17 × 3 cm, with three centrally attached vessels and 5 cm long umbilical cord. The umbilical cord shows no knots or gross abnormalities (cassette 1). The membranes are tan and opaque and show no significant exudates, nodules, or green discoloration (cassette 2). The fetal surface of placenta shows a normal vascular pattern. The maternal surface features multiple intact cotyledons. No significant adherent blood clot or cotyledon compression is seen. Sectioning reveals dark red to purple spongy parenchyma without significant scarlike areas or masses. Representative sections of central and peripheral placenta are submitted in cassettes 3 and 4, respectively (two separate specimens, placenta and umbilical cord).

MICROSCOPIC DIAGNOSIS: Sections are umbilical cord showing three vessels. No significant inflammatory infiltrates are seen. Sections of membranes feature intact chorionic and amnionic membranes. Focal mild neutrophilic infiltrates are identified within chorionic membranes. Sections of placenta show multiple chorionic villi with villous architecture consistent with 32 weeks' gestational age. Villous vascularity is within normal limits. There is mild intervillous fibrin deposition. No significant large vessels lesions are seen. Minimal neutrophilic infiltrates are present within the fibrin beneath the chorionic plate.

DIAGNOSIS: Placenta, delivery; early third-trimester placenta, membranes, and umbilical cord showing mild early placentitis.

COMMENTS: While no gross pathologic changes of placental abruption are seen, acute abruption may not be accompanied by demonstrable placental changes at the time of pathologic examination.

CPT Code(s): _____

ICD-9-CM Code(s): _____

Abstracting Questions

1. How many specimens were examined? _____

2. According to the notes in the CPT manual before 88300, the unit of services for codes 88300 through 88309 is the what? _____

3. Also in the notes of the CPT manual before 88300, a specimen is defined as tissue(s) submitted for individual and separate attention, requiring individual examination and pathologic _____

Practice Exercise 3-54: Cervical Disc

LOCATION: Outpatient, Hospital

PATIENT: Sally Reagon

ATTENDING PHYSICIAN: Timothy Pleasant, MD

SURGEON: Timothy Pleasant, MD

PATHOLOGIST: Grey Lonewolf, MD

CLINICAL HISTORY: Severe cervical spinal stenosis.

SPECIMEN RECEIVED: Cervical disc.

GROSS DESCRIPTION: The specimen is labeled with the patient's name and "cervical disc" and consists of approximately 5 grams of tan fibrous fragments.

MICROSCOPIC DIAGNOSIS: Sections show disc tissue.

DIAGNOSIS: Disc tissue (cervical).

CPT Code(s): _____

ICD-9-CM Code(s): _____

Abstracting Question

1. What statement in the code description for 88304 identifies cervical disc pathological examination? _____

Practice Exercise 3-55: Cerebral Hematoma

LOCATION: Inpatient, Hospital

PATIENT: Daniel Smithson

ATTENDING PHYSICIAN: Timothy Pleasant, MD

SURGEON: Timothy Pleasant, MD

PATHOLOGIST: Grey Lonewolf, MD

CLINICAL HISTORY: Nontraumatic cerebral bleeding.

SPECIMEN RECEIVED: Cerebral hematoma.

GROSS DESCRIPTION: Submitted in formalin and labeled with the patient's name and "cerebral hematoma" are fragments of reddish brown blood clot measuring approximately 4.5 × 3.5 × 1.5 cm in aggregate. Representative fragments are submitted in one cassette.

MICROSCOPIC DIAGNOSIS: Sections show fragments of fresh blood clot and a single fragment of brain parenchyma featuring intact cortex and underlying white matter and mild-to-moderate edema. No neoplasm is identified.

DIAGNOSIS: Cerebral hematoma, evacuation: Recent blood clot and benign brain parenchyma.

CPT Code(s): _____

ICD-9-CM Code(s): _____

Abstracting Question

---

1. How many cassettes were submitted? _____

■ MEDICINE SECTION (90281-99607)

Most procedures noninvasive (not entering body)

Contains invasive procedures

Example: 92973, Percutaneous thrombectomy

Many specialized tests

Example: Audiology and biofeedback

Special lightning bolt icon (⚡)

- Indicates substances pending FDA (Food and Drug Administration) approval

Immunizations

Often used

Two types of immunizations

- Active and passive

Correct coding includes

- Supply injected

- Administration of injection

Active—Bacteria or Virus

Bacteria that cause disease made nontoxic (toxoid)

- Injected to build immunity

Small dose active virus injected (vaccine)

- Injected to build immunity

Example: Poliovirus

Passive Immunization

Does not cause immune response

Contains antibodies against certain diseases—immune globulins

Immune Globulins (90281-90399)

Identifies immune globulin product

Example: Botulism antitoxin

Report administration separately

Immune Globulin Codes Divided by

Type
e.g., rabies, hepatitis B

Method
e.g., intramuscular, intravenous, subcutaneous

Dose
e.g., full dose, minidose

Immunization Administration (90460-90474)

Administration (giving of substance)

- Reported in addition to substance given

- 90460, 90461 Patients through age 18 when counseled regarding immunization

- 90471-90474 Patients over 18

- 90471, +90472 = Percutaneous, intradermal, subcutaneous, or intramuscular injection

- 90473, +90474 = Oral or intranasal

Methods of Administration

- Percutaneous

- Intradermal

- Subcutaneous

- Intramuscular

- Intranasal

- Oral

Report Administration for Each Dose—Single or Combination

Example: 10-year-old patient receives 3 separate injections

- 90471 administration tetanus

- 90472 administration rubella

- 90472 administration diphtheria

OR depending on payer:

- 90471 administration tetanus

- 90472 × 2 administration rubella and diphtheria

Vaccines, Toxoids (Vaccine Product Codes) (90476-90749)

Many codes age-specific

Example: 90658, influenza vaccine, for ages 3 and over

Codes for products for single diseases

Example: 90703, tetanus

Codes for combination diseases

Example: 90700, diphtheria, tetanus toxoids, and acellular pertussis (DTaP)

Some vaccines given on schedule

Example: 90633, 2-dose hepatitis A vaccine

- 1st dose, 1st visit

- 2nd dose, 2nd visit

Caution: There Are Multiple Diphtheria Codes

- 90696-90702, 90719-90723 diphtheria and diphtheria with other substances

  Example: 90719, diphtheria for IM use

  Example: 90698, diphtheria, tetanus toxoids, and acellular pertussis (synthetic form of pertussis) (DTaP), *Haemophilus influenza* Type B (HiB), and inactivated poliovirus (IPV) for IM use

---

Remember
Third-party payers do not usually require modifier -51 used with Vaccine/Toxoid codes
Rather, depending on payer:
- List each code multiple times or
- Use times (×) symbol and indicate number

Important Reporting Rule. If vaccine administered during an office visit that was not related to the E/M

- Report E/M service (with modifier -25) + Vaccine + administration

Office visit for vaccine only: Report only vaccine and the administration (no E/M service)

Routine Vaccinations

Influenza
Substance (vaccine) 90653-90668 and 90685-90688

Administration for patients age 19 years and over

- G0008 HCPCS National Level II for Medicare patients
- 90471/90472

Pneumococcal
Substance (vaccine) 90732

Administration

- G0009 HCPCS National Level II for Medicare
- 90471/90472 administration

Psychiatry (90785-90899)

Psychiatric Diagnostic Evaluation

Involved assessment to identify patient diagnosis and develop treatment plan

Codes for evaluation (90791) and evaluation with medical service (90792)

Psychotherapy

Therapeutic treatment of psychological disorder or behavior

Services reported with codes 90832-90838

- Time based codes (30, 45, or 60 minutes)
- Codes subdivided based on if psychotherapy provided in addition to a primary procedure
- Provided to patient and/or family member(s)

Other Psychotherapy

- Crisis psychotherapy provides treatment for a patient's experiencing a reaction to a more specific event or situation (90839, 90840)

Codes 90845-90853 report services for

- Psychoanalysis

- Family, multiple-family, and group psychotherapy

Biofeedback (90901, 90911)

Used to help patients gain control over body processes

>   *Example:* Elevated BP (blood pressure) or manage chronic pain

Patient training in biofeedback by professional

- Continues on own

Services often part psychophysiologic (mind/body) therapy

Dialysis (90935-90999)

Cleanses blood

- Temporary (non-ESRD [end-stage renal disease])

- Permanent (ESRD)

Two parts to report ESRD dialysis services

- Physician service

- Hemodialysis procedure

Hemodialysis Service (90935-90940)

Hemodialysis is the procedure

Used for ESRD and non-ESRD

Billed per day for inpatients receiving hemodialysis and also for outpatient non-ESRD

Includes all physician E/M services related to procedure

- Use modifier -25 if separate E/M service provided

Miscellaneous Dialysis Procedures (90945-90947)

Describes other dialysis procedures

>   *Example:* Peritoneal dialysis in which toxins are passively absorbed into dialysis fluid

Services billed on per-day basis for inpatient ESRD patients

ESRD Physician Services (90951-90970)

Include

- Establishment of dialyzing cycle

- Physician services

- E/M outpatient dialysis visits

- Telephone calls

- Patient management during dialysis

Reported per month: 90951-90966
Month is defined as 30 days

Less than full month of service 90967-90970 per day

Codes divided by age and number of encounters

Codes are used to report outpatient dialysis services for ESRD patients

Other Diagnosis Procedures (90989-90999)
Patients can receive training in self-dialysis (90989, 90993)

Codes divided by complete or partial training program

Gastroenterology (91010-91299)

For tests and treatments of esophagus, stomach, and intestine

Codes usually reported with E/M or consultation service code

• **Caution:** Many bundled services

Ophthalmology (92002-92499)

Contains E/M "eye" codes

Definitions for new and established patients same as for E/M section

Codes are for bilateral services

• If only one eye, use modifier -52 (reduced service)

Special Ophthalmologic Services (92015-92287)

For special evaluations of visual system

Goes beyond those usually provided in evaluation

May be reported in addition to basic visual service

Special Otorhinolaryngologic Services (92502-92700)

Special treatments and diagnostic services

Example: Nasal function tests (rhinomanometry) or audiometric tests

All hearing tests bilateral unless one ear indicated in description

Cardiovascular in Medicine Section (See pg 393 for details)

Services can be

• Invasive or noninvasive

• Diagnostic or therapeutic

Subheadings

• Therapeutic Services and Procedures

• Cardiography

• Cardiovascular Monitoring Services

• Implantable and Wearable Cardiac Device Evaluations

• Echocardiography

• Cardiac Catheterization

• Intracardiac Electrophysiologic Procedures/Studies

• Peripheral Arterial Disease Rehabilitation

• Noninvasive Physiologic Studies and Procedures

• Other Procedures

• Other Studies

Noninvasive Vascular Diagnostic Studies (93880-93998)

Vascular codes for procedures on noncoronary veins and arteries

Include

- Patient care

- Supervision and interpretation (S&I)

- Copy of results

Pulmonary (94002-94799)

For ventilation management therapies and diagnostic tests

Includes procedure and interpretation of test results

- Additional E/M service reported separately

Allergy and Clinical Immunology (95004-95199)

Divided into three subheadings

1. Allergy Testing (95004-95071)

2. Ingestion Challenge Testing (95076-95079)

3. Allergen Immunotherapy (95115-95199)

Allergy Testing (95004-95071)

Sensitivity testing using various types of tests with type and number of tests based on physician's judgment

> *Example:* Percutaneous, intracutaneous, inhalation

> *Example:* Extracts, venoms, biologics, and foods

Medical record will indicate

- Number and type of tests

- Method testing

Ingestion Challenge Testing (95076-95079)

- Sensitivity to food, drugs, and other substances

- 95076 initial 120 minutes; 95079 each additional 60 minutes

- Services less than 60 minutes, report E/M code

Allergen Immunotherapy (95115-95199)

Codes divided into three types of services:

1. Injection only

2. Prescription and injection

3. Provision of antigen (substance) only

Physician service bundled into immunotherapy codes

If separate E/M service provided, report separately

Neurology and Neuromuscular Procedures (95782-96020)

Contains codes to report tests, such as

- Sleep tests

- Muscle tests (electromyography)

- Range-of-motion measurements

- Electroencephalogram (EEG)

- Electromyography (EMG)

- Analysis and programming of neurostimulators

- Motion analysis

- Functional brain mapping

Many bundled services

Services usually provided in addition to E/M service

Medical Genetics and Genetic Counseling Services (96040)

Trained genetic counselors assess risk of genetic defects in offspring

Includes

- Pedigree construction

- Obtaining structured genetic history

- Analysis of risk

- Counseling

Central Nervous System (CNS) Assessments/Tests (96101-96125)

Used to report

- Psychological tests

- Speech/Language assessments

- Developmental progress assessments

- Thinking/Reasoning examinations

Standardized cognitive performance testing

Codes based on per-hour basis

- Includes written report of results

Health and Behavior Assessment/Intervention (96150-96155)

- Identify psychological behavior, emotional, cognitive, or social factors important to treatment or management of physical health problems

Hydration, Therapeutic, Prophylactic, Diagnostic Injections and Infusions, and Chemotherapy and Other Highly Complex Drug or Highly Complex Biologic Agent Administration (96360-96549)

Infusion: Therapeutic procedure to introduce fluid into body

Hydration: Infusion for purpose of rehydration; includes prepackaged fluid

Injection: Subcutaneous (Sub-Q, SC), intramuscular (IM), intra-arterial (IA), and intravenous (IV)

Codes report the physician work related to the infusion, hydration, or injection

- Affirmation of treatment plan
- Direct supervision of staff
- Significant, separately identifiable E/M is reported with -25

Codes include

- Local anesthesia
- Intravenous start
- Access to indwelling intravenous catheter or port
- Flush at conclusion
- Standard tubing, syringes, and supplies

Multiple drug administrations in same session are reported separately

Use only one initial code to report multiple infusions or injections or combinations

> For the physician, assign initial code based on primary reason for encounter
>
> The secondary infusion/injection is reported with a subsequent or concurrent code, unless the protocol requires two separate IV sites
>
> > *Example:* If three different agents were administered in the same session, report one initial code and two additional sequential codes
>
> Determination of initial code is based on primary reason for encounter

Some codes are time based, so medical documentation must indicate time infusion begins and ends

Time is defined as the actual time used to administer the drug/substance

Hydration (96360, 96361)

IV infusion for hydration and includes prepackaged fluid/electrolytes

- 96360 IV infusion for hydration up to 1 hour
- 96361 IV infusion for hydration, each additional hour
  - Report for hydration intervals greater than 30 minutes beyond 1 hour
  - Start infusion time over if a different bag is started
  - Do not report hydration codes when the fluid is used to administer a drug (incidental hydration)
  - Do not report hydration codes for infusion of <30 minutes

Therapeutic, Prophylactic, and Diagnostic Injections and Infusions (Excludes Chemotherapy and Other Highly Complex Drug or Highly Complex Biologic Agent Administration) (96365-96379)

Types of drug administration

- Therapeutic
- Prophylactic
- Diagnostic

Codes divided by administration method

- Subcutaneous
- Intramuscular
- Intra-arterial
- Intravenous push

A push is defined as when a health care professional is needed to administer the drug/substance and monitor the patient or an infusion that takes 15 minutes or less to administer

Also report the substance administered

96365-96368 report therapeutic, prophylactic, or diagnostic IV infusions, other than hydration and chemotherapy

- Typically require direct physician supervision
- Special consideration for preparing, dosing, or disposing
- Trained staff who administer infusion
- Monitoring of vital signs during infusion

Chemotherapy and Other Highly Complex Drug or Highly Complex Biologic Agent Administration (96401-96549)

Represents only preparation and administration of chemotherapy

- If separate E/M service provided, report E/M code + -25

Report all drugs/substances separately

Codes are not limited to patients with diagnosis of cancer

Codes also include infusion of antineoplastic agents, monoclonal antibody agents, and biological response modifiers for treatment of noncancer diagnoses

Chemical can be administered (injected) into

- Lesion
- Vein
- Tissue
- Muscle
- Artery
- Cavity
- Nerve

Intravenously injected chemicals: Two methods of delivery of chemical

1. IV push quickly delivers substance/medication into vein (15 minutes or less)

2. IV infusion delivers over longer period of time

Codes often divided by time the infusion/injection procedure takes

Example: 96413 chemotherapy administration, intravenous, infusion up to 1 hour

Report the initial code that represents the main reason why the patient was being treated, even though it might not be the first drug/substance infused

Example: Patient received 1 hour of hydration first, then 2 hours of chemotherapy intravenously. Code the initial chemotherapy infusion 96413 for the first hour of chemo, 96415 for the second hour, then code 96360 for the hydration

Special supplies (e.g., special needles) reported separately using 99070 or HCPCS National Level II code

Report any intra-arterial catheter placement with 36620-36640

Injections with chemotherapy

- Report separately any analgesic or antiemetic (for vomiting)

- Given before or after chemotherapy

Use code J0881 to report injection of darbepoetin alfa and J0885 to report injection of epoetin alfa

---

Photodynamic Therapy (96567-96571)

Used in addition to bronchoscopy or endoscopy codes

Injected agent remains in cancerous cells longer than normal cells

- After agent dissipates from normal cells, patient exposed to laser light

- Agent absorbs light

- Light produces oxygen and cancer cells destroyed

Special Dermatologic Procedures (96900-96999)

Usually specialized procedures provided on consultation basis

- Separate E/M consultation code would then be appropriate

Treatment of skin conditions:

Actinotherapy—with ultraviolet light

Photochemotherapy—with light-sensitive chemicals and light rays

Physical Medicine & Rehabilitation (97001-97799)

Used by physicians and therapists to report a variety of services

Treatments
Traction

Modalities

Electrical stimulation (used to help heal fractures)

Therapeutic procedures

Gait training

Functional activities

Patient Training

Codes often have time components

> *Example:* 97761 reports prosthetic training, extremity, each 15 minutes

Active Wound Care Management (97597-97610)

Debridement

Debridement without anesthesia with removal of devitalized tissue by different techniques, such as water pressure, sharp selective debridement with scissors, scalpel, and forceps

97597 and 97598 include total surface area of all wounds

Codes based on centimeters treated

Nonselective debridement (97602): Healthy tissue removed along with necrotic tissue, with wet-to-moist dressings, enzymatic or abrasive methods

Negative pressure wound therapy (NPWT) (97605, 97606)

- Vacuuming of drainage and tissue from wound
  - Then negative pressure draws the edges of the wound together
- Application of topical medications/ointments
- Assessment of wound
- Directions to patient on continued care of wound
- Each code for ongoing care reported on per-session basis

Osteopathic and Chiropractic Services (98925-98943)

Both inpatient and outpatient settings

Physician services bundled into codes

Codes divided by body area

Education and Training for Patient Self-Management (98960-98962)

- Use of standardized curriculum for education to individual or group for management of illness

Non–Face-to-Face Nonphysician Services (98966-98969)

Reports nonphysician E/M services using telephone/Internet

Established patient, family member of the patient, or a guardian

98966-98968 telephone E/M services

98969 online E/M services

To report physician services, see 99441-99443

Special Services, Procedures, and Reports (99000-99091)

Handling and conveyance of laboratory specimens

• 99000-99002

Postoperative follow-up visits included in surgical package

• 99024

Office visits after posted hours or in locations other than office

• 99050-99060

Supplies and materials

• 99070

Hospital mandated on-call services

• 99026, 99027

Moderate (Conscious) Sedation (99143-99150)

Type of sedation in which the patient can respond to verbal commands

• Appendix G of the CPT manual contains summary of codes that include moderate (conscious) sedation

The bullseye symbol ⊙ indicates these codes in the CPT manual

Do not report sedation services with codes marked with bullseye when sedation is provided by same physician performing procedure

• Second physician provides sedation, report with 99148-99150

Included in service is:

• Patient assessment

• IV establishment

• Administration of agent

• Maintenance of sedation

• Monitoring of vital signs

• Recovery

Codes divided based on patient age (under 5 and 5 and over) and time (30 minutes and each 15 minutes over)

■ PRACTICE EXERCISES

Practice Exercise 3-56: Cardiac Catheterization

CARDIAC CATHETERIZATION REPORT

LOCATION: Inpatient, Hospital

PATIENT: Wade Land

REFERRING PHYSICIAN: James Noonar, MD

CARDIOLOGIST: Marvin Elhart, MD

INDICATION: Unstable angina.

PROCEDURE: Right iliofemoral angiography, left heart catheterization, selective coronary angiography, and left ventriculography.

COMPLICATIONS: None.

RESULTS: Hemodynamics: The left ventricular pressure before the LV gram was 133/7 with an LVEDP of 11. After the LV gram it was 130/8 with an LVEDP of 12. The aortic pressure on pullback was 130/59.

Left Ventriculography: Showed that the left ventricle is normal in size. It was hard to assess segmental wall motion because of the frequency of PVCs; however, the overall left ventricular systolic function was normal. There might be some distal anterior wall hypokinesis.

Selective Coronary Angiography
1. Right coronary artery: This was a medium-size dominant artery that has mild diffuse atherosclerotic changes. After the PDA there was about 30% narrowing.
2. Left main coronary artery: This has 80-90% eccentric narrowing in the midportion.
3. Left circumflex artery: This was a medium-size artery that has mild atherosclerotic changes proximally. It gave rise to a medium-size bifurcating first obtuse marginal that has 99% proximal narrowing. The inferior of the two branches, which was a smaller size artery, has 90% proximal narrowing.
4. Left anterior descending coronary artery: This was a medium-size artery that has mild diffuse atherosclerotic changes. The first diagonal was a small artery that had 90% proximal narrowing. The second diagonal was a larger artery that has about 60% narrowing in the midportion. Immediately after that diagonal, the left anterior descending artery has about 50% narrowing. There was moderate diffuse disease after that. Please note that the visualization of the diagonals and the left anterior descending artery was rather limited as we tried not to inject in a strong way into the left main.

CONCLUSION
1. Normal overall left ventricular systolic function.
2. Severe left main disease.
3. Severe left circumflex and first diagonal disease.

RECOMMENDATIONS
1. Maximum medical treatment.
2. Intra-aortic balloon pump.
3. Consult CT surgery to evaluate the patient for bypass surgery.

CPT Code(s): _____

ICD-9-CM Code(s): _____

Abstracting Questions

1. What are the three categories bundled into the code reported for cardiac catheterization? _____

2. What was the approach for this procedure? _____

3. Was a modifier required on the catheterization code and if a modifier was required, which one would it be? _____

4. For what two procedures were injections provided? _____

Practice Exercise 3-57: Saphenous Vein Mapping

RADIOLOGY REPORT

LOCATION: Outpatient, Hospital

PATIENT: Mirta Hubert

ORDERING PHYSICIAN: James Noonar, MD

ATTENDING/ADMIT PHYSICIAN: James Noonar, MD

RADIOLOGIST: Morton Monson, MD

PERSONAL PHYSICIAN: Alma Naraquist, MD

EXAMINATION: Saphenous vein mapping.

CLINICAL SYMPTOMS: Pre-coronary artery bypass graft; atherosclerotic heart disease of native coronary arteries, chest pain.

FINDINGS: The left greater saphenous vein was mapped from midthigh through the proximal calf. Measurements above the knee were 1.0×0.92 cm, at the knee 0.73×0.73 cm, and below the knee 0.54×0.54 cm. The multiple branches encountered were not evaluated.

CPT Code(s): _____

ICD-9-CM Code(s): _____

Abstracting Question

1. What type of scan was used for mapping of vessels? _____

Practice Exercise 3-58: Venous Ultrasound

RADIOLOGY REPORT

LOCATION: Inpatient, Hospital

PATIENT: Dave James

ORDERING PHYSICIAN: Frank Gaul, MD

ATTENDING/ADMIT PHYSICIAN: Frank Gaul, MD

RADIOLOGIST: Morton Monson, MD

PERSONAL PHYSICIAN: Frank Gaul, MD

EXAMINATION: Bilateral lower extremity venous ultrasound.

CLINICAL SYMPTOMS: Leg pain and swelling. Rule out deep venous thrombosis.

FINDINGS: This examination was somewhat limited as a result of the patient being recently out of surgery and unable to be moved at all. As visualized, both the right and the left common femoral, superficial femoral, popliteal, and posterior tibial veins are fully compressible and demonstrate the presence of normal spontaneous, phasic, and augmented flow.

IMPRESSION: No evidence for deep venous thrombosis is seen within either of the lower extremities. Please see above comments.

CPT Code(s): _____

ICD-9-CM Code(s): _____

Abstracting Question

1. What is a deep venous thrombosis? _____

Practice Exercise 3-59: Extremities Ultrasound

RADIOLOGY REPORT

LOCATION: Outpatient, Hospital

PATIENT: Eric Tayes

ORDERING PHYSICIAN: Frank Gaul, MD

ATTENDING/ADMIT PHYSICIAN: Frank Gaul, MD

RADIOLOGIST: Morton Monson, MD

EXAMINATION: Ultrasound of both lower extremities; abdomen ultrasound.

CLINICAL SYMPTOMS: Lower extremity swelling, difficulty breathing.

FINDINGS: Ultrasound examination of the deep venous system of both lower extremities is negative. No evidence of deep venous thrombosis in either lower extremity. The posterior tibial, greater saphenous, and popliteal through the femoral veins are patent and negative for thrombus bilaterally. Normal phasicity.

Abdomen Ultrasound: Diffusely coarsened echotexture of the liver with some nodularity consistent with fatty infiltration. Cirrhotic configuration of the liver. Small calcified granuloma in the spleen. The spleen is otherwise negative. There is ascites in all four quadrants. No bile duct dilatation. No gallbladder wall thickening or cholelithiasis. Small amount of fluid adjacent to the gallbladder is likely related to the ascites. The pancreas is obscured by bowel gas. The abdominal aorta is of normal caliber. The right kidney measures approximately 9 cm in length and shows no evidence of hydronephrosis, calculi, or mass. The left kidney measures approximately 9.9 cm in length and shows no evidence of hydronephrosis, calculi, or mass.

CPT Code(s): _____

ICD-9-CM Code(s): _____

Abstracting Questions

1. How was the scan for the abdomen different than the scan for the extremities? _____

2. How would the "cirrhotic configuration of the liver" diagnosis be reported?

_____

Practice Exercise 3-60: Renal Dialysis Progress Note

RENAL DIALYSIS PROGRESS NOTE

LOCATION: Outpatient, Clinic

PATIENT: Jyl Couts

PHYSICIAN: Ira Avila, MD

The 45-year-old patient presents today for regular monthly visit. She has been slightly tired. She denies any shortness of breath or chest pain. No constipation. The patient complains of some weakness in her legs when she walks to the grocery store.

PHYSICAL EXAMINATION: Her blood pressure at home has been in the 130s/80s. On exam today, her weight is 152.5 pounds. Regular heart rate at 79 per minute. The lungs are clear bilaterally without crackles. No edema in the extremities. Catheter condition is good, and the exit site is clean and dry. No evidence of infection.

IMPRESSION/PLAN

The patient is on CAPD, two bag sizes of 1.5% and 2.5%; doing well with that.

She is on 4000 units of EPO once a week due to anemia due to end-stage renal disease with hemoglobin of 12. We will continue that at this time.

The patient has possibility of claudication. She has history of an aneurysm, which was measured at 6.1 cm on a CT scan done in the transverse section. We will obtain an ultrasound to follow up on her abdominal aortic aneurysm and do ABIs on the lower extremities.

The patient requested a handicap permit, and I will hold that for now until we do her studies.

The patient seems to agree with the plan.

CPT Code(s): _____

ICD-9-CM Code(s): _____

Abstracting Questions

1. Does the type of dialysis the patient receives affect code selection?

   _____

2. What is end-stage renal disease? _____

■ HCPCS CODING

Developed by Centers for Medicare and Medicaid Services (CMS)

- Formerly HCFA

HCPCS developed in 1983
CPT did not contain all codes necessary for Medicare services reporting

---

One of Two Levels of Codes

1. Level I, CPT

2. Level II, HCPCS, also known as national codes

Phased Out Level III, Local Codes

Developed by Medicare and other carriers for use at local level

Varied by locale

Discontinued October 2002 due to HIPAA code set regulations

Some codes incorporated into HCPCS Level I and Level II

Level II, National Codes

Codes for wide variety of providers

- Physicians

- Dentists

- Orthodontists

Codes for wide variety of services

- Specific drugs

- Durable medical equipment (DME)

- Ambulance services

Code book published every January, but codes are added and deleted throughout the year and providers are notified through carrier bulletins

Format

Begins with letter, followed by four digits

> *Example:* E0605, vaporizer, room type

Each letter represents group codes

> *Example:* "J" codes used to report drugs, J0585, onabotulinumtoxina, 1 unit

Temporary Codes

Certain letters indicate temporary codes

> *Example:* K0552, Supplies for external drug infusion pump

- K codes are temporary codes

HCPCS National Level II Index

Directs coder to specific codes

Do not code directly from index

Reference main portion of text before assigning code

Alphabetical order

Table of Drugs

Listed by generic name, not brand name

■ AN OVERVIEW OF THE ICD-9-CM

INTRODUCTION

Morbidity (illness)

Mortality (death)

CM = Clinical Modification

Provides continuity of data

World Health Organization's (WHO) ICD-9 used globally; many countries already use ICD-10

1977: United States develops ICD-9 version

• Has more code subsets

• Data collapse back to ICD-9 for uniformity of data

Medicare

Medicare Catastrophic Act of 1988

Required use of ICD-9-CM codes for outpatient claims

Act abolished but codes still used

Uses of ICD-9-CM

Facilities track patient use through codes

Fiscal entities track health care costs

Research

• Health care quality

• Future needs

• Newer cancer center built if patient use warrants

ICD-9-CM on CMS-1500

Diagnoses establish medical necessity

Services and diagnoses must correlate

CMS-1500 example (Fig. 3-15)

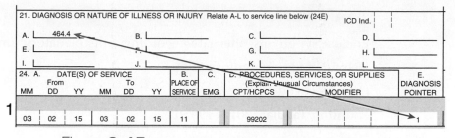

Figure **3-15** Diagnosis code and service must correlate.

Ethics

Documentation must support diagnosis and match procedures or service performed

Example:
- Services provided
- Diagnosis justifies services

If in doubt, check it out; don't make assumptions

Your Job: Translate documentation into ICD-9-CM codes

FORMAT OF ICD-9-CM

Volume 1, Diseases, Tabular

Volume 2, Diseases, Index

Volume 1, Diseases, Tabular

Contains code numbers

001.0-999.9 Diagnosis codes describe condition

Factors Influencing Health Status and External Cause codes (V & E codes) = supplemental information

Volume 2, Diseases, Index

Appears before Tabular in book

Refers coder to code numbers in Volume 1

Never code directly from Index!

ICD-9-CM CONVENTIONS

Symbols, abbreviations, punctuation, and notations

NEC: Not elsewhere classifiable

- No more-specific code exists

NOS: Not otherwise specified

- Unspecified in documentation

[ ] Brackets

Enclose synonyms, alternative wording, or explanatory phrases

Helpful, additional information

Can affect code

Found in Tabular (001.0-999.9)

( ) Parentheses

Contain nonessential modifiers

• Take them or leave them

Found in Tabular and Index

Do not affect code assignment

Colon & Brace

: **Colon:** Tabular, completes statement with one or more modifiers

} **Brace:** Tabular, modifying statements to right of brace

Lozenge, Section Mark, & Bold Type

□ **Lozenge:** Can indicate code unique to ICD-9-CM

§ **Section mark:** Can be footnote indicator

Bold type: Codes and code titles in Tabular, Volume 1

Italicized Type

All excludes notes

Codes NOT used as principal diagnosis

Slanted Brackets [ ]

Enclose manifestations of underlying condition

Code underlying condition first

Includes, Excludes, Use Additional Code

Includes notes: In chapter, section, or category

Excludes notes: Conditions are coded elsewhere

Use Additional Code: Assignment of other code(s) is necessary

And/With

And: Means and/or

With: One condition with (in addition to) another condition

Code, If Applicable, Any Causal Condition First

May be first-listed diagnosis if no causal condition applicable or known

> ***Example:*** 707.10, Ulcer of lower limb, except decubitus; states
>
> • Chronic venous hypertension with ulcer (459.31)

If ulcer caused by chronic venous hypertension

• **First:** 459.31 chronic venous hypertension

• **Second:** 707.10 ulcer of lower limb

VOLUME 2, INDEX

Nonessential modifiers: Have no effect on code selection

Enclosed in parentheses

Clarify diagnosis

> ***Example:*** Ileus (adynamic) (bowel) . . .

Terms

Main terms (bold typeface)

• Subterms

• Indented two spaces to right

• Not bold

Cross References

Directs you: *see, see also*

• "*see*" directs you to specific term, must be referenced

> ***Example:*** Panotitis—*see* Otitis media

• "*see also*" directs you to another term for more information, may also be referenced

> ***Example:*** Perivaginitis (*see also* Vaginitis)

• "*see category*" Volume 1, Tabular, specific information about use of code

> ***Example:*** Mesencephalitis (*see also* Encephalitis) 323.9; late effect—*see* category 326

Notes

Define terms

Give further coding instructions

> ***Example:*** Index: "Melanoma"
>
> **Note:** "Except where otherwise indicated . . ."

Mandatory fifth digits also appear as notes (one reason to never code from Index)

Eponyms

Disease or syndrome named for person

> *Example:* Arnold-Chiari (*see also* Spina bifida)

Etiology and Manifestation of Disease

Etiology = cause of disease

Manifestation = symptom

Combination codes = etiology and manifestation in one code

Neoplasm

In Volume 2, Index, locate Neoplasm Table under the alphabetic entry "N"

SECTIONS

Section 1, Index to Diseases and Injuries

Section 2, Table of Drugs and Chemicals

Section 3, Index to External Causes of Injuries and Poisonings (E Codes)

Section 1, Index to Diseases

Largest part of Volume 2—Index

First step in coding, locate main term in Index

Subterms indented two spaces to right

May have more than one subterm

Section 2, Table of Drugs and Chemicals

Located after the Index to Diseases

Contains classification of drugs and substances to identify poisoning and adverse effects

- Adverse effect occurs when substance is taken correctly but patient has a negative reaction to substance

  Condition E-code for drug found under therapeutic column

- Poisoning occurs when substance is incorrectly taken

  > *Example:* Amoxicillin prescribed for bronchitis causes rash (adverse effect). Rather than one tablet of prescribed amoxicillin, patient takes 4 tablets and nausea results (poisoning)

Drug name placed alphabetically on left under heading "Substance" (Fig. 3-16)

First column: "Poisoning" code for substance involved if not related to an adverse effect

E codes identify how poisoning occurred

> *Example:* If alkaline antiseptic solution poisoning occurred by accident, E858.7

TABLE OF DRUGS AND CHEMICALS / Adjunct, pharmaceutical

Substance	Poisoning	External Cause (E Code)				
		Accident	Therapeutic Use	Suicide Attempt	Assault	Undetermined
Acetylcholine (chloride)	971.0	E855.3	E941.0	E950.4	E962.0	E980.4
Acetylcysteine	975.5	E858.6	E945.5	E950.4	E962.0	E980.4
Acetyldigitoxin	972.1	E858.3	E942.1	E950.4	E962.0	E980.4

Figure **3-16** Section 2, Table of Drugs and Chemicals.

- Accidental poisoning by alkaline antiseptic solution: 976.6 (substance) and E858.7 (how it occurred)
- Identify agent condition E code for occurrence
- Code any resulting condition (e.g., coma)

Headings

Accident: Unintentional

Therapeutic: Correct dosage, correctly administered, with adverse effects

Suicide attempt: Self-inflicted

Assault: Intentionally inflicted by another person

Undetermined: Unknown cause

Section 3, E Codes

Index to External Causes of Injuries and Poisonings

Provides additional information about the nature of the injury/poisoning and locality

Never principal (inpatient), sole, or primary (outpatient) diagnosis

Separate Index to External Causes

- Alphabetical, main terms in bold
- Subterms are indented 2 spaces to right under main term

A Word of Caution about the Index

Some words in Index do not appear in Tabular—saves space

Exact word may not be in code description in Tabular

- Usually found in Index
- Must locate the term in the Index, then locate in Tabular
- Additional coding instructions found in Tabular

VOLUME 1, TABULAR

Two Major Divisions

1. Classification of Diseases and Injuries (codes 001.0-999.9)
2. Supplementary Classification (V codes and E codes)

Classification of Diseases and Injuries

Main portion of ICD-9-CM

Codes from 001.0 to 999.9

Most chapters are body systems

Example:

- Digestive System
- Respiratory System

Divisions of Classification of Diseases and Injuries

Chapters 1 through 17

- *Section:* A group of related conditions
- *Category:* Represents single disease/condition
- *Subcategory:* More specific
- *Subclassification:* Most specific

Remember
Assign to highest level of specificity, based on documentation
If 4-digit code exists, do not report 3-digit code
If 5-digit code exists, do not report 4-digit code

■ USING THE ICD-9-CM

Guidelines developed by Cooperating Parties

- American Hospital Association (AHA)
- American Health Information Management Association (AHIMA)
- Centers for Medicare and Medicaid Services (CMS)
- National Center for Health Statistics (NCHS)

GENERAL GUIDELINES

Appendix A of this text contains resources to view the *ICD-9-CM Official Guidelines for Coding and Reporting*

You must know and follow the Guidelines when assigning diagnoses codes

- All certification examinations adhere to the Guidelines
- As you review this ICD-9-CM material, locate the information in the Guidelines of your ICD-9-CM
- In this way, you will become familiar with the location of Guidelines content to be able to quickly reference the Guidelines during the examination

Outpatient coders primarily use Sections I and IV

Diagnostic Coding and Reporting Guidelines do NOT cover all situations

• Outpatient coders also use many Section II and III guidelines

STEPS TO DIAGNOSIS CODING

Identify MAIN term(s) in diagnosis

Locate MAIN term(s) in Index

Review subterms

Follow cross-reference instructions (e.g., *see, see also*)

Verify code(s) in Tabular

• Read Tabular notes

• Code to highest specificity

• Never code from Index!

Level of Detail in Coding

Assign diagnosis (dx) to highest level of specificity

Do NOT use 3-digit code if there is 4th

Do NOT use 4-digit code if there is 5th

Acute and Chronic Conditions

Exists alone or together

May be separate or combination codes

If two codes, code acute first

　Example: acute (577.0) and chronic (577.1) pancreatitis

Combination code: Both acute and chronic condition

• Diarrhea (acute) (chronic) 787.91, Acute and subacute bacterial endocarditis 421.0

• Otitis acute, chronic, and subacute 382.9

Combination Code

Always use combination code if one exists

　Example: encephalomyelitis (dx) due to rubella (manifestation), 056.01

Multiple Coding for Single Condition

Etiology (cause)

Manifestation (symptom)

• Slanted brackets [ ]

　Example: Retinopathy, diabetic 250.5 *[362.01]*

• Must check Tabular notes to assign correct 5th digit for diabetes

- Tabular: 362.0, Diabetic retinopathy, instructs to "Code first diabetes 249.5, 250.5"

SELECTION OF PRIMARY DIAGNOSIS

Condition for encounter

Documented in medical record

Condition that is responsible for services provided

Also list coexisting condition(s) or comorbidity(ies)

Diagnosis and procedure MUST correlate

- Medical necessity established
- No correlation = no reimbursement

Codes in Brackets

Never sequence as primary diagnosis

Always sequence in order listed in Index

> ***Example:***

- Index lists: Diabetes, gangrene 250.7 *[785.4]*
- 785.4 = gangrene
- Tabular, 785.4 indicates "Code first any associated underlying condition: diabetes (250.7-) . . ."
- Code first diabetes, then gangrene
- 250.7- = diabetes (- = 5th digit)
- 785.4 = gangrene

Two or More Interrelated Conditions

When two or more interrelated conditions exist and either could be primary diagnosis, either may be sequenced first

> ***Example:*** Patient with mitral valve stenosis and coronary artery disease (two interrelated conditions)

- Either can be primary diagnosis and sequenced first
- Resource intensiveness affects choice

V CODES

Located after 999.9 in Tabular

Two digits before decimal (e.g., V10.10)

Index for V codes, Index to Diseases and Injuries

Main terms: contraception, counseling, dialysis, status, examination

Uses of V Codes

Not sick BUT receives health care (e.g., vaccination)

Services for known disease/injury (e.g., chemotherapy)

A circumstance/problem that influences patient's health BUT NOT current illness/injury

> *Example:* Organ transplant status

> *Example:* Birth status and outcome of delivery (newborn)

Section I.C.18.e. of the *Official Guidelines for Coding and Reporting* contains the V Code Table

- Identifies how V codes are listed (first, first/additional, additional only)

Special Note about "History of"
Index to Disease, MAIN term "History"
Entries between "family" and "visual loss V19.0" = "Family history of"
Entries before "family" and after "visual loss V19.0" = "Personal history of"

History V Code Categories in Tabular

V10 Personal history of malignant neoplasm

V11 Personal history of mental disorder

V12 Personal history of certain other diseases

V13 Personal history of other diseases

Except: V13.4 Personal history of arthritis, and V13.6 Personal history of congenital malformations. These conditions are life-long so are not true history codes

V14 Personal history of allergy to medicinal agents

V15 Other personal history presenting hazards to health

Except: V15.7 Personal history of contraception

V16 Family history of malignant neoplasm

V17 Family history of certain chronic disabling diseases

V18 Family history of certain other specific conditions

V19 Family history of other conditions

LATE EFFECTS

Late effect residual of (remaining from) previous illness/injury, e.g., burn that leaves scar

Residual coded first (scar)

Cause (burn) coded second

Late effect codes are not in a separate chapter; rather, throughout Tabular

Reference the term "Late" in the Index

There is no time limit on developing a residual

There may be more than one residual

Example: Patient has a stroke (434.91) and develops paralysis on dominant side (hemiparesis, 438.21) and loss of ability to communicate (aphasia, 438.11)

DIAGNOSTIC CODING AND REPORTING GUIDELINES FOR OUTPATIENT SERVICES

Physician's office

Hospital-based outpatient services

Part of *ICD-9-CM Official Guidelines for Coding and Reporting*, Section IV

Guideline A

The term *first-listed diagnosis* is used rather than *principal diagnosis*

Outpatient Surgery: Reason for surgery

Observation Stay: Medical condition that occasioned admission

Guideline B

Use codes 001.0 through V91.99 to code dx, symptoms, conditions, problems, complaints, or other reason(s) for visit

Guideline C

Documentation should describe patient's condition, using terminology that includes specific diagnoses as well as symptoms, problems, or reasons for encounter

Guideline D

Selection of codes 001.0 through 999.9 (Chapters 1-17) will frequently be used to describe reason for encounter

Guideline E

Codes that describe symptoms and signs, as opposed to diagnoses, acceptable for reporting purposes when an established dx has NOT been confirmed by physician

Guideline F

V codes deal with encounters for circumstances other than disease or injury

  Example: Well-baby checkup (V20.2)

Guideline G

Codes have either three, four, or five digits

4th and/or 5th digit codes provide greater specificity

Three-digit code used ONLY if there is NO 4th or 5th digit

Where 4th and/or 5th digits provided, must be assigned

Diagnoses NOT coded to full digits available are invalid

Guideline H

List first code for dx, condition, problem, or other reason for encounter/visit shown in medical record to be chiefly responsible for services provided

List additional codes that describe any coexisting conditions

Guideline I

Do NOT code diagnoses documented as probable, suspected, questionable, ruled out, or working diagnoses

Rather, code condition(s) to highest degree of certainty for that encounter/visit, such as symptoms, signs, abnormal test results, or other reason for visit

Example: Cough and fever, probably pneumonia

- Code as cough (786.2) and fever (780.6-) (in this order)

Guideline J

Chronic diseases treated on an ongoing basis may be coded and reported as many times as patient receives treatment and care for condition(s)

Guideline K

Code all documented conditions that coexist at time of visit, that require or affect patient care, treatment, or management

Do NOT code conditions previously treated, no longer existing

"History of" codes (V10-V19) may be used as secondary codes if

- Impacts current care or treatment

Guidelines L and M

For patients receiving diagnostic or therapeutic services ONLY

Sequence first

- Diagnosis,
- Condition,
- Problem, or
- Other reason shown in medical record to be chiefly responsible for encounter

Codes for other diagnoses (e.g., chronic conditions)

- May be sequenced as secondary diagnoses

   Exception:

Patients receiving chemotherapy (V58.11), radiation therapy (V58.0), or rehabilitation (code depends on type)

- V code first; dx or problem for which service being performed second

Guideline N

For patients receiving preoperative evaluations ONLY

- Code from category V72.8 (Other specified examinations)

- Assign secondary code for reason for surgery
- Code also any findings related to preoperative evaluation

Guideline O

Code dx that required ambulatory surgery

If postoperative dx different

- Code postoperative dx

Guideline P

Code routine prenatal visits with no complications

- V22.0 (Supervision of normal first pregnancy)
- V22.1 (Supervision of other normal pregnancy)
- Do NOT use these codes with pregnancy complication codes

ICD-9-CM, CHAPTER 1, INFECTIOUS AND PARASITIC DISEASES

Divided based on etiology (cause of disease)

Many Combination Codes

Example: 112.0 candidiasis infection of mouth, which reports both organism and condition with one code

Multiple Codes

Sequencing must be considered

- UTI due to *Escherichia coli*
- 599.0 (UTI) etiology
- 041.4- *(E. coli)* organism (in this order)

Human Immunodeficiency Virus

Code HIV or HIV-related illness ONLY if stated as confirmed in diagnostic statement

- 042 HIV or HIV-related illness
- V08 Asymptomatic HIV status
- 795.71 Nonspecific HIV serology

Previously Diagnosed HIV-Related Illness

Code prior dx HIV-related disease 042 (HIV)

NEVER assign these patients to:

- V08 (Asymptomatic) or
- 795.71 (Nonspecific serologic evidence of HIV)

HIV Sequencing

Sequence first that reason most responsible for encounter, if HIV (042)

Followed by secondary dx that affects encounter or patient care

HIV and Pregnancy

This is an exception to HIV sequencing

During pregnancy, childbirth, or puerperium, code

- 647.6- (Other specified infectious and parasitic diseases), followed by 042 (HIV)

Asymptomatic HIV during pregnancy, childbirth, or puerperium

- 647.6- (Other specified infections and parasitic diseases) and
- V08 (Asymptomatic HIV infection status)
- Reporting asymptomatic HIV varies by state
  - Check the state's reporting laws

Inconclusive Laboratory Test for HIV

795.71 (Inconclusive serologic test for HIV)

- Reporting inconclusive laboratory HIV tests varies by state
  - Check the state's reporting laws

HIV Screening

Code V73.89 (Screening for other specified viral disease)

- Patient in high-risk group for HIV
- V69.8 (Other problems related to lifestyle)

Patients returning for HIV screening results = V65.44 (HIV counseling)

Caution

Incorrectly applying these HIV coding rules can cause patient hardship and may be a violation of law

- Insurance claims for patients with HIV usually need patient's written agreement for disclosure

---

Section I.C.1.b. Septicemia, Systemic Inflammatory Response Syndrome (SIRS), Sepsis, Severe Sepsis, and Septic Shock

Sepsis: Assign systemic infection code as first listed when sepsis is present

- Assign a sepsis code as secondary when sepsis develops during encounter

Septicemia/Sepsis: Usually an 038 septicemia code and a 995.9- SIRS code (in this order)

- Code the organ system dysfunction followed by the SIRS (e.g., 518.81 respiratory failure followed by 995.92)

Septic Shock: Organ dysfunction associated with severe sepsis

• Code underlying systemic infection (e.g., 038.--) followed by the SIRS code (995.92), followed by septic shock (785.52)

ICD-9-CM, CHAPTER 2, NEOPLASMS

Two steps for coding neoplasms

• Incorrectly applying these neoplasm codes can also cause patient hardship

Index

1. Locate histologic type of neoplasm (e.g., sarcoma, melanoma)

   • Review all instructions

2. Locate code identified by body site

   • Usually in Neoplasm Table in Index under "N"

   • Neoplasm Table divided into columns:

     · Malignant (Primary, Secondary, Ca in situ)

     · Benign

     · Uncertain behavior

     · Unspecified

   Example: Pathology report confirmed diagnosis stated in operative report of primary malignant neoplasm of the bladder neck. ICD-9-CM Index, Neoplasm Table, bladder, neck, under Primary column, 188.5. Code then referenced in Tabular to ensure accurate assignment.

Treatment directed at malignancy: Neoplasm is principal dx

Except for Chemotherapy or Radiotherapy:

• Therapy (treatment) followed by neoplasm code

  · Chemotherapy: V58.11

  · Radiotherapy: V58.0

Surgical removal of neoplasm and subsequent chemotherapy or radiotherapy

• Code malignancy as principal dx

Surgery to determine extent of malignancy

• Code malignancy as principal dx

  • V10, "Personal history of malignant neoplasm" if

    1. Neoplasm was previously destroyed and/or

    2. No longer being treated

If patient receives treatment for secondary neoplasm (metastasis)

• Secondary neoplasm is documented principal dx

• Even though primary is still present

Patient treated for anemia or dehydration due to neoplasm or therapy code

• Anemia or dehydration followed by neoplasm

Patient admitted to repair complication of surgery for an intestinal malignancy

- Complication principal dx

- Complication is reason for encounter

- Malignancy secondary dx

Patient receiving chemotherapy or radiotherapy post-op removal of neoplasm

- Code: Therapy followed by active neoplasm

- Do NOT report H/O (history of) neoplasm until treatment is completed

ICD-9-CM, CHAPTER 3, ENDOCRINE, NUTRITIONAL, AND METABOLIC DISEASES AND IMMUNITY DISORDERS

Disorders of Other Endocrine Glands

Diabetes Mellitus 250 coded frequently

Subterms in Index often have two codes

Example:

- Diabetic iritis 250.5- for diabetes (etiology)

- [364.42] for iritis (manifestation)

5th digit indicates type of diabetes

0 type II or unspecified type, not stated as uncontrolled

Fifth-digit 0 is for use for type II patients, even if the patient requires insulin

1 type I [juvenile type], not stated as uncontrolled

2 type II or unspecified type, uncontrolled

Fifth-digit 2 is for use for type II diabetic patients, even if the patient requires insulin

3 type I [juvenile type], uncontrolled

V58.67 used in addition to diabetes code to report long-term use of insulin

If type is not indicated, code type II diabetes

Patient with type II diabetes can receive insulin for periods when diabetes is uncontrolled

Type I diabetic is one who is insulin-dependent

- Unnecessary to report V58.67 with type I diabetes

Other Metabolic and Immunity Disorders Section

Disorders such as gout and dehydration

Disorders often have many names

Example: 242.0- Toxic diffuse goiter, also known as

- Basedow's disease

- Graves' disease

- Primary thyroid hyperplasia

ICD-9-CM, CHAPTER 4, DISEASES OF BLOOD AND BLOOD-FORMING ORGANS

Short chapter with 10 sections

Includes anemia, blood disorders, coagulation defects

Often used code, anemia

Many different types of anemia

- Hereditary hemolytic (282)
- Iron deficiency (280)
- Acquired hemolytic (283)
- Aplastic (284)
- Other and Unspecified (285)

Multiple coding often necessary

Identify underlying disease condition

ICD-9-CM, CHAPTER 5, MENTAL, BEHAVIORAL, AND NEURODEVELOPMENTAL DISORDERS

Includes codes for

- Personality disorders
- Stress disorders
- Neuroses
- Psychoses
- Sexual deviation/dysfunction, etc.

5th digit = status of episode

> ***Example:*** 304.2, cocaine dependence, is assigned the following 5th digits:
>
> - 0 unspecified (episode)
> - 1 continuous
> - 2 episodic
> - 3 in remission

ICD-9-CM, CHAPTER 6, DISEASES OF NERVOUS SYSTEM AND SENSE ORGANS

Central Nervous System

Peripheral Nervous System

Disorders of Eye

Diseases of Ear

Pain—Category 338

Acute or chronic pain not elsewhere classified due to:

- Trauma
- Neoplasm
- Postoperative
- Psychosocial dysfunction

Principal/Primary diagnosis

- When definitive diagnosis not established
- Pain management is reason for encounter/admission

ICD-9-CM, CHAPTER 7, DISEASES OF CIRCULATORY SYSTEM

Three types of hypertension

1. Malignant accelerated, severe, poor prognosis
2. Benign continuous, mild (BP elevated) controllable
3. Unspecified NOT indicated as either malignant or benign

Hypertension (401-405)

Hypertension table located in Index of ICD-9-CM

- Under "H," Hypertension
- Codes divided based on type (Malignant, Benign, Unspecified)

Hypertension, Essential, or NOS

Assign hypertension (arterial, essential, primary, systemic, NOS) to 401

4th digit indicates type

- 0 Malignant
- 1 Benign
- 9 Unspecified

Hypertension with Heart Disease

402 Category

Certain heart conditions when stated "due to hypertension" or implied ("hypertensive")

Add 4th digit for type

Use additional code to specify type of heart failure (428)

Hypertensive Chronic Kidney Disease

Cause-and-effect relationship assumed in chronic kidney disease (CKD) with hypertension

Category 403, Hypertensive chronic kidney disease, used when following present:

- Chronic kidney disease (585.-)

5th digit assignment required for stage of CKD

- 0 CKD stage I through IV
- 1 CKD stage V or end stage

Use additional code to identify stage of chronic kidney disease

Hypertensive Heart and Chronic Kidney Disease

Assign 404 when both hypertensive chronic kidney disease and hypertensive heart disease stated

Assume cause-and-effect relationship

Assign 5th digit for mention of stage of chronic kidney disease and/or heart failure

- Use additional code to specify type of heart failure (428)

Hypertensive Cerebrovascular Disease

Code

- Cerebrovascular disease (430-438)
- Type of hypertension (401-405)

Hypertensive Retinopathy

Code

- Hypertensive retinopathy (362.11)
- Type of hypertension (401-405)

Hypertension, Secondary

Hypertension caused by an underlying condition

- Code
  - Underlying condition
  - Type of hypertension (405)

Hypertension, Transient

Transient hypertension: Temporary elevated BP

Do NOT assign 401-405, Hypertensive Disease

- Hypertension dx is NOT established
- Use
  - 796.2, Elevated blood pressure or
  - 642.3-, Transient hypertension of pregnancy

Hypertension, Controlled

Hypertension controlled by therapy

- Assign code from 401-405

Hypertension, Uncontrolled

Untreated or uncontrolled hypertension

- Assign code from 401-405

Documentation must state malignant hypertension to use 404

Elevated Blood Pressure

Elevated blood pressure coded 796.2

- Elevated BP reading without hypertension is dx
- Hypertension NOT stated, NOT coded to 401

ICD-9-CM, CHAPTER 8, DISEASES OF RESPIRATORY SYSTEM

Watch for "Use additional code to identify infectious organism"

Some codes indicate specific organism and do not need an additional code

Respiratory failure sequencing

If the respiratory failure is due to an acute condition (such as MI [myocardial infarction]) or acute exacerbation of a chronic condition (such as COPD [chronic obstructive pulmonary disease]), sequence the acute condition first

Example: MI (acute condition) and respiratory failure

- Sequence MI first and respiratory failure second

If the respiratory failure (acute condition) is due to a chronic nonrespiratory condition (such as myasthenia gravis), sequence the respiratory failure first

Example: Acute respiratory failure (acute) and myasthenia gravis (chronic)

- Sequence acute respiratory failure first and myasthenia gravis second

Acute Respiratory Infection Section

Frequently used codes, such as

- Common cold (460, acute nasopharyngitis)
- Sore throat (462, acute pharyngitis)
- Acute tonsillitis (463)
- Bronchitis (490-491)
- Acute upper respiratory infection (465, URI)
- Influenza (487, flu)
- Pneumonia (480-486)

ICD-9-CM, CHAPTER 9, DISEASES OF DIGESTIVE SYSTEM

Mouth to anus + accessory organs

Extensive subcategories

- 574 Cholelithiasis (10 subcategories)
- Each has 5th digit subclassification

Commonly used codes

- Ulcers (531-534)
  - Gastric (531)
  - Duodenal (532)
  - Peptic (533)
  - Gastrojejunal (534)
- Hernias (550-553)

ICD-9-CM, CHAPTER 10, DISEASES OF GENITOURINARY SYSTEM

Commonly used codes

- Urinary tract infection (599.0)
- Inflammation of prostate (601.-)
- Disorders of female genitalia organs (625-627)

Stages of chronic kidney disease

- Stage I: Blood flow through kidney increases, kidney enlarges (585.1)
- Stage II: (mild) Small amounts of blood protein (albumin) leak into urine (microalbuminuria) (585.2)
- Stage III: (moderate) Albumin and other protein losses increase. Patient may develop high blood pressure and kidney loses ability to filter waste (585.3)
- Stage IV: (severe) Large amounts of urine pass through kidney, blood pressure increases (585.4)
- Stage V: Ability to filter waste nearly stops (585.5)
- End-stage renal failure (585.6)

    When documentation indicates chronic renal disease (CKD) and ESRD, report ESRD

- Unspecified 585.9

Status post kidney transplant, assign V42.0

- Patient may still have CKD

ICD-9-CM, CHAPTER 11, COMPLICATIONS OF PREGNANCY, CHILDBIRTH, AND THE PUERPERIUM

Extensive multiple coding with many 5th digit assignments and notes

Admission for pregnancy, complication

- Obstetric complication = primary dx

Chapter 11 ICD-9-CM codes take precedence over codes from other chapters

Codes 640-676.9 share same 5th digit subclassification

- Denotes current episode of care
- 0 Unspecified as to episode of care or not applicable
- 1 Delivered, with or without mention of antepartum condition

- 2 Delivered, with mention of postpartum complication
- 3 Antepartum condition or complication
- 4 Postpartum condition or complication

General Rules

Not all encounters are pregnancy-related

Example: Pregnant woman, broken ankle (medial malleolus, open)

- Broken ankle (824.1)
- V22.2 Pregnant state incidental; must be documented in medical record that condition being treated not affecting pregnancy

Complications of Pregnancy, Childbirth, and Puerperium

Chapter 11 codes (630-679)

Used only on mother's medical record

Not on newborn medical record

Selection of Primary Diagnosis

Routine prenatal visits, no complications:

- V22.0, Supervision, normal **first** pregnancy or
- V22.1, Supervision, **other** normal pregnancy

Prenatal outpatient visits for high-risk pregnancies:

- V23, Supervision of high-risk pregnancy

Fifth Digit

All categories EXCEPT 650 (Normal delivery)

Requires 5th digit for

- Antepartum
- Postpartum
- If delivery has occurred

Appropriate 5th digit listed under each code

Example: 640.0, Threatened abortion

- 0 unspecified episode
- 1 delivered with or without complication
- 3 antepartum condition or complication

Note that NOT all 5th digits are applicable (640.0, cannot assign 2 or 4)

Postpartum Period

After delivery +6 weeks

Abortions

Codes 634-637 require 5th digits

- 0 unspecified

- 1 incomplete; POC (product of conception) NOT expelled

- 2 complete; all POC expelled prior to care

Abortions with Liveborn Fetus
Attempted abortion results in liveborn fetus

- 644.21 (Early onset of delivery)

- Use V27.- (Outcome of delivery)

- Attempted abortion code also assigned

ICD-9-CM, CHAPTER 12, DISEASES OF SKIN AND SUBCUTANEOUS TISSUE

Skin

Epidermis

Dermis

Subcutaneous tissue

Infectious skin/subcutaneous tissue

Scar tissue

Accessory Organs

Sweat glands

Sebaceous glands

Nails

Hair and hair follicles

Other

Multiple Codes Often Necessary

Example: Cellulitis due to *Staphylococcus*, report

- Cellulitis 682.-

- Staph 041.-

ICD-9-CM, CHAPTER 13, DISEASES OF MUSCULOSKELETAL SYSTEM AND CONNECTIVE TISSUE

Bone

Bursa

Cartilage

Fascia

Ligaments

Muscle

Synovia

Tendons

Chapter 13 Sections

Extensive notes and 5th digits

- Arthropathies (joint disease) and related disorders
- Dorsopathies (curvature of spine)
- Rheumatism, Excluding Back
- Osteopathies, Chondropathies, and Acquired Musculoskeletal Deformities

ICD-9-CM, CHAPTERS 14 AND 15, CONGENITAL ANOMALIES AND CONDITIONS ORIGINATING IN PERINATAL PERIOD

Congenital Anomalies (abnormalities at birth), 740-759

Conditions Originating in Perinatal Period

- Perinatal period through 28th day following birth
- Codes can be used after 28th day if documented that condition originated during perinatal period

Chapter 17 codes are only for the newborn record; never on the maternal record

Assign V30-V39 as first listed according to type of birth

ICD-9-CM, CHAPTER 16, SYMPTOMS, SIGNS, AND ILL-DEFINED CONDITIONS

Do NOT code a sign or symptom if

- Definitive dx made (symptoms are part of disease)

Used only if no specific dx made

ICD-9-CM, CHAPTER 17, INJURY AND POISONING

Section Examples

Fractures

Dislocations

Sprains and Strains

Intracranial Injury

Internal Injury

Crushing Injury

Foreign Body

Burns

Late Effects

Poisoning

Acute fracture care vs. aftercare

Use aftercare codes after completion of active treatment

- Cast change/removal (V53.7)

- Removal of external/internal devices (V54.0-)

- Medication adjustments

- Follow-up visits following fracture treatment

E Codes

Provide supplemental information

Never principal diagnosis

Index and Tabular

E code Index located in Section III

    Directly before the Tabular

    Not in the Index to Disease, Volume 2

E codes are located after the V codes in the Tabular

Identify

- Cause of an injury or poisoning

- Intent (unintentional or intentional)

- Place it occurred

General E Code Guidelines

Use with any code in Volume 1

Initial encounter

- Use E code

Subsequent encounter

- Use late effects E codes, if appropriate

Intent

Unknown, Undetermined (E980-E989)

Unspecified, Undetermined (E980-E989)

Questionable, Undetermined (E980-E989)

Table of Drugs and Chemicals

Alphabetic listing with codes (see Fig. 3-16)

Do NOT code directly from Table

Always reference Tabular

Two or more substances involved

If two or more substances involved

- Code each unless combination code exists

- Code substance more closely related to principal dx

510

- Include one code from each category (cause, intent, place)

Interaction of drug(s) and alcohol

- Use poisoning and E codes for both

Unknown or suspected intent
Unknown

Unspecified

Questionable

Undetermined cause
Intent known, cause unknown, use

- E928.9, Unspecified accident

- E958.9, Suicide and self-inflicted injury by unspecified means

- E968.9, Assault by unspecified means

Late effects of external cause
Should be used with late effect of a previous injury/poisoning

Should NOT be used with related current injury code

Coding of Burns
Multiple injuries and burns
Sequence most severe injury first (physician determined)

Current burns
Sequence highest-degree burn first

Current burns (940-948) classified by

- Depth (severity)

- Extent (% body surface)

- Agent (if necessary)

Depth of burn (Fig. 3-17)
1st degree: Erythema

2nd degree: Blistering

3rd degree: Full-thickness involvement

Burns classified
- According to extent of body surface involved

Category 948
- 4th digits = % body surface involved

- 5th digits = % body surface involved in 3rd-degree burns

- Rule of Nines applies

Burn Example: 3rd-degree burn of abdomen (10%) and 2nd-degree burn of thigh (5%) by hot water

- 942.33 Burn, abdomen, 3rd degree

- 945.26 Burn, thigh, 2nd degree

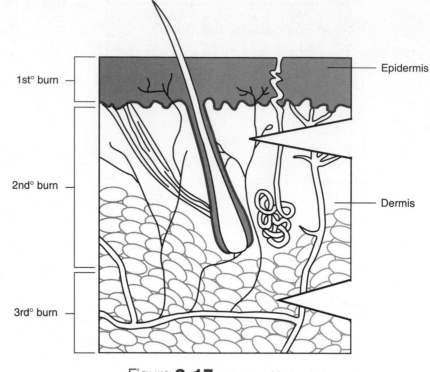

Figure **3-17** Degree of burns.

- 948.11 15% total burn area and 10% 3rd degree
- E924.0 Burn by hot liquid

Coding for multiple injuries
Separate code for each injury

Sequence most serious injury first

Vessel and nerve damage
Code primary injury first

- Use additional code if minor nerve damage

Primary injury = nerve damage

- Code nerve damage first

Multiple fractures
Same coding principles as multiple injuries

Code multiple fractures by site

Sequenced by severity

Fractures
Not indicated as closed or open = closed

Same bone fractured AND dislocated:

- Code fracture ONLY (highest level of injury)

UNIT 4

Preparing for Practice Examinations

Some of the CPT code descriptions for physician services include physician extender services. Physician extenders, such as nurse practitioners, physician assistants, and nurse anesthetists, etc., provide medical services typically performed by a physician. Within this educational material the term "physician" may include "and other qualified health care professionals" depending on the code. Refer to the official CPT® code descriptions and guidelines to determine codes that are appropriate to report services provided by non-physician practitioners.

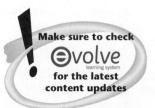

Make sure to check
evolve
learning system
**for the latest
content updates**

EXAMINATIONS

> **DISCLAIMER:** Every effort has been made to ensure that the content of the practice exams in Unit 4 and on the companion Evolve website resemble the format and content of current certification examinations. However, the examinations may be revised at any time and it is your responsibility to review all certification information published by the certifying organization.

You have three opportunities to practice taking an examination:

• Pre-Examination (before study)

• Post-Examination (after study)

• Final Examination (at the end of your complete program of study)

You should have a current edition of the following texts:

• ICD-9-CM (*International Classification of Diseases,* 9th Edition, Clinical Modification), Volumes 1 and 2

• HCPCS *(Healthcare Common Procedure Coding System)*

• CPT *(Current Procedural Terminology)*

No other reference material is allowed for any of the examinations.

• For the Pre-Examination and Post-Examination, you will need a computer and the three coding references listed above (ICD-9-CM [Vols. 1 and 2], HCPCS, CPT).

• For the Final Examination, you will need paper, pencils, and an eraser, along with the three coding references.

• Each organization's certification examination has different scoring requirements, but as you take the examinations with this text, you should strive for 80% to 90% on the Post-Examination and 70% as a minimum on the Final Examination. AAPC's standard for passing is usually about 70%.

> **NOTE:** To enable the learner to calculate an examination score, minimums have been identified as "passing" within this text; however, this may or may not be the percentage identified by the certifying organization as a "passing" grade. It is your responsibility to review all certification information published by the certifying organization.

> **NOTE:** It is expected that the examiner is able to assign key components when reporting evaluation and management services. See updated E/M questions for examples of the new format. All categories of codes (I, II, and III) are potentially on the examination.

PRE-EXAMINATION AND POST-EXAMINATION

The Pre-Examination contains 150 questions and is located on the companion Evolve website. The purpose of the Pre-Examination is only to assess your beginning level of knowledge and skill—your starting place. Based on your scores, you can tailor your study to target your weakest areas and increase your scores. Take the Pre-Examination before you begin your studies.

Your score will automatically be calculated for you. A passing score for the examinations in this text requires 70%.

The software will calculate and retain your scoring information.

Immediately on completion of your study, you should complete the Post-Examination on Evolve. After you are finished, the program on Evolve will automatically compare your Pre-Examination scores with your Post-Examination scores and will store your results. By comparing the results of the Pre-Examination and the Post-Examination (the same examination will be taken twice), the software illustrates the improvements you have achieved or the areas that you will need to practice more on before taking the Final Examination.

Rationales for each question are available for review after you complete the Post-Examination. Study the questions for which you did not choose the right response. Did you misread the question, did you not know the material well enough to answer correctly, or did you run out of time? Knowing why you missed a question is an important step toward improving your skill level.

Ideally, you should complete each examination in one sitting (5 hours and 40 minutes, or 340 minutes); if time does not allow, spread the examination times over several periods. There are no time extensions during an actual examination setting, and learning how to judge the amount of time you should spend on each question is an important part of this learning experience to prepare you for the real certification examination.

FINAL EXAMINATION

If you scored well on all areas of the Post-Examination (80% to 90%), you are ready to move on to the Final Examination, located in Unit 4 of the text.

There is an answer sheet on which to place your answers; it is located directly before the examination. Remove your answer sheet from this text, and enter your answer for each of the 150 questions using paper and pencil.

NOTE: The real AAPC certification examination is currently paper and pencil.

Once you have completed the Final Examination, go to Evolve to enter your answers on the electronic score sheet. The software will then provide you with the answers and compare your scores to illustrate your improvement.

A passing score for the Final Examination is the same as for the Pre/Post-Examination—70%.

If you did not attain a minimum score on each section, you should develop a plan to restudy those particular areas where the examination indicates you are having difficulties. There are rationales for each question in the Final Examination, and you should review that information as well as material in the text. You can take any of the practice examinations again after your additional study.

FINAL EXAMINATION ANSWER SHEET

Medical Terminology
1. (A) (B) (C) (D)
2. (A) (B) (C) (D)
3. (A) (B) (C) (D)
4. (A) (B) (C) (D)
5. (A) (B) (C) (D)
6. (A) (B) (C) (D)
7. (A) (B) (C) (D)
8. (A) (B) (C) (D)

Anatomy
9. (A) (B) (C) (D)
10. (A) (B) (C) (D)
11. (A) (B) (C) (D)
12. (A) (B) (C) (D)
13. (A) (B) (C) (D)
14. (A) (B) (C) (D)
15. (A) (B) (C) (D)
16. (A) (B) (C) (D)

ICD-9-CM
17. (A) (B) (C) (D)
18. (A) (B) (C) (D)
19. (A) (B) (C) (D)
20. (A) (B) (C) (D)
21. (A) (B) (C) (D)
22. (A) (B) (C) (D)
23. (A) (B) (C) (D)
24. (A) (B) (C) (D)
25. (A) (B) (C) (D)
26. (A) (B) (C) (D)

HCPCS
27. (A) (B) (C) (D)
28. (A) (B) (C) (D)
29. (A) (B) (C) (D)
30. (A) (B) (C) (D)
31. (A) (B) (C) (D)

Practice Management
32. (A) (B) (C) (D)
33. (A) (B) (C) (D)
34. (A) (B) (C) (D)
35. (A) (B) (C) (D)
36. (A) (B) (C) (D)
37. (A) (B) (C) (D)

Coding Guidelines
38. (A) (B) (C) (D)
39. (A) (B) (C) (D)
40. (A) (B) (C) (D)
41. (A) (B) (C) (D)
42. (A) (B) (C) (D)
43. (A) (B) (C) (D)

10000 Integumentary System
44. (A) (B) (C) (D)
45. (A) (B) (C) (D)
46. (A) (B) (C) (D)
47. (A) (B) (C) (D)
48. (A) (B) (C) (D)
49. (A) (B) (C) (D)
50. (A) (B) (C) (D)
51. (A) (B) (C) (D)
52. (A) (B) (C) (D)
53. (A) (B) (C) (D)

20000 Musculoskeletal System
54. (A) (B) (C) (D)
55. (A) (B) (C) (D)
56. (A) (B) (C) (D)
57. (A) (B) (C) (D)
58. (A) (B) (C) (D)
59. (A) (B) (C) (D)
60. (A) (B) (C) (D)
61. (A) (B) (C) (D)
62. (A) (B) (C) (D)
63. (A) (B) (C) (D)

30000 Respiratory and Cardiovascular System
64. (A) (B) (C) (D)
65. (A) (B) (C) (D)
66. (A) (B) (C) (D)
67. (A) (B) (C) (D)
68. (A) (B) (C) (D)
69. (A) (B) (C) (D)
70. (A) (B) (C) (D)
71. (A) (B) (C) (D)
72. (A) (B) (C) (D)
73. (A) (B) (C) (D)

40000 Digestive System
74. (A) (B) (C) (D)
75. (A) (B) (C) (D)
76. (A) (B) (C) (D)
77. (A) (B) (C) (D)
78. (A) (B) (C) (D)
79. (A) (B) (C) (D)
80. (A) (B) (C) (D)
81. (A) (B) (C) (D)
82. (A) (B) (C) (D)
83. (A) (B) (C) (D)

50000 Urinary, Male Genital System, Female Genital System, and Maternity Care and Delivery
84. (A) (B) (C) (D)
85. (A) (B) (C) (D)
86. (A) (B) (C) (D)
87. (A) (B) (C) (D)
88. (A) (B) (C) (D)
89. (A) (B) (C) (D)
90. (A) (B) (C) (D)
91. (A) (B) (C) (D)
92. (A) (B) (C) (D)
93. (A) (B) (C) (D)

60000 Endocrine System, Nervous System, Eye and Ocular Adnexa
94. (A) (B) (C) (D)
95. (A) (B) (C) (D)
96. (A) (B) (C) (D)
97. (A) (B) (C) (D)
98. (A) (B) (C) (D)
99. (A) (B) (C) (D)
100. (A) (B) (C) (D)
101. (A) (B) (C) (D)
102. (A) (B) (C) (D)
103. (A) (B) (C) (D)

Evaluation and Management (E/M)
104. (A) (B) (C) (D)
105. (A) (B) (C) (D)
106. (A) (B) (C) (D)
107. (A) (B) (C) (D)
108. (A) (B) (C) (D)
109. (A) (B) (C) (D)
110. (A) (B) (C) (D)
111. (A) (B) (C) (D)
112. (A) (B) (C) (D)
113. (A) (B) (C) (D)

Anesthesia
114. (A) (B) (C) (D)
115. (A) (B) (C) (D)
116. (A) (B) (C) (D)
117. (A) (B) (C) (D)
118. (A) (B) (C) (D)
119. (A) (B) (C) (D)
120. (A) (B) (C) (D)
121. (A) (B) (C) (D)

70000 Radiology
122. (A) (B) (C) (D)
123. (A) (B) (C) (D)
124. (A) (B) (C) (D)
125. (A) (B) (C) (D)
126. (A) (B) (C) (D)
127. (A) (B) (C) (D)
128. (A) (B) (C) (D)
129. (A) (B) (C) (D)
130. (A) (B) (C) (D)

80000 Pathology and Laboratory
131. (A) (B) (C) (D)
132. (A) (B) (C) (D)
133. (A) (B) (C) (D)
134. (A) (B) (C) (D)
135. (A) (B) (C) (D)
136. (A) (B) (C) (D)
137. (A) (B) (C) (D)
138. (A) (B) (C) (D)
139. (A) (B) (C) (D)
140. (A) (B) (C) (D)

90000 Medicine
141. (A) (B) (C) (D)
142. (A) (B) (C) (D)
143. (A) (B) (C) (D)
144. (A) (B) (C) (D)
145. (A) (B) (C) (D)
146. (A) (B) (C) (D)
147. (A) (B) (C) (D)
148. (A) (B) (C) (D)
149. (A) (B) (C) (D)
150. (A) (B) (C) (D)

FINAL EXAMINATION

Direction: Report only the professional component unless specifically directed to do otherwise within the question.

Subject Area: Medical Terminology

1. This term means the surgical removal of the fallopian tube:
   A. ligation
   B. hysterectomy
   C. salpingostomy
   D. salpingectomy

2. This combining form means "thirst":
   A. dips/o
   B. acr/o
   C. cortic/o
   D. somat/o

3. This term is also known as a homograft:
   A. autograft
   B. allograft
   C. xenograft
   D. zenograft

4. Which of the following terms means "taste"?
   A. Meissner
   B. pacinian
   C. gustatory
   D. astrocytes

5. This suffix means "removal":
   A. -penia
   B. -ectomy
   C. -itis
   D. -pexy

6. Which of the following terms does NOT describe a receptor of the body?
   A. mechanoreceptor
   B. proprioceptor
   C. thermoreceptor
   D. endoreceptor

7. This term means abnormal thickening of the skin:
   A. ductus
   B. dermatofibroma
   C. dermatitis
   D. pachyderma

8. The term that defines the relaxation phase of the heartbeat is:
   A. systole
   B. sinoatrial
   C. diastole
   D. septa

Subject Area: Anatomy

9. This is the first portion of the small intestine:
   A. jejunum
   B. ileum
   C. duodenum
   D. cecum

10. This is a part of the inner ear:
    A. vestibule
    B. malleus
    C. incus
    D. stapes

11. This is the area behind the cornea:
    A. anterior chamber
    B. choroid layer
    C. ciliary body
    D. fundus

12. Which of the following is a covering of the chamber walls of the heart?
    A. endocardium
    B. myocardium
    C. pericardium
    D. epicardium

13. The shaft of a long bone:
    A. diaphysis
    B. epiphysis
    C. metaphysis
    D. periosteum

14. The act of turning upward, such as the hand turned palm upward:
    A. supination
    B. adduction
    C. pronation
    D. circumduction

15. The middle layer of the skin, also known as the corium or true skin, is the:
    A. epidermis.
    B. stratum corneum.
    C. dermis.
    D. subcutaneous.

16. This is the collarbone:
    A. patella
    B. tibia
    C. scapula
    D. clavicle

Subject Area: ICD-9-CM

17. Three-week-old female with obstructive apnea.
    A. 770.8
    B. 770.82
    C. 769
    D. 770.83

18. Mild intellectual disabilities due to congenital iodine-deficiency hypothyroidism.
    A. 243, 317
    B. 244.8, 317
    C. 243, 318.0
    D. 317, 243

19. Admission for hemodialysis because of acute renal failure.
    A. V56.31, 584.9
    B. V56, 584
    C. V56.0, 584.9
    D. 584.9, V56.0

20. Glomerulonephritis due to viral hepatitis.
    A. 580.9, 070
    B. 070, 580.9
    C. 580.81, 070.9
    D. 070.9, 580.81

21. Initial encounter to repair a laceration of left hand.
    A. 882.0
    B. 883.0
    C. 887.2
    D. 882.2

22. Mr. Hallberger is 62 and has multiple problems. I am examining him in the intensive critical care unit. I understand he has fluid overload with acute renal failure and was started on ultrafiltration by the nephrologist on duty. He has an abnormal chest x-ray. He has preexisting type II diabetes mellitus and sepsis. We are left with a patient now who is still sedated and on a ventilator because of acute respiratory failure. Code the diagnoses only.
    A. 782.3, 585.9, 792, 250.40, 039.9, 518.81
    B. 789.59, 584.7, 793.19, 250.4, 039.9, 518.81
    C. 276.50, 587, 793.19, 250.00, 038.9, 518.81, 99223
    D. 038.9, 995.92, 584.9, 518.81, 250.00, 793.19

23. Bloody stool.
    A. 772.4
    B. 792.1
    C. 578.1
    D. 578.0

24. A lethargic patient presents with vomiting and severe cramping, and the physician determines during the initial encounter that the condition was caused by the ingestion of five tablets of Tylenol With Codeine and half a bottle of whiskey.
    A. 965.01, 965.4, 980.0, 780.79, 787.03, 789.00, E980.0, E980
    B. 965.09, 965.61, 980.0, 780.79, 787.03, 789.00, E980.0
    C. 966.09, 965.4, 980.0, 780.71, 787.03, 789.00, E980.4, E980.9
    D. 965.09, 965.4, 980.0, 780.79, 787.03, 789.00, E980.0, E980.9

25. Initial encounter to treat a fracture of the right patella with abrasion.
    A. 822.0, 916.0
    B. 822.0
    C. 916.0, 822.1
    D. 823.00

26. Sarcoidosis causing cardiomyopathy.
    A. 135, 517.8
    B. 135, 425.8
    C. 425.8, 135
    D. 135, 425.8, V71.7

Subject Area: HCPCS

27. A patient is issued a 22-inch seat cushion for his wheelchair.
    A. E2601
    B. E0950
    C. E0190
    D. E2602

28. A patient with chronic lumbar pain previously purchased a TENS and now needs replacement batteries.
    A. E1592
    B. A5082
    C. A4772
    D. A4630

29. A patient presents for trimming of 10 dystrophic toenails.
    A. G0127 × 2, 703.8
    B. G0127, G0127 × 9, 703.0
    C. G0127, 703.8
    D. G0127 × 5, G0127 × 5, 703.9

30. A patient with chronic obstructive pulmonary disease is issued a medically necessary nebulizer with a compressor and humidifier for extensive use with oxygen delivery.
    A. E0570, E0550
    B. E0555, E0574
    C. E0580, E0550
    D. E0575, E0550

31. Which HCPCS modifier indicates the great toe of the right foot?
    A. -T1
    B. -T3
    C. -T4
    D. -T5

Subject Area: Practice Management

32. This entity develops and publishes an annual plan that outlines the Medicare monitoring program.
    A. MAC
    B. FI
    C. OIG
    D. CMS

33. This program was developed by CMS to promote national correct coding methods and to control inappropriate payment of Part B claims and hospital outpatient claims.
    A. NCCI
    B. NFS
    C. HIPAA
    D. MA-PA

34. What is an NPI?
    A. National Payer Incentive
    B. National Provider Identification
    C. National Provider Index
    D. National Payer Identification

35. The RBRVS is a
    A. payment reform implemented in 1992
    B. listing of the customary charge for services
    C. payment list that indicates the prevailing charge in a locality
    D. listing of the physician's individual charges for a service

36. Which of the following is NOT considered fraud or abuse?
    A. Lack of documentation of medical necessity for services reported
    B. Accepting a $20 gift card from a shoe repair representative for each Medicare patient referred to his store
    C. Referring patients to a radiology center in which your physician is a partner
    D. Going to lunch with a pharmaceutical representative

37. This document is a notification in advance of services that Medicare probably will not pay for and the estimated cost to the patient.
    A. Wavier of Liability
    B. Coordination of Benefits
    C. Advanced Beneficiary Notice
    D. UPIN

Subject Area: Coding Guidelines

38. Which punctuation mark between codes in the index of the CPT manual indicates a range of codes is available?
    A. period
    B. comma
    C. semicolon
    D. hyphen

39. Which of the following most accurately describes the designation "(Separate procedure)"? The procedure is:
    A. incidental to another procedure.
    B. reported if it is the only procedure performed.
    C. reported if the procedure is unrelated to a more major procedure performed at the same time on the same site.
    D. All of the above

40. Specific coding guidelines in the CPT manual are located in:
    A. the index.
    B. the introduction.
    C. the beginning of each section.
    D. Appendix A.

41. The symbol that indicates an add-on code in the CPT manual is:
    A. ▲
    B. ●
    C. +
    D. ►◄

42. When you see the symbol "⊘" next to a code in the CPT manual, you know that:
    A. the code is a new code.
    B. the code contains new or revised text.
    C. the code is a modifier -51 exempt code.
    D. FDA approval is pending.

43. The term that indicates this is the type of code for which the full code description can be known only if the common part of the code (the description preceding the semicolon) of a preceding entry is referenced:
    A. stand-alone
    B. indented
    C. independent
    D. add-on

Subject Area: 10000 Integumentary System

44. **OPERATIVE REPORT**

    OPERATIVE PROCEDURE: Excision of back lesion.

    INDICATIONS FOR SURGERY: The patient has an enlarging lesion on the upper midback.

    FINDINGS AT SURGERY: There was a 5-cm, upper midback lesion.

    OPERATIVE PROCEDURE: With the patient prone, the back was prepped and draped in the usual sterile fashion. The skin and underlying tissues were anesthetized with 30 mL of 1% lidocaine with epinephrine.

    Through a 5-cm transverse skin incision, the lesion was excised. Hemostasis was ensured. The incision was closed using 3-0 Vicryl for the deep layers and running 3-0 Prolene subcuticular stitch with Steri-Strips for the skin.

    The patient was returned to the same-day surgery center in stable postoperative condition. All sponge, needle, and instrument counts were correct. Estimated blood loss is 0 mL.

PATHOLOGY REPORT LATER INDICATED: Dermatofibroma, skin of back. Assign code(s) for the physician service only.
A. 11406, 12002, 216.5
B. 11424, 215.7
C. 11406, 12032, 216.5
D. 11606, 232.5

45. What CPT and ICD-9-CM codes would be used to code a subsequent encounter in which a split-thickness skin graft, both thighs to the abdomen, measuring 45 × 21 cm, is performed on a patient who has third-degree burns of the abdomen? Documentation stated 20% of the body surface was burned, with 9% third degree. The patient also sustained second-degree burns of the upper back.
A. 15100 × 2, 949.3, 949.2, 948.00
B. 15100, 15101 × 9, 942.33, 942.24, 948.20
C. 15100, 15101-51 × 9, 946.3, 949.2, 948.02
D. 15100, 15101 × 8, 948.01, 942.29

46. **EMERGENCY DEPARTMENT REPORT CHIEF COMPLAINT:** Nasal bridge laceration.

SUBJECTIVE: The patient is a 74-year-old male who presents to the emergency department with a laceration to the bridge of his nose. He fell in the bathroom tonight. He recalls the incident. He just sort of lost his balance. He denies any vertigo. He denies any chest pain or shortness of breath. He denies any head pain or neck pain. There was no loss of consciousness. He slipped on a wet floor in the bathroom and lost his balance; that is how it happened. He has not had any blood from the nose or mouth.

PAST MEDICAL HISTORY:
1. Parkinson's.
2. Back pain.
3. Constipation.

MEDICATIONS: See the patient record for a complete list of medications.

ALLERGIES: NKDA.

REVIEW OF SYSTEMS: Per HPI. Otherwise, negative.

PHYSICAL EXAMINATION: The exam showed a 74-year-old male in no acute distress. Examination of the HEAD showed no obvious trauma other than the bridge of the nose, where there is approximately a 1.5- to 2-cm laceration. He had no bony tenderness under this. Pupils were equal, round, and reactive. EARS and NOSE: OROPHARYNX was unremarkable. NECK was soft and supple. HEART was regular. LUNGS were clear but slightly diminished in the bases.

PROCEDURE: The wound was draped in a sterile fashion and anesthetized with 1% Xylocaine with sodium bicarbonate. It was cleansed with sterile saline and then repaired using interrupted 6-0 Ethilon sutures (Dr. Barney Teller, first-year resident, assisted with the suturing).

ASSESSMENT: Nasal bridge laceration, status post fall.

PLAN: Keep clean. Sutures out in 5 to 7 days. Watch for signs of infection.
A. 12051, 873.20, E885.9
B. 12011, 873.20, E885.9
C. 12011, 873.32, E888.8
D. 12011, 11000, 873.32, E929.9

47. The patient is brought to surgery for repair of an accidentally inflicted open wound of the left thigh, the total extent measuring approximately 40 × 35 cm.

    DESCRIPTION OF PROCEDURE: The legs were prepped with Betadine scrub and solution and then draped in a routine sterile fashion. Split-thickness skin grafts measuring about a 10,000th inch thick were taken from both thighs, meshed with a 3:1 ratio mesher, and stapled to the wounds. The donor sites were dressed with scarlet red, and the recipient sites were dressed with Xeroform, Kerlix fluffs, and Kerlix roll, and a few ABD pads were used for absorption. Estimated blood loss was negligible. The patient tolerated the procedure well and left surgery in good condition.
    A. 15120, 15121 × 12, 891.0, E929.9
    B. 15100, 15101, 11010, 891.0, E928.9
    C. 15220, 15221 × 13, 890.0, E928.9
    D. 15100, 15101 × 13, 890.0, E928.9

48. What CPT and ICD-9-CM codes would be used to code the destruction of a malignant lesion on the skin of the female genitalia measuring 1.6 cm using cryosurgery?
    A. 17272, 184.4
    B. 11602, 199.0
    C. 11420, 198.82
    D. 11622, 184.4

49. **SAME-DAY SURGERY**

    DIAGNOSIS: Inverted nipple with mammary duct ectasia, left.

    OPERATION: Excision of mass deep to left nipple.
    With the patient under general anesthesia, a circumareolar incision was made with sharp dissection and carried down into the breast tissue. The nipple complex was raised up using a small retractor. We gently dissected underneath to free up the nipple entirely. Once this was done, we had the nipple fully unfolded, and there was some evident mammary duct ectasia. An area 3 × 4 cm was excised using electrocautery. Hemostasis was maintained with the electrocautery, and then the breast tissue deep to the nipple was reconstructed using sutures of 3-0 chromic. Subcutaneous tissue was closed using 3-0 chromic, and then the skin was closed using 4-0 Vicryl. Steri-Strips were applied. The patient tolerated the procedure well and was returned to the recovery area in stable condition. At the end of the procedure, all sponges and instruments were accounted for.
    A. 19120-RT, 610.4
    B. 11404-LT, 611.1
    C. 19112, 610.4
    D. 19120-LT, 610.4

50. This patient returns today for palliative care to her feet. Her toenails have become elongated and thickened, and she is unable to trim them on her own. She states that she has had no problems and no acute signs of any infection or otherwise to her feet. She returns today strictly for trimming of her toenails.

    EXAMINATION: Her pedal pulses are palpable bilaterally. The nails are mycotic, 1 through 4 on the left, and 1 through 3 on the right.

    ASSESSMENT: Onychomycosis, 1 through 4 on the left and 1 through 3 on the right.

    PLAN: Mild debridement of mycotic nails × 7. This patient is to return to the clinic in 3 to 4 months for follow-up palliative care.
    A. 11721 × 7, 117.9
    B. 99212, 11721, 110.1
    C. 11719, 110.1
    D. 11721, 110.1

51. **OPERATIVE REPORT**
    With the patient having had a wire localization performed by radiology, she was taken to the operating room and, under local anesthesia of the left breast, was prepped and draped in a sterile manner. A breast line incision was made through the entry point of the wire, and a core of tissue surrounding the wire (approximately 1 × 2 cm) was removed using electrocautery for hemostasis. The specimen, including the wire, was then submitted to radiology, and the presence of the lesion within the specimen was confirmed. The wound was checked for hemostasis, and this was maintained with electrocautery. The breast tissue was reapproximated using 2-0 and 3-0 chromic. The skin was closed using 4-0 Vicryl in a subcuticular manner. Steri-Strips were applied. The patient tolerated the procedure well and was discharged from the operating room in stable condition. At the end of the procedure, all sponges and instruments were accounted for. Pathology report later indicated: Benign tissue, breast.
    A. 11602-LT, 238.3
    B. 11400-LT, 174.9
    C. 19125-LT, 217
    D. 19125-LT, 239.3

52. What CPT and ICD-9-CM codes would be assigned to report an initial encounter for treatment of a 40 sq cm debridement of an open anterior abdominal laceration, including subcutaneous tissue and muscle, with grit and rubble? The patient fell while speed walking and landed on a sharp rock, injuring the epigastric region of the abdomen.
    A. 11000, 879.2, E880.1, E920.8
    B. 11010, 879.6, E880.1
    C. 11042, 11045, 879.2
    D. 11043, 11046, 879.3, E888.0, E920.8, E001.0

53. What code(s) is used by the radiologist when performing ultrasound preoperative placement of a needle localization wire of a single lesion of the breast? The patient was diagnosed with adenocarcinoma of the upper outer quadrant of the right breast, primary site.
   A. 19285-RT, 19125, 174.5
   B. 19125-RT, 174.4
   C. 19285-RT, 174.4
   D. 19286-RT, 174.5

Subject Area: 20000 Musculoskeletal System

54. A small incision was made over the left proximal tibia, and a traction pin was inserted through the bone to the opposite side. Weights were then affixed to the pins to stabilize the closed tibial fracture temporarily until fracture repair could be performed. Assign codes for the physician service.
   A. 20650-LT, 823.00
   B. 20663-LT, 823.92
   C. 20690-LT, 823.40
   D. 20692-LT, 823.92

55. **OPERATIVE REPORT**

PREOPERATIVE DIAGNOSIS: Left thigh abscess.

PROCEDURE PERFORMED: Incision and drainage of left thigh abscess.

OPERATIVE NOTE: With the patient under general anesthesia, he was placed in the lithotomy position. The area around the anus was carefully inspected, and we saw no evidence of communication with the perirectal space. This appears to have risen in the crease at the top of the leg, extending from the posterior buttocks region up toward the side of the base of the penis. In any event, the area was prepped and draped in a sterile manner. Then we incised the area in fluctuation. We obtained a lot of very foul-smelling, almost stool-like material (it was not stool, but it was brown and very foul-smelling material). This was not the typical pus one sees with a *Staphylococcus aureus*–type infection. The incision was widened to allow us to probe the cavity fully. Again, I could see no evidence of communication to the rectum, but there was extension down the thigh and extension up into the groin crease. The fascia was darkened from the purulent material. I opened some of the fascia to make sure the underlying muscle was viable. This appeared viable. No gas was present. There was nothing to suggest a necrotizing fasciitis. The patient did have a very extensive inflammation within this abscess cavity. The abscess cavity was irrigated with peroxide and saline and packed with gauze vaginal packing. The patient tolerated the procedure well and was discharged from the operating room in stable condition.
   A. 26990-LT, 682.6
   B. 27301-LT, 682.6
   C. 27301-LT, 682.60
   D. 27025-LT, 682.6

56. **OPERATIVE REPORT**

PREOPERATIVE DIAGNOSIS: Compound fracture, left humerus, with possible loss of left radial pulse.

PROCEDURE PERFORMED: Open reduction internal fixation, left compound humerus fracture.

PROCEDURE: While under a general anesthetic, the patient's left arm was prepped with Betadine and draped in sterile fashion. We then created a longitudinal incision over the anterolateral aspect of his left arm and carried the dissection through the subcutaneous tissue. We attempted to identify the lateral intermuscular septum and progressed to the fracture site, which was actually fairly easy to do because there was some significant tearing and rupturing of the biceps and brachialis muscles. These were partial ruptures, but the bone was relatively easy to expose through this. We then identified the fracture site and thoroughly irrigated it with several liters of saline. We also noted that the radial nerve was easily visible, crossing along the posterolateral aspect of the fracture site. It was intact. We carefully detected it throughout the remainder of the procedure. We then were able to strip the periosteum away from the lateral side of the shaft of the humerus both proximally and distally from the fracture site. We did this just enough to apply a 6-hole plate, which we eventually held in place with six cortical screws. We did attempt to compress the fracture site. Due to some comminution, the fracture was not quite anatomically aligned, but certainly it was felt to be very acceptable.

Once we had applied the plate, we then checked the radial pulse with a Doppler. We found that the radial pulse was present using the Doppler, but not with palpation. We then applied Xeroform dressings to the wounds and the incision. After padding the arm thoroughly, we applied a long-arm splint with the elbow flexed about 75 degrees. He tolerated the procedure well, and the radial pulse was again present on Doppler examination at the end of the procedure.

A. 24515-RT, 812.30, E887
B. 24500-LT, 812.20, E888.9
C. 24515-LT, 812.31, E887
D. 24505-LT, 812.20, E888.9

57. John, an 84-year-old male, tripped while on his morning walk. He stated he was thinking about something else when he inadvertently tripped over the sidewalk curb and fell to his knees. X-ray indicated a fracture of his right patella. With the patient under general anesthesia, the area was opened and extensively irrigated. The left aspect of the patella was severely fragmented, and a portion of the patella was subsequently removed. The remaining patella fragments were wired. The surrounding tissue was repaired, thoroughly irrigated, and closed in the usual manner.

A. 27524-RT, 822.0, E880.1
B. 27520-RT, 822.0, E880.1
C. 27524-RT, 822.1, E888.9
D. 27524-RT, 822.0, E888.9

58. Libby was thrown from a horse while riding along the side of the road; a truck that honked the horn as it passed her startled her horse. The horse reared up, and Libby was thrown to the ground. The condyle of her left tibia was fractured and required insertion of multiple pins to stabilize the defect area. A Monticelli multiplane external fixation system was then attached to the pins. Code the placement of the fixation device and diagnosis(es) only.
   A. 20661-LT, 823.82, E828.9
   B. 20692-LT, 823.00, E828.2
   C. 20692-LT, 823.82, E828.2
   D. 20690-LT, 823.00, E828.2

59. Maryann received a blow to her right tibial shaft while moving a large stuffed chair up a flight of stairs when the person in front of the chair slipped and released his hold on the chair. The full weight of the chair was pushed against her; when she was unable to hold the chair in place, both she and the chair fell to the landing a dozen steps below. The chair tipped on its side and landed on her tibia. On x-ray, the right tibia shaft was fractured in three places. Screws and pins were placed through the skin to secure the fracture sites.
   A. 27750-RT, 823.80, E917.3
   B. 27756-RT, 823.80, E917.3
   C. 27756-RT, 823.20, E917.3
   D. 27750-RT, 823.20, E917.3

60. The physician applies a Minerva-type fiberglass body cast from the hips to the shoulders and to the head. Before application, a stockinette is stretched over the patient's torso, and further padding of the bony areas with felt padding was done. The patient was diagnosed with Morquio-Brailsford kyphosis. Assign codes for the physician service only.
   A. 29040, 277.5, 737.41
   B. 29710, 737.41
   C. 29025, 737.41, 277.5
   D. 29000, 737.10, 277.5

61. Mary tells her physician that she has been having pain in her left wrist for several weeks. The physician examines the area and palpates a ganglion cyst of the tendon sheath. He marks the injection sites, sterilizes the area, and injects corticosteroid into two areas.
   A. 20550-LT × 2, 727.42
   B. 20551-LT, 727.41
   C. 20551-LT × 2, 727.43
   D. 20612-LT, 727.42

62. Darin was a passenger in an automobile rollover accident and was not wearing a seat belt at the time. He was thrown from the automobile and was pinned under the rear of the overturned vehicle. He sustained craniofacial separation, Le Forte III fracture that required complicated internal and external fixation using an open approach to repair the extensive damage. A halo device was used to hold the head immobile.
   A. 21435, 20661
   B. 21435
   C. 21432
   D. 21436, 20661

63. Carl Ostrick, a 21-year-old male, slipped on a patch of ice on his sidewalk while shoveling snow. When he fell, his left hand was wedged under his body and his carpometacarpal joint was dislocated. After manipulating the joint back into normal alignment, the surgeon on the following day fixed the dislocation by placing a wire through the skin at the tip of the finger and on through the carpometacarpal joint to maintain alignment. Code the subsequent procedure and diagnoses.
A. 26608-F1, 833.01, E886.0
B. 26650-FA, 833.14, E888.9
C. 26706-LT, 833.00, E885.9
D. 26676-LT, 833.04, E885.9

Subject Area: 30000 Respiratory and Cardiovascular System

64. **OPERATIVE PROCEDURE**

PREOPERATIVE DIAGNOSIS: 68-year-old male in a coma.

POSTOPERATIVE DIAGNOSIS: 68-year-old male in a coma.

PROCEDURE PERFORMED: Placement of a triple lumen central line in right subclavian vein.

    With the usual Betadine scrub to the right subclavian vein area and with a second attempt, the subclavian vein was cannulated and the wire was threaded. The first time the wire did not thread right, and so the attempt was aborted to make sure we had good identification of structures. Once the wire was in place, the needle was removed and a tissue dilator was pushed into position over the wire. Once that was removed, then the central lumen catheter was pushed into position at 17 cm and the wire removed. All three ports were flushed. The catheter was sewn into position, and a dressing applied.
A. 36011, 780.09
B. 36011, 780.01
C. 36556, 780.09
D. 36556, 780.01

65. What CPT and ICD-9-CM codes report a percutaneous insertion of a dual-lead pacemaker by means of the subclavian vein? The diagnosis is sick sinus syndrome, tachy-brady.
A. 33249, 427.0, 427.81
B. 33217, 427.81
C. 33208, 427.81
D. 33240, 426.12, 427.0

66. **OPERATIVE REPORT**

PREOPERATIVE DIAGNOSIS: Atelectasis of the left lower lobe.

PROCEDURE PERFORMED: Fiberoptic bronchoscopy with brushings and cell washings.

PROCEDURE: The patient was already sedated, on a ventilator, and intubated; so his bronchoscopy was done through the ET tube. It was passed easily down to the carina. About 2 to 2.5 cm above the carina, we could see the trachea, which appeared good, as was the carina. In the right lung, all segments were patent and entered, and no masses were seen. The left lung, however, had petechial ecchymotic areas scattered throughout the airways. The tissue was friable and swollen, but no mucous plugs were noted, and all the airways were open, just somewhat swollen. No abnormal secretions were noted at all. Brushings were taken as well as washings, including some with Mucomyst to see whether we could get some distal mucous plug, but nothing really significant was returned. The specimens were sent to appropriate cytological and bacteriological studies. The patient tolerated the procedure fairly well.

A. 31622, 31623-51, 518.0
B. 31623, 770.4
C. 31623-LT, 518.0
D. 31624, 770.4

67. **OPERATIVE REPORT**

PREOPERATIVE DIAGNOSIS:
1. Hypoxia.
2. Pneumothorax.

POSTOPERATIVE DIAGNOSIS:
1. Hypoxia.
2. Pneumothorax.

PROCEDURE: Chest tube placement.

DESCRIPTION OF PROCEDURE: The patient was previously sedated with Versed and paralyzed with Nimbex. Lidocaine was used to numb the incision area in the midlateral left chest at about nipple level. After the lidocaine, an incision was made, and we bluntly dissected to the area of the pleural space, making sure we were superior to the rib. On entrance to the pleural space, there was immediate release of air noted. An 18-gauge chest tube was subsequently placed and sutured to the skin. There were no complications for the procedure, and blood loss was minimal.

DISPOSITION: Follow-up, single-view, chest x-ray showed significant resolution of the pneumothorax except for a small apical pneumothorax that was noted.

A. 32556, 799.02, 512.89
B. 32551, 71010, 799.00, 512.89
C. 32551, 512.89, 799.02
D. 32556, 799.00, 512.0

68. **OPERATIVE REPORT**

PREOPERATIVE DIAGNOSIS: Atherosclerotic heart disease.

POSTOPERATIVE DIAGNOSIS: Atherosclerotic heart disease.

OPERATIVE PROCEDURE: Coronary bypass grafts × 2 with a single graft from the aorta to the distal left anterior descending and from the aorta to the distal right coronary artery.

PROCEDURE: The patient was brought to the operating room and placed in a supine position. Under general intubation anesthesia, the anterior chest and legs were prepped and draped in the usual manner. A segment of greater saphenous vein was harvested from the left thigh, utilizing the endoscopic vein harvesting technique, and prepared for grafting. The sternum was opened in the usual fashion, and the left internal mammary artery was taken down and prepared for grafting. The flow through the internal mammary artery was very poor. The patient did have a 25-mm difference in arterial pressure between the right and left arms, the right arm being higher. The left internal mammary artery was therefore not used. The pericardium was incised sharply and a pericardial well created. The patient was systemically heparinized and placed on bicaval to aortic cardiopulmonary bypass with the stump in the main pulmonary artery for cardiac decompression. The patient was cooled to 26°C, and on fibrillation an aortic cross-clamp was applied and potassium-rich cold crystalline cardioplegic solution was administered through the aortic root with satisfactory cardiac arrest. Subsequent doses were given down the vein grafts as the anastomoses were completed and via the coronary sinus in a retrograde fashion. Attention was directed to the right coronary artery. The end of the greater saphenous vein was then anastomosed thereto with 7-0 continuous Prolene distally. The remaining graft material was then grafted to the left anterior descending at the junction of the middle and distal third. The aortic cross-clamp was removed after 149 minutes with spontaneous cardioversion. The usual maneuvers to remove air from the left heart were then carried out using transesophageal echocardiographic technique. After all the air was removed and the patient had returned to a satisfactory temperature, he was weaned from cardiopulmonary bypass after 213 minutes utilizing 5 g per kilogram per minute of dopamine. The chest was closed in the usual fashion. A sterile compression dressing was applied, and the patient returned to the surgical intensive care unit in satisfactory condition.

A. 33511, 33517, 440.9
B. 33511, 33508, 414.01
C. 33534, 33508, 414.00
D. 33511, 33517, 414.01

69. **OPERATIVE REPORT:** The patient is in for a bone marrow biopsy. The patient was sterilized by standard procedure. Bone marrow core biopsies were obtained from the left posterior iliac crest with minimal discomfort. At the end of the procedure, the patient denied discomfort, without evidence of complications. The patient has diffuse, malignant lymphoma. Assign codes for the physician service only.

A. 20225, 229.0
B. 38221, 202.80
C. 38230, 200.10
D. 38220, 202.80

70. Patient is a 40-year-old male who was involved in a motor vehicle crash. He is having some pulmonary insufficiency.

PROCEDURE: Bronchoscope was inserted through the accessory point on the end of the ET tube and was then advanced through the ET tube. The ET tube came pretty close down to the carina. We selectively intubated the right mainstem bronchus with the bronchoscope. There were some secretions here, and these were aspirated. We then advanced this selectively into first the lower and then the middle and upper lobes. Secretions were present, more so in the middle and lower lobes. No mucous plug was identified. We then went into the left mainstem and looked at the upper and lower lobes. There was really not much in the way of secretions present. We did inject some saline and aspirated this out. We then removed the bronchoscope and put the patient back on the supplemental O_2. We waited a few minutes. The oxygen level actually stayed pretty good during this time. We then reinserted the bronchoscope and went down to the right side again. We aspirated out all secretions and made sure everything was clear. We then removed the bronchoscope and pulled back on the ET tube about 1.5 cm. We then again placed the patient on supplemental oxygenation.

FINDINGS: No mucous plug was identified. Secretions were found mainly in the right lung and were aspirated. The left side looked pretty clear.
A. 31646, 518.52, E819.9
B. 32654, 518.82, E812
C. 31645-50, 518.52, E819.9
D. 31645-RT, 518.52, E988.5

71. This 52-year-old male has undergone several attempts at extubation, all of which failed. He also has morbid obesity and significant subcutaneous fat in his neck. The patient is now in for a flap tracheostomy and cervical lipectomy. The cervical lipectomy is necessary for adequate exposure and access to the trachea and also to secure tracheotomy tube placement. Assign code(s) for the physician service only.
A. 31610, 15839-51
B. 31610
C. 31610, 15838
D. 31603, 15839-51

72. Connie was brought to the operating room for repair of an acute, traumatic diaphragmatic hernia.
A. 39540, 862.0
B. 39503, 756.6
C. 39541, 862.0
D. 39540, 756.6

73. This patient returns to the operating room for placement of an additional chest tube for an anterior pneumothorax due to a contusion lung injury. The same physician had just placed a chest tube 4 days earlier.
A. 32551, 860.0
B. 32554, 861.21
C. 32551-58, 861.21
D. 32551, 861.3

Subject Area: 40000 Digestive System

74. What CPT code would you use if the physician performs a pyloroplasty and vagotomy in the same surgical session?
A. 43865
B. 50400
C. 43635
D. 43640

75. This 43-year-old female comes in with a peritonsillar abscess. The patient is brought to same-day surgery and given general anesthetic. On examination of the peritonsillar abscess, an incision was made and fluid was drained. The area was examined again, saline was applied, and then the area was packed with gauze. The patient tolerated the procedure well.
A. 42825, 475
B. 42700, 475
C. 42825, 463
D. 42700, 474.0

76. **OPERATIVE REPORT**

    PREOPERATIVE DIAGNOSIS: Abdominal pain.

    POSTOPERATIVE DIAGNOSIS: Normal endoscopy.

    PROCEDURE: The flexible video therapeutic endoscope was passed without difficulty into the oropharynx. The gastroesophageal junction was seen at 40 cm. Inspection of the esophagus revealed no erythema, ulceration, varices, or other mucosal abnormalities. The stomach was entered and the endoscope advanced to the second duodenum. Inspection of the second duodenum, first duodenum, duodenal bulb, and pylorus revealed no abnormalities. Retroflexion revealed no lesions along the curvature. Inspection of the antrum, body, and fundus of the stomach revealed no abnormalities. The patient tolerated the procedure well. The patient complained of abdominal pain and weight loss.
    A. 45378, 789.00, 783.21
    B. 43235, 789.00, 783.21
    C. 49320, 783.0, 789.00
    D. 43255, 278.01, 789.01

77. This 70-year-old male is brought to the operating room for a biopsy of the pancreas. A wedge biopsy is taken and sent to pathology. The report comes back immediately indicating that primary malignant cells were present in the specimen. The decision was made to perform a total pancreatectomy. Code the operative procedure(s) and diagnosis only.
    A. 48100, 197.8
    B. 48155, 157.8
    C. 48155, 48100-51, 157.9
    D. 48155, 48100-51, 88309, 157.9

78. This patient is taken to the operating room from the intensive care unit (ICU). The area of the stoma appears to be necrotic, and on this basis the surgeon indicates that the patient has been taken back to the operating room. The stoma was originally created 4 months ago by her previous surgeon.

    PROCEDURE PERFORMED: Revision ileostomy stoma.

    OPERATIVE NOTE: With the patient moved onto the operating table, the abdomen was prepped and draped. The segment of bowel that was serving as the ileostomy was freed up. Going in through this large open wound, we were able to identify which segment of bowel this was. We resected the end of the bowel that was necrotic and freed up enough of the distal small bowel so that we could bring it out through a new stoma that was placed lateral to the original stoma. The stoma was created, the bowel was brought out, and the mucosa was sewn onto the skin. With this accomplished, we appeared to have a viable stoma. The patient tolerated this procedure and was returned to the ICU in stable condition.
    A. 44310, 560.1, E878.1
    B. 45136, 009.0, E878.0
    C. 44312, 569.62, 557.0, E878.3
    D. 44314, 557.0

79. This patient is brought back to the operating room during the postoperative period by the same physician to repair an esophagogastrostomy leak, transthoracic approach, done 2 days ago. The patient is status post esophagectomy for esophageal cancer, and is still undergoing chemotherapy. Code the procedure and the diagnosis for the complication.
    A. 43320-78, 530.10
    B. 43340-78, 578.9
    C. 43341, 997.49, 239.0
    D. 43415-78, 997.49, 150.9

80. The patient was taken to the operating room for a repair of a strangulated inguinal hernia. This hernia was previously repaired 4 months ago.
    A. 49521, 550.11
    B. 49520, 550.10
    C. 49492, 550.90
    D. 49521-78, 550.93

81. The physician is using an abdominal approach to perform a proctopexy combined with a sigmoid resection; the patient was diagnosed with colon cancer, primary site sigmoid flexure of the colon:
    A. 45540, 153.3
    B. 45541, 153.7
    C. 45550, 153.3
    D. 45345, 154.0

82. What code would you use to report a rigid proctosigmoidoscopy with removal of two nonadenomatous polyps of the rectum by snare technique?
    A. 45320, 569.0
    B. 45383, 211.3
    C. 45309 × 2, M8210/0
    D. 45315, 569.0

83. **OPERATIVE REPORT**

    PREOPERATIVE DIAGNOSIS: Leaking from intestinal anastomosis.

    POSTOPERATIVE DIAGNOSIS: Leaking from intestinal anastomosis.

    PROCEDURE PERFORMED: Proximal ileostomy for diversion of colon. Oversew of right colonic fistula.

    OPERATIVE NOTE: This patient was taken back to the operating room from the intensive care unit. She was having acute signs of leakage from an anastomosis I performed 3 days previously. We took down some of the sutures holding the wound together. We basically exposed all of this patient's intestine. It was evident that she was leaking from the small bowel as well as from the right colon. I thought the only thing we could do would be to repair the right colon. This was done in two layers, and then we freed up enough bowel to try to make an ileostomy proximal to the area of leakage. We were able to do this with great difficulty, and there was only a small amount of bowel to be brought out. We brought this out as an ileostomy stoma, realizing that it was of questionable viability and that it should be watched closely. With that accomplished, we then packed the wound and returned the patient to the intensive care unit.
    A. 44310, 998.31
    B. 44310-78, 997.49, E878.2
    C. 45136, 996.5, E878.2
    D. 45136-78, 998.32, E879.1

Subject Area: 50000 Urinary, Male Genital System, Female Genital System, and Maternity Care and Delivery

84. This patient is 35 years old at 36 weeks' gestation. She presented in spontaneous labor. Because of her prior cesarean section, she is taken to the operating room to have a repeat lower-segment transverse cesarean section performed. The patient also desires sterilization, and so a bilateral tubal ligation will also be performed. A single, liveborn infant was the outcome of the delivery.
A. 59510, 58600-51, V25.2
B. 59620, 58615-51, 644.21, V27.0
C. 59514, 58605-51, V27.0, 644.21
D. 59514, 58611, 654.21, 644.21, V27.0, V25.2

85. The pediatric physician takes this newborn male to the nursery to perform a clamp circumcision.
A. 54160, V50.2
B. 54150, V50.21
C. 54160, V50.21
D. 54150, V50.2

86. **OPERATIVE REPORT**

PREOPERATIVE DIAGNOSIS: Possible recurrent transitional cell carcinoma of the bladder.

POSTOPERATIVE DIAGNOSIS: No evidence of recurrence.

PROCEDURE PERFORMED: Cystoscopy with multiple bladder biopsies.

PROCEDURE NOTE: The patient was given a general mask anesthetic, prepped, and draped in the lithotomy position. The 21-French cystoscope was passed into the bladder. There was a hyperemic area on the posterior wall of the bladder, and a biopsy was taken. Random biopsies of the bladder were also performed. This area was fulgurated. A total of 7 sq cm of bladder was fulgurated. A catheter was left at the end of the procedure. The patient tolerated the procedure well and was transferred to the recovery room in good condition. The pathology report indicated no evidence of recurrence.
A. 52224, 596.7, V10.51
B. 51020, 52204, V16.52
C. 52234, V10.51
D. 52224 × 4, 236.7

87. This 1-year-old boy has a midshaft hypospadias with a very mild degree of chordee. He also has a persistent right hydrocele. The surgeon brought the boy to surgery to perform a right hydrocele repair and one-stage repair of hypospadias with preputial onlay flap.
A. 54322, 55040, 752.61, 752.63
B. 54322, 55041-51, 752.61, 752.63, 603.9
C. 54324, 55060-51, 752.61, 752.63, 603.9
D. 54324, 55060, 752.63, 603.9

88. This gentleman has worsening bilateral hydronephrosis. He did not have much of a post void residual on bladder scan. He is taken to the operating room to have a bilateral cystoscopy and retrograde pyelogram. The results come back as gross prostatic hyperplasia as the cause of the hydronephrosis.
    A. 52005, 600.3
    B. 52000, 591, 600.9
    C. 52005-50, 600.91, 591
    D. 52000-50, 591, 600.9

89. This patient is a 42-year-old female who has been having prolonged and heavy bleeding during menstruation.

    SURGICAL FINDINGS: On pelvic exam under anesthesia, the uterus was normal size and firm. The examination revealed no masses. She had a few small endometrial polyps in the lower uterine segment.

    DESCRIPTION OF PROCEDURE: After induction of general anesthesia, the patient was placed in the dorsolithotomy position, after which the perineum and vagina were prepped, the bladder straight catheterized, and the patient draped. After bimanual exam was performed, a weighted speculum was placed in the vagina and the anterior lip of the cervix was grasped with a single tooth tenaculum. An endocervical curettage was then done with a Kevorkian curet. The uterus was then sounded to 8.5 cm. The endocervical canal was dilated to 7 mm with Hegar dilators. A 5.5-mm Olympus hysteroscope was introduced using a distention medium. The cavity was systematically inspected, and the preceding findings noted. The hysteroscope was withdrawn and the cervix further dilated to 10 mm. Polyp forceps was introduced, and a few small polyps were removed. These were sent separately. Sharp endometrial curettage was then done. The hysteroscope was then reinserted, and the polyps had essentially been removed. The patient tolerated the procedure well and was returned to the recovery room in stable condition. Pathology confirmed benign endometrial polyps.
    A. 58558, 57460-51, 626.2, 621.0
    B. 58558, 626.2, 621.0
    C. 58558, 57558-51, 626.2, 621.0
    D. 58558, 626.6, 239.5

90. **OPERATIVE REPORT**

    PREOPERATIVE DIAGNOSIS: Missed abortion with fetal demise, 11 weeks.

    POSTOPERATIVE DIAGNOSIS: Missed abortion with fetal demise, 11 weeks.

    PROCEDURE: Suction D&C.

    The patient was prepped and draped in a lithotomy position under general mask anesthesia, and the bladder was straight catheterized; a weighted speculum was placed in the vagina. The anterior lip of the cervix was grasped with a single-tooth tenaculum. The uterus was then sounded to a depth of 8 cm. The cervical os was then serially dilated to allow passage of a size 10 curved suction curette. A size 10 curved suction curette was then used to evacuate the intrauterine contents. Sharp curette was used to gently palpate the uterine wall with negative return of tissue, and the suction curette was again used with negative return of tissue. The tenaculum was removed from the cervix. The speculum was removed from the vagina.

All sponges and needles were accounted for at completion of the procedure. The patient left the operating room in apparent good condition having tolerated the procedure well.
A. 59812, 634.92
B. 59812, 638.90
C. 59820, 632
D. 59856, 632

91. **OPERATIVE REPORT**

    PREOPERATIVE DIAGNOSIS: Right ureteral stricture.

    POSTOPERATIVE DIAGNOSIS: Right ureteral stricture.

    PROCEDURE PERFORMED: Cystoscopy, right ureteral stent change.

    PROCEDURE NOTE: The patient was placed in the lithotomy position after receiving IV sedation. He was prepped and draped in the lithotomy position. The 21-French cystoscope was passed into the bladder, and urine was collected for culture. Inspection of the bladder demonstrated findings consistent with radiation cystitis, which has been previously diagnosed. There is no frank neoplasia. The right ureteral stent was grasped and removed through the urethral meatus; under fluoroscopic control, a guidewire was advanced up the stent, and the stent was exchanged for a 7-French 26-cm stent under fluoroscopic control in the usual fashion. The patient tolerated the procedure well.
    A. 51702-LT, 593.3
    B. 52005-RT, 595.9
    C. 52332-RT, 595.9
    D. 52332-RT, 593.3

92. This 41-year-old female presented with a right labial lesion. A biopsy was taken, and the results were reported as VIN III, cannot rule out invasion. The decision was therefore made to proceed with wide local excision of the right vulva.

    PROCEDURE: The patient was taken to the operating room, and general anesthesia was administered. The patient was then prepped and draped in the usual manner in lithotomy position, and the bladder was emptied with a straight catheter. The vulva was then inspected. On the right labium minora at approximately the 11 o'clock position, there was a multifocal lesion. A marking pen was then used to mark out an elliptical incision, leaving a 1-cm border on all sides. The skin ellipse was then excised using a knife. Bleeders were cauterized with electrocautery. A running locked suture of 2-0 Vicryl was then placed in the deeper tissue. The skin was finally reapproximated with 4-0 Vicryl in an interrupted fashion. Good hemostasis was thereby achieved. The patient tolerated this procedure well. There were no complications.
    A. 56605, 184.4
    B. 56625, 233.32
    C. 56620, 233.32
    D. 11620, 184.4

93. This 32-year-old female presents with an ectopic pregnancy. The physician elects to remove the entire fallopian tube with the products of conception laparoscopically.
    A. 59120, 633.90
    B. 59151, 633.90
    C. 58943, 633.10
    D. 59120, 633.80

Subject Area: 60000 Endocrine System, Nervous System, Eye and Ocular Adnexa

94. **OPERATIVE REPORT**

    PREOPERATIVE DIAGNOSIS: FUO.

    PROCEDURE PERFORMED: Lumbar puncture.

    DESCRIPTION OF PROCEDURE: The patient was placed in the lateral decubitus position with the left side up. The legs and hips were flexed into the fetal position. The lumbosacral area was sterilely prepped. It was then numbed with 1% Xylocaine. I then placed a 22-gauge spinal needle on the first pass into the intrathecal space between the L4 and L5 spinous processes. The fluid was minimally xanthochromic. I sent the fluid for cell count for differential, protein, glucose, Gram stain, and culture. The patient tolerated the procedure well without apparent complication. The needle was removed at the end of the procedure. The area was cleansed, and a Band-Aid was placed.
    A. 62272, 780.91
    B. 62268, 780.60
    C. 62272, 782.3, 780.60
    D. 62270, 780.60

95. **OPERATIVE REPORT**

    PREOPERATIVE DIAGNOSIS: Mechanical ectropion, left lower eye.

    PROCEDURE PERFORMED: Medial tarsorrhaphy, left lower eye.

    In the operating room, after intravenous sedation, the patient was given a total of about 0.5 mL of local infiltrative anesthetic. The skin surfaces on the medial area of the lid, medial to the punctum, were denuded. A bolster had been prepared and double 5-0 silk suture was passed through the bolster, which was passed through the inferior skin and raw lid margin, then through the superior margin, and out through the skin. A superior bolster was then applied. The puncta were probed with wire instrument and found not to be obstructed. The suture was then fully tied and trimmed. Bacitracin ointment was placed on the surface of the skin. The patient left the operating room in stable condition, without complications, having tolerated the procedure well.
    A. 67875-LT, 374.12
    B. 67710-LT, 374.11
    C. 67882-LT, 374.10
    D. 67880-LT, 374.12

96. Marginal laceration involving the left lower eyelid and laceration of the left upper eyelid involving the tarsus. Both required full-thickness repair. Also, there were multiple stellate lacerations above the left eye, totaling 24.2 cm and requiring full-thickness layered repair. Assign code(s) for the physician service only.
    A. 67935-E2, 12017
    B. 67930-E2, 13152-51, 13153
    C. 67935-E2, 67935-E1-51, 12056-51
    D. 67935-E2, 12017-51

97. This 66-year-old male has been diagnosed with a senile cataract of the posterior subcapsular and is scheduled for a cataract extraction by phacoemulsification of the right eye. The physician has taken the patient to the operating room to perform a posterior subcapsular cataract extraction with IOL placement, diffuse of the right eye.
    A. 66982-RT, 366.09
    B. 66984-RT, 366.14
    C. 66983-RT, 366.12
    D. 66830-RT, 366.14

98. **OPERATIVE REPORT**

    PREOPERATIVE DIAGNOSIS: Brain tumor versus abscess.

    PROCEDURE: Craniotomy.

    DESCRIPTION OF PROCEDURE: Under general anesthesia, the patient's head was prepped and draped in the usual manner. It was placed in Mayfield pins. We then proceeded with a craniotomy. An inverted U-shaped incision was made over the posterior right occipital area. The flap was turned down. Three burr holes were made. Having done this, I then localized the tumor through the burr holes and dura. We then made an incision in the dura in an inverted U-shaped fashion. The cortex looked a little swollen but normal. We then used the localizer to locate the cavity. I separated the gyrus and got right into the cavity and saw pus, which was removed. Cultures were taken and sent for pathology report, which came back later describing the presence of clusters of gram-positive cocci, confirming that this was an abscess. We cleaned out the abscessed cavity using irrigation and suction. The bed of the abscessed cavity was cauterized. Then a small piece of Gelfoam was used for hemostasis. Satisfied that it was dry, I closed the dura. I approximated the scalp. A dressing was applied. The patient was discharged to the recovery room.
    A. 61154, 324.0
    B. 61154, 239.6
    C. 61320, 324.0, 041.89
    D. 61150, 239.6

99. This patient is in for a recurrent herniated disc at L5-S1 on the left. The procedure performed is a repeat laminotomy and foraminotomy at the L5-S1 interspace.
    A. 63030-LT, 722.10
    B. 63030-LT, 722.11
    C. 63042-LT, 722.11
    D. 63042-LT, 722.10

100. **OPERATIVE REPORT**

PREOPERATIVE DIAGNOSIS: Herniated disc L4-5 on the left.

PROCEDURE PERFORMED: Laminotomy, foraminotomy, removal of herniated disc L4-5 on the left.

PROCEDURE: Under general anesthesia, the patient was placed in the prone position and the back was prepped and draped in the usual manner. An incision was made in the skin extending through subcutaneous tissue. Lumbodorsal fascia was divided. The erector spinae muscles were bluntly dissected from the lamina of L4-5 on the left. The interspace was localized. I then performed a generous laminotomy and foraminotomy here, and retracted on the nerve root. It was obvious there was a herniated disc. I removed it, entered the space, and removed degenerating material, satisfied that I had decompressed the root well. There were free fragments lying around beneath the nerve root. We removed all of these. I was able to pass a hockey stick down the foramen across the midline, satisfied I had taken out the large fragments from the interspace at L4-5, and decompressed it well. I irrigated the wound well, put a Hemovac drain in the wound, and then closed the wound in layers using double-knotted 0 chromic on the lumbodorsal fascia with Vicryl 2-0 plain, in the subcutaneous tissue, and surgical staples on the skin. A dressing was applied. The patient was discharged to the recovery room.
A. 63030-LT, 722.10
B. 63012-LT, 722.32
C. 63047-LT, 722.92
D. 63047-LT, 63048-LT, 722.10

101. This patient came in with an obstructed ventriculoperitoneal shunt. The procedure performed was to be a revision of shunt. After inspecting the shunt system, the entire cerebrospinal fluid shunt system was removed and a similar replacement shunt system was placed. Patient has normal pressure hydrocephalus (NPH).
A. 62180, 996.1, 331.3
B. 62258, 996.2, 331.5
C. 62256, 996.2, 331.4
D. 62190, 996.2, 331.5

102. Burr hole for a left frontal ventricular puncture for implanting catheter, layered repair of 8-cm scalp laceration, and repair of multiple facial and eyelid lacerations with an approximate total length of 12 cm. Assign code(s) for the physician service only.
A. 61020, 12015-51
B. 61107, 12034-51, 12015-51
C. 61215, 12015-51
D. 61107, 12034-51

103. What CPT and ICD-9-CM codes would you assign to report the removal of 30% of the left thyroid lobe, with isthmusectomy? The diagnosis was benign growth of the thyroid.
A. 60210, 226
B. 60220, 237.4
C. 60212, 239.7
D. 60225, 226, 239.7

Subject Area: Evaluation and Management (E/M)

104. Dr. Black admits a patient with an 8-day history of a low-grade fever, tachycardia, tachypnea, and possible radiologic evidence of basal consolidation of the lung and limited pleural effusion on the left side, per patient as seen at outside clinic several days prior. The patient has also been experiencing swelling of the extremities. The pulse is rapid and thready, as checked by patient on her own during the past couple days. A complete ROS of constitutional factors, ophthalmologic, otolaryngologic, cardiovascular, respiratory, gastrointestinal, genitourinary, musculoskeletal, integumentary, neurologic, psychiatric, endocrine, hematologic, lymphatic, allergic, and immunologic was performed and negative except for the symptoms described above. Past history includes tachycardia and pneumonia. Family history includes heart disease, hypertension, and high cholesterol in both parents. The patient drinks only occasionally and quit smoking 4 years ago. The comprehensive examination was performed and diminished bowel sounds were noted. The physician orders laboratory tests and radiographic studies, including a follow-up chest x-ray, as he considers the extensive diagnostic options, the medical decision-making complexity is high for this patient.
    A. 99233, 780.60, 785.0, 786.06, 511.9, 787.5, V15.82
    B. 99233, 780.60, 427.0, 786.06, 486, 511.9
    C. 99223, 780.60, 785.0, 786.06
    D. 99223, 780.60, 785.0, 786.06, 511.9, 787.5, V15.85, V17.49

105. Bill, a retired U.S. Air Force pilot, was on observation status 12 hours to assess the outcome of a fall from the back of a parked pickup truck into a gravel pit.
    History of Present Illness: The patient is a 42-year-old gentleman who works at the local garden shop. He explained that yesterday he fell from his pickup truck as he was loading gravel for a landscaping project. He lost his footing when attempting to climb from the pickup bed and fell approximately 4 feet and landed on a rock that was protruding from the ground 4 inches, striking his head on the rock. He did not lose consciousness, but was dizzy. He subsequently developed a throbbing headache (8/10) and swelling at the point of impact. The duration of the dizziness was approximately 10 minutes. The headache persisted for 26 hours after the fall. He did take ibuprofen without significant improvement in the pain level. Review of Systems: Constitutional, eyes, ears, nose, throat, lungs, cardiovascular, gastrointestinal, skin, neurologic, lymphatic, and immunologic negative except for HPI statements. PFSH: He is married and has 2 children. He has been working at the garden shop for 4 years. He currently smokes one pack of cigarettes a day and has smoked for 10 years. His father died of heart disease when he was 52. He has one brother with ankylosing spondylitis and one sister who is healthy as far as he knows. His mother died when he was 14 years old. He is currently on no prescribed medications. A comprehensive exam is documented and rendered. The medical decision making is of low complexity.
    The physician discharged Bill from observation that same day after 10 hours, after determining that no further monitoring of his condition was necessary. The physician provided a detailed examination and indicated that the medical decision making was of low complexity.
    A. 99218, 784.0, E888.8
    B. 99234, V71.4, E884.9
    C. 99217, V71.4, E888.8
    D. 99234, 99217, 784.0, E884.9

106. A gynecologist admits an established patient, a 35-year-old female with dysfunctional uterine bleeding, after seeing her in the clinic that day. During the course of the history, the physician notes that the patient has a history of infrequent periods of heavy flow. She has had irregular heavy periods and intermittent spotting for 4 years. The patient has been on a 3-month course of oral contraceptives for symptoms with no relief. The patient states that she has occasional headaches. A complete ROS was performed, consisting of constitutional factors, ophthalmologic, otolaryngologic, cardiovascular, respiratory, gastrointestinal, genitourinary, musculoskeletal, integumentary, neurologic, psychiatric, endocrine, hematologic, lymphatic, allergic, and immunologic which were all negative, except for the symptoms described above. The family history is positive for endometrial cancer, with mother, two aunts, and two sisters who had endometrial cancer. The patient has a personal history of cervical and endometrial polyp removal 3 years prior to admission. The patients states that she does not smoke and only drinks socially. As a part of the comprehensive examination, the physician notes the patient has a large amount of blood in the vault and an enlarged uterus. The prolonged hemorrhaging has resulted in a very thin and friable endometrial lining. The physician orders the patient to be started on intravenous Premarin and orders a full laboratory workup. The medical decision making is of moderate complexity.
    A. 99215, 99222, V13.29, V16.49
    B. 99222, 626.8, V13.29, V16.49
    C. 99215, 99222, 623.8, V13.29, V16.4
    D. 99222, 626.1, V16.49

107. Karra Hendricks, a 37-year-old female, is an established patient who presents to the office with right lower quadrant abdominal pain with fever. The patient states she has had the pain for 3 days. She has taken Tylenol for her fever with some relief. The patient does have occasional diarrhea and headaches. She smokes approximately 5-10 cigarettes a day and drinks socially. The physician performs a detailed examination. The medical decision making is noted to be of a moderate complexity.
    A. 99203, 789.03
    B. 99213, 789.04, 780.60
    C. 99214, 789.03, 780.60
    D. 99221, 789.05, 780.60

108. A neurological consultation in the emergency department of the local hospital is requested by the ED physician for a 25-year-old male with suspected closed head trauma. The neurologist saw the patient in the ED. The patient had a loss of consciousness this morning after receiving a blow to the head in a basketball game. He presents to the emergency department with a headache, dizziness, and confusion. During the course of the history, the patient relates that he has been very irritable, confused, and has had a bit of nausea since the incident. All other systems reviewed and are negative: Constitutional, ophthalmologic, otolaryngologic, cardiovascular, respiratory, genitourinary, musculoskeletal, integumentary, psychiatric, endocrine, hematologic, lymphatic, allergic, and immunologic. The patient states that he does have a history of headaches and that both parents have hypertension, also a grandfather with heart disease. He also states that he does drink beer on the weekends and does not smoke. Physical examination reveals the patient to be unsteady and exhibiting difficulty in concentration when stating months in reverse. The pupils dilate unequally

(anisocoria). The physician continues with a complete comprehensive examination involving an extensive review of neurological function. The neurologist orders a stat CT and MRI. The physician suspects a subdural hematoma or an epidural hematoma and the medical decision-making complexity is high. The neurologist admits the patient to the hospital. Assign codes for the neurologist's services only.

A. 99285, 780.09, 780.4, 784.0
B. 99253, 784.0, 780.09, 780.4
C. 99255, 379.41, 784.0, 298.9, 780.4, E917.0, E007.6
D. 99245, 784.0, 780.09, 780.4, E917.0, E007.6

109. Dr. Stephanopolis makes subsequent hospital visits to Salanda Ortez, who has been in the hospital for primary viral pneumonia. She was experiencing severe dyspnea, rales, fever, and chest pain for over a week. The patient states that this morning she had nausea and her heart was racing while she was experiencing some dyspnea and SOB. The chest radiography showed patchy bilateral infiltrates and basilar streaking. Sputum microbiology was positive for a secondary bacterial pneumonia. An expanded problem-focused physical examination was performed. The medical decision making was moderate. The patient was given intravenous antibiotic as treatment for the bacterial pneumonia.

A. 99233, 786.09, 786.7, 780.60, 729.1, 786.50, 793.19, 795.39
B. 99232, 482.9, 480.9
C. 99221, 786.09, 786.7, 780.60, 729.1, 786.50, 793.19, 795.39
D. 99234, 482.89

110. An obstetrician is requested to provide an office consultation to a 23-year-old female with first-trimester bleeding from Dr A. The patient presents with a history of brownish discharge and occasional pinkish discharge. During the history, the patient relates that she has had suprapubic pain in the past week and cramping. She states her pain is 8/10. She has felt nausea and has vomited on three occasions. On one occasion, the nausea was accompanied by dizziness and vertigo. All other systems are negative at this time and included: Constitutional factors, ophthalmologic, otolaryngologic, cardiovascular, respiratory, musculoskeletal, integumentary, neurologic, psychiatric, endocrine, hematologic, lymphatic, allergic, and immunologic. The PFSH included patient history of tonsillectomy with family history of breast cancer on her mother's side. The patient does not smoke or drink. The physician conducts a comprehensive examination focused on the chief complaint and related systems. The uterus is found to be soft and involuted. There is cervical motion tenderness and significant abdominal tenderness on palpation. A left pelvic mass is palpated in the left quadrant. The physician orders a pelvic ultrasound, a complete CBC, and differential. Considering the range of possible diagnoses, the medical decision-making complexity is high.

A. 99255, 634.91, 719.65
B. 99242, 634.90, 719.65
C. 99245, 640.93, 789.34
D. 99245, 649.53, 789.34

111. Dr. Martin admits a 65-year-old female patient to the hospital to rule out acute pericarditis following a severe viral infection. The patient has complained of retrosternal, sharp, intermittent pain of 2 days' duration that is reduced by sitting up and leaning forward, accompanied by tachypnea. ROS: She does not currently have chest pain but is complaining of

shortness of breath. She states that her legs and feet have been swollen of late. She reports no change in her vision or her hearing, and she has not had a rash. No dyspnea stated. PFSH: She states that she has had an echocardiogram in the past when she complained of chest tightness and her family physician gave her some medication, but she is not certain what it was. She has three adult children, all healthy. Her husband is deceased. She does not smoke or consume alcohol. Her father died at age 69 from congestive heart failure and her mother died of influenza at 70. Refer to the admission form for a list of current medications. The examination was detailed. The medical decision making was of high complexity.

A. 99236, 786.51, 786.06, 786.05
B. 99223, 420.91, 411.1, 442.9, 415.19, 530.9
C. 99245, 420.91, 411.1, 442.9, 415.19, 530.9
D. 99221, 786.51, 786.06, 786.05

112. A 57-year-old male was sent by his family physician to a urologist for an office consultation due to hematuria. The patient has had bright red blood in his urine sporadically for the past 3 weeks. His family physician gave him a dose of antibiotic therapy for urinary tract infection; however, the symptom still persists. The patient states that he does experience some lower back discomfort when urinating, with no fever, chills, or nausea. The patient is currently taking Lotrel 10/20 for his hypertension, which is stable at this time, and has allergies to Sulfa. The urologist performs a detailed history and physical examination. The urologist recommends a cystoscopy to be scheduled for the following day and discusses the procedure and risks with the patient. The urologist also contacted the family physician with the recommendations and is requested to proceed with the cystoscopy and any further follow-up required. The medical decision making is of moderate complexity. A report was sent to attending physician. Report only the office service.

A. 99243, 599.70, 724.2
B. 99244-57, 52000, 599.0, 724.2
C. 99253, 599.9, 724.2
D. 99221, 599.70, 724.2

113. A 56-year-old established male patient presents to his family physician for a preventive checkup at the local outpatient clinic. The physician conducts a multisystem history and physical examination, and the checkup takes 45 minutes.

A. 99214, V70.4
B. 99403, V70.7
C. 99386, V70.0
D. 99396, V70.0

Subject Area: Anesthesia

114. Which HCPCS modifier indicates an anesthesia service in which the anesthesiologist medically directs one CRNA?

A. -QX
B. -QY
C. -QZ
D. -QK

115. This is the anesthesia formula:
    A. B + M + P
    B. B + P + M
    C. B + T + M
    D. B + T + N

116. Anesthesia service for a needle biopsy of the pleura, 32400.
    A. 00528
    B. 00500
    C. 00520
    D. 00522

117. If the anesthesia service were provided to a patient who had severe systemic disease, what would the physical status modifier be?
    A. P1
    B. P2
    C. P3
    D. P4

118. This type of anesthesia is also known as a nerve block.
    A. Local
    B. Epidural
    C. Regional
    D. MAC

119. The following is the anesthesia formula:
    A. BTC
    B. TBC
    C. BTQ
    D. BTM

120. Anesthesia service includes the following care:
    A. Preoperative, intraoperative
    B. Preoperative, intraoperative, postoperative
    C. Intraoperative, postoperative
    D. Preoperative, postoperative

121. What qualifying circumstances code would be used to identify the administration of anesthesia that is complicated by an emergency condition?
    A. 99100
    B. 99116
    C. 99135
    D. 99140

Subject Area: 70000 Radiology

122. **EXAMINATION OF:** Right hip.

    DIAGNOSIS: Primary unilateral osteoarthritis right hip.

    ONE-VIEW RIGHT HIP: A single frontal view is obtained of the right hip. No previous studies are available for comparison. Right hip arthroplasty is seen. Alignment appears grossly unremarkable on this single view. There are skin staples present. Air is seen in the soft tissues, likely due to recent surgery. There appear to be two drains present. The tip of one overlies the soft tissues superolateral to the greater trochanter. The second one is more inferior. The tip overlies the right proximal femoral prosthesis.

IMPRESSION: Single view of the right hip with findings consistent with recent right total hip arthroplasty.
A. 72100, 719
B. 73500-RT, 715.95
C. 72100-26, 715.9
D. 73500-26-RT, 715.95, V43.64

123. **EXAMINATION OF:** Cervical spine.

CLINICAL SYMPTOMS: Herniated disc.

FINDINGS: A single spot fluoroscopic film from the operating room is submitted for interpretation. The cervical spine is not well demonstrated above the level of the inferior aspect of C6. There is a metallic surgical plate seen anterior to the cervical spine. The cephalic portion of the plate is at the level of C6 at its superior endplate. That extends in an inferior direction, presumably anterior to C7; however, there is not adequate visualization of C7 to confirm location. Density overlies the C6-7 intervertebral disc space, suggesting the presence of a bone plug in this area; however, again visualization is not adequate in this area. Further evaluation with plain radiographs is recommended.
A. 72100-26, 722.10
B. 72020-26, 722.0
C. 72100-52-26, 722.0
D. 72020-52-26, 722.11

124. This patient undergoes a gallbladder sonogram due to epigastric pain. The report indicates that the visualized portions of the liver are normal. No free fluid noted within Morison's pouch. The gallbladder is identified and is empty. No evidence of wall thickening or surrounding fluid is seen. There is no ductal dilatation. The common hepatic duct and common bile duct measure 0.4 and 0.8 cm, respectively. The common bile duct measurement is at the upper limits of normal.
A. 76700-26, 789.07
B. 76705-26, 789.06
C. 76775-26, 789.05
D. 76705, 789.07

125. **EXAMINATION OF:** Chest.

CLINICAL SYMPTOMS: Pneumonia.

PA AND LATERAL CHEST X-RAY WITH FLUOROSCOPY.

CONCLUSION: Ventilation within the lung fields has improved compared with previous study.
A. 71020-26, 482.89
B. 71034, 482.83
C. 71023-26, 486
D. 71023, 486

126. **EXAMINATION OF:** Abdomen and pelvis.

    CLINICAL SYMPTOMS: Ascites.

    CT OF ABDOMEN AND PELVIS: Technique: CT of the abdomen and pelvis was performed without oral or IV contrast material per physician request. No previous CT scans for comparison.

    FINDINGS: No ascites. Moderate-sized pleural effusion on the right.
    A. 74160-26, 789.59
    B. 74176-26, 511.9
    C. 74150, 511.9
    D. 74160, 789.59

127. Report the professional component of the following service: This 68-year-old male is seen in Radiation Oncology Department for prostate cancer. The oncologist performs a complex clinical treatment planning, approves a dosimetry calculation, manages a complex isodose plan and orders treatment devices which include blocks, special shields, and wedges. He also performs treatment management. The patient had 5 days of radiation treatments for 2 weeks, a total of 10 days of treatment.
    A. 77263, 77300-26, 77315-26, 77334, 185
    B. 77300, 77315, 77334, 77427 × 2, 185
    C. 77263, 77300-26, 77315-26, 77334-26, 77427 × 2, 185
    D. 77263, 77427 × 2, 185

128. This 69-year-old female is in for a magnetic resonance examination of the brain because of new seizure activity. After imaging without contrast, contrast was administered and further sequences were performed. Examination results indicated no apparent neoplasm or vascular malformation.
    A. 70543-26, 780.31
    B. 70543-26, 780.39
    C. 70553-26, 780.39
    D. 70553, 345.90

129. **EXAMINATION OF:** Brain.

    CLINICAL FINDING: Acute onset, severe headache.

    COMPUTED TOMOGRAPHY OF THE BRAIN was performed without contrast material.

    FINDINGS: There is blood within the third ventricle. The lateral ventricles show mild dilatation with small amounts of blood.

    IMPRESSION: Acute subarachnoid hemorrhage.
    A. 70460-26, 784.0
    B. 70250, 784.0
    C. 70450-26, 430
    D. 70450-26, 784.0

130. This patient is suffering from primary lung cancer and is in for a follow-up CT scan of the thorax with contrast material. Code the physician component only.
    A. 71250-26, 197.0
    B. 71260, 162.9
    C. 71260-26, 162.9
    D. 71270-26, 239.1

Subject Area: 80000 Pathology and Laboratory

131. This 69-year-old female presents to the laboratory after her physician ordered quantitative and qualitative assays for troponin to assist in the diagnosis of her chief complaint of acute onset of chest pain.
    A. 84484, 80299, 786.51
    B. 84512, 84484, 80299, 786.59
    C. 84484, 84512, 786.50
    D. 84484, 84512, 786.59

132. **Report the global service.**

    CLINICAL HISTORY: Mass, left atrium.

    SPECIMEN RECEIVED: Left atrium.

    GROSS DESCRIPTION: The specimen is labeled with patient's name and "left atrial myxoma" and consists of a 4 × 4 × 2-cm ovoid mass with a partially calcified hemorrhagic white-tan tissue.

    INTRAOPERATIVE FROZEN SECTION DIAGNOSIS: Myxoma

    MICROSCOPIC DESCRIPTION: Sections show a well-circumscribed mass consisting of fibromyxoid tissue showing numerous vascular channels. Areas of superficial ulceration and chronic inflammatory infiltrate are noted. Areas of calcification are also present.

    DIAGNOSIS: Myxoma, benign, left atrium.
    A. 88305, 239.89
    B. 88307-26, 88331-26, 212.7
    C. 88307, 88331-26, 212.7
    D. 88305, 212.7

133. **CLINICAL HISTORY:** Boil, left groin.

    SPECIMEN RECEIVED: Necrotic fascia left groin and leg (anterior and posterior).

    GROSS DESCRIPTION: The specimen is labeled with the patient's name and "fascia left groin and leg" and consists of multiple segments of skin and soft tissue measuring up to 30 cm in greatest dimension. The skin is unremarkable, with the soft tissue being hemorrhagic and friable and foul smelling.

    MICROSCOPIC DESCRIPTION: Sections of skin and soft tissue show coagulative necrosis with neutrophilic exudates.

    DIAGNOSIS: Skin and soft tissue, left groin and leg, anterior and posterior showing coagulative necrosis and acute inflammation.
    A. 88304, 680.9
    B. 88305-26, 709.8
    C. 88304-26, 709.8, 680.2
    D. 88305, 682.2

134. This 34-year-old established female patient is in for her yearly physical and lab. The physician orders a comprehensive metabolic panel, automated hemogram and manual differential WBC count (CBC), and a thyroid-stimulating hormone. Code the lab only.
    A. 99395, 80050
    B. 80050-52
    C. 80069, 80050
    D. 80050

135. **CLINICAL HISTORY:** Necrotic soleus muscle, right leg.

    SPECIMEN RECEIVED: Soleus muscle, right leg.

    GROSS DESCRIPTION: Submitted in formalin, labeled with the patient's name and "soleus muscle right leg," are multiple irregular fragments of tan, gray, and brown soft tissue measuring 8 × 8 × 2.5 cm in aggregate. Multiple representative fragments are submitted in four cassettes.

    MICROSCOPIC DESCRIPTION: The slides show multiple sections of skeletal muscle showing severe coagulative and liquefactive necrosis. Patchy neutrophilic infiltrates are present within the necrotic tissue.

    DIAGNOSIS: Soft tissue, soleus muscle, right leg debridement; necrosis and patchy acute inflammation, skeletal muscle—infective myositis.
    A. 88305-26, 728.2
    B. 88304-26, 728.0
    C. 88307-26, 785.4
    D. 88304-26, 728.2

136. This patient is in for a kidney biopsy (50200) because a mass was identified by ultrasound. The specimen is sent to pathology for gross and microscopic examination. Report the technical and professional components for this service. The results are pending.
    A. 88305-26, 593.9
    B. 88307-26, 593.89
    C. 88307, 593.9
    D. 88305, 593.9

137. This patient presented to the laboratory yesterday to have blood drawn for a creatinine measurement. The results came back at higher than normal levels; therefore, the patient was asked to return to the laboratory today for a repeat creatinine blood test before the nephrologist is consulted. Report the second day of test only.
    A. 82540 × 2, 790.6
    B. 82550, 790.6
    C. 82550, 790.91
    D. 82540, 790.6

138. Code a pregnancy test, urine.
    A. 84702
    B. 84703
    C. 81025
    D. 84702 × 2

139. This is a patient with atrial fibrillation who comes to the clinic laboratory routinely for a quantitative digoxin level. This test was performed today.
    A. 80101, 80102, 428.0
    B. 81001, V58.83, V58.69, 427.41
    C. 80162, V58.83, V58.69, 427.31
    D. 80162, 785.0

140. What CPT code would you use to report a bilirubin, total (transcutaneous)?
    A. 82252
    B. 82247
    C. 82248
    D. 88720

Subject Area: 90000 Medicine

141. What CPT code would be used to code the technical aspect of an evaluation of swallowing by video recording using a flexible fiberoptic endoscope?
    A. 92611
    B. 92612
    C. 92610
    D. 92613

142. The patient presented for a spontaneous nystagmus test that included gaze, fixation, and recording and used vertical electrodes. Assign code(s) for the physician service only.
    A. 92541
    B. 92547
    C. 92541, 92544, 92547
    D. 92541, 92547

143. How would you report a screening hearing test in which no abnormalities are reported?
    A. 92551, V72.19
    B. 92555, V72.19
    C. 92553, V72.19
    D. 92620, V80.3

144. This 40-year-old patient who is a type II diabetic is seen in an inpatient setting for psychotherapy. The doctor spends 50 minutes face to face with the patient. The patient is seen for depression.
    A. 90834, 311, 250.90
    B. 90832, 311, 250.90
    C. 90834, 311
    D. 90832, 311

145. A patient presents for a pleural cavity chemotherapy session with 10 mg doxorubicin HCl that requires a thoracentesis to be performed.
    A. 96446, J9000
    B. 96440, 32554, J9000
    C. 96440, J9000
    D. 96446, 32554, J9000

146. What CPT code would be used to report a home visit for a respiratory patient to care for the mechanical ventilation?
A. 99503
B. 99504
C. 99505
D. 99509

147. Which code would be used to report an EEG (electroencephalogram) provided during carotid surgery?
A. 95816
B. 95819
C. 95822
D. 95955

148. **INDICATION:** Pulmonary hypertension secondary to newly diagnosed acute myocardial infarction.

PROCEDURE PERFORMED: Insertion of Swan-Ganz catheter.

DESCRIPTION OF PROCEDURE: The right internal jugular and subclavian area was prepped with antiseptic solution. Sterile drapes were applied. Under usual sterile precautions, the right internal jugular vein was cannulated. A 9-French introducer was inserted, and a 7-French Swan-Ganz catheter was inserted without difficulty. Right atrial pressures were 2 to 3, right ventricular pressures 24/0, and pulmonary artery 26/9 with a wedge pressure of 5. This is a Trendelenburg position. The patient tolerated the procedure well.
A. 93451, 93503-51, 410.91
B. 93451, 416.8
C. 93503, 93452, 410.91
D. 93503, 410.91, 416.8

149. **DIALYSIS INPATIENT NOTE:** This 24-year-old male patient is on continuous ambulatory peritoneal dialysis (CAPD) using 1.5%. He drains more than 600 mL. He is tolerating dialysis well. He continues to have some abdominal pain, but his abdomen is not distended. He has some diarrhea. His abdomen does not look like acute abdomen. His vitals, other than blood pressure in the 190s over 100s, are fine. He is afebrile.

At this time, I will continue with 1.5% dialysate. Because of diarrhea, I am going to check stool for white cells, culture. Next we will see what the primary physician says today. His HIDA scan was normal. The patient suffers from ESRD and has had 6 encounters this month. Code this service.
A. 90947, 90960, 585.6, 787.91, V45.11
B. 90945, 585.6, 787.91, V45.11
C. 90960, 585.6, V45.11
D. 90945, 585.6

150. **DIAGNOSIS:** Atrial flutter.

PROCEDURE PERFORMED: Electrical cardioversion.

DESCRIPTION OF PROCEDURE: The patient was sedated with Versed and morphine. She was given a total of 5 mg of Versed. She was cardioverted with 50 joules into sinus tachycardia.

The patient was given a 20-mg Cardizem IV push. Her heart rate went down to the 110s, and she was definitely in sinus tachycardia.

CONCLUSION: Successful electrical cardioversion of atrial flutter into sinus tachycardia.
A. 92961, 427.61
B. 92960, 427.32
C. 92960, 92973, 427.32
D. 92960, 427.89

Figure Credits

1-34   From Kumar V, Abbas AK, Aster J: *Robbins and Cotran Pathologic Basis of Disease*, ed 8, Philadelphia, 2010, Saunders.

1-41   From Damjanov I: *Pathology for the Health Professions*, ed 4, St. Louis, 2012, Saunders.

1-42   From Kissane JM, editor: *Anderson's Pathology*, ed 9, St. Louis, 1990, Mosby.

1-46   From Canale ST, Beaty JH, *Campbell's Operative Orthopaedics*, ed 11, Philadelphia, 2008, Mosby.

1-47   From Thibodeau GA, Patton KT: *Anatomy & Physiology*, ed 8, St. Louis, 2013, Mosby.

1-53   From Yanoff M, Duker J: *Ophthalmology*, ed 3, St. Louis, 2009, Mosby.

2-2   From *Federal Register*, January 10, 2013, Vol 78, No. 7, Rules and Regulations.

3-1   Courtesy U.S. Department of Health and Human Services, Centers for Medicare and Medicaid Services.

3-4   Courtesy U.S. Department of Health and Human Services, Centers for Medicare and Medicaid Services.

3-16   Modified from Buck CJ: *2014 ICD-9-CM, Volumes 1, 2, and 3, Professional Edition*, St. Louis, 2014, Saunders.

Resources

The most current coding guidelines and code system updates are posted to the Evolve website at **http://evolve.elsevier.com/Buck/physicianexam.**

Once registered for your free Evolve resources, go to the ***Course Documents*** section, then select ***Coding Updates, Tips, and Links*** to reference the following:

- *Official Guidelines for Coding and Reporting*
- 1995 Guidelines for E/M Services
- 1997 Documentation Guidelines for Evaluation and Management Services

- CPT Updates
- ICD-9-CM Updates
- HCPCS Updates

- Study Tips
- WebLinks

Some of the CPT code descriptions for physician services include physician extender services. Physician extenders, such as nurse practitioners, physician assistants, and nurse anesthetists, etc., provide medical services typically performed by a physician. Within this educational material the term "physician" may include "and other qualified health care professionals" depending on the code. Refer to the official CPT® code descriptions and guidelines to determine codes that are appropriate to report services provided by non-physician practitioners.

Medical Terminology

ablation	removal or destruction by cutting, chemicals, or electrocautery
abortion	termination of pregnancy
absence	without
actinotherapy	treatment of acne using ultraviolet rays
adenoidectomy	removal of adenoids
adipose	fatty
adrenals	glands, located at the top of the kidneys, that produce steroid hormones
albinism	lack of color pigment
allograft	homograft, same species graft
alopecia	condition in which hair falls out
amniocentesis	percutaneous aspiration of amniotic fluid
amniotic sac	sac containing the fetus and amniotic fluid
A-mode	one-dimensional ultrasonic display reflecting the time it takes a sound wave to reach a structure and reflect back; maps the structure's outline
anastomosis	surgical connection of two tubular structures, such as two pieces of the intestine
aneurysm	abnormal dilation of vessels, usually an artery
angina	sudden pain
angiography	radiography of the blood vessels
angioplasty	procedure in a vessel to dilate the vessel opening
anhidrosis	deficiency of sweat
anomaloscope	instrument used to test color vision
anoscopy	procedure that uses a scope to examine the anus
antepartum	before childbirth
anterior (ventral)	in front of
anterior segment	those parts of the eye in the front of and including the lens (cornea, iris, ciliary body, aqueous humor)

anteroposterior	from front to back
antigen	a substance that produces a specific response
aortography	radiographic recording of the aorta
apex cardiography	recording of the movement of the chest wall over the end of the heart
aphakia	absence of the lens of the eye
apicectomy	excision of a portion of the temporal bone
apnea	cessation of breathing
arthrocentesis	injection and/or aspiration of joint
arthrodesis	surgical immobilization of joint
arthrography	radiography of joint
arthroplasty	reshaping or reconstruction of joint
arthroscopy	use of scope to view inside joint
arthrotomy	incision into a joint
articular	pertains to joint
asphyxia	lack of oxygen
aspiration	use of a needle and a syringe to withdraw fluid
assignment	Medicare's payment for the service, which participating physicians agree to accept as payment in full
asthma	shortage of breath caused by contraction of bronchi
astigmatism	condition in which the refractive surfaces of the eye are unequal
atelectasis	incomplete expansion of lung, collapse
atherectomy	removal of plaque by percutaneous method
atrophy	wasting away
audiometry	hearing test
aural atresia	congenital absence of the external auditory canal
auscultation	listening to sounds within the body
autograft	from patient's own body
avulsion	ripping or tearing away of part either surgically or accidentally
axillary nodes	lymph nodes located in the armpit
bacilli	plural of bacillus, a rod-shaped bacterium
barium enema	radiographic contrast medium
beneficiary	person who benefits from health or life insurance
bifocal	two focuses in eyeglasses, one usually for close work and the other for improvement of distance vision
bilaminate skin	skin substitute usually made of silicone-covered nylon mesh
bilateral	occurring on two sides
biliary	refers to gallbladder, bile, or bile duct
bilobectomy	surgical removal of two lobes of a lung
biofeedback	process of giving a person self-information

biometry	application of a statistical measure to a biologic fact
biopsy	removal of a small piece of living tissue for diagnostic purposes
block	frozen piece of a sample
brachytherapy	therapy using radioactive sources that are placed inside the body
bronchiole	smaller division of bronchial tree
bronchography	radiographic recording of the lungs
bronchoplasty	surgical repair of the bronchi
bronchoscopy	inspection of the bronchial tree using a bronchoscope
B-scan	two-dimensional display of tissues and organs
bulbocavernosus	muscle that constricts the vagina in a female and the urethra in a male
bulbourethral	gland with duct leading to the urethra
bundle of His	muscular cardiac fibers that provide the heart rhythm to the ventricles; blockage of this rhythm produces heart block
bundled codes	one code that represents a package of services
bunion	hallux valgus, abnormal increase in size of metatarsal head that results in displacement of the great toe
burr	drill used to create an entry into the cranium
bursa	fluid-filled sac that absorbs friction
bursitis	inflammation of bursa (joint sac)
bypass	to go around
calcaneal	pertaining to the heel bone
calculus	concretion of mineral salts, also called a stone
calycoplasty	surgical reconstruction of a recess of the renal pelvis
calyx	recess of the renal pelvis
cancellous	lattice-type structure, usually of bone
cardiopulmonary	refers to the heart and lungs
cardiopulmonary bypass	blood bypasses the heart through a heart-lung machine
cardioversion	electrical shock to the heart to restore normal rhythm
cardioverter-defibrillator	surgically placed device that directs an electrical shock to the heart to restore rhythm
carotid body	located on each side of the common carotid artery, often a site of tumor
cartilage	connective tissue
cataract	opaque covering on or in the lens
catheter	tube placed into the body to put fluid in or take fluid out
caudal	same as inferior; away from the head, or the lower part of the body

causalgia	burning pain
cauterization	destruction of tissue by the use of cautery
cavernosa	connection between the cavity of the penis and a vein
cavernosography	radiographic recording of a cavity, e.g., the pulmonary cavity or the main part of the penis
cavernosometry	measurement of the pressure in a cavity, e.g., the penis
central nervous system	brain and spinal cord
cervical	pertaining to the neck or to the cervix of the uterus
cervix uteri	rounded, cone-shaped neck of the uterus
cesarean	surgical opening through abdominal wall for delivery
cholangiography	radiographic recording of the bile ducts
cholangiopancreatography	ERCP, radiographic recording of the biliary system or pancreas
cholecystectomy	surgical removal of the gallbladder
cholecystoenterostomy	creation of a connection between the gallbladder and intestine
cholecystography	radiographic recording of the gallbladder
cholesteatoma	tumor that forms in middle ear
chondral	referring to the cartilage
chordee	condition resulting in the penis being bent downward
chorionic villus sampling	CVS, biopsy of the outermost part of the placenta
circumflex	a coronary artery that circles the heart
Cloquet's node	also called a gland; it is the highest of the deep groin lymph nodes
closed fracture repair	not surgically opened with/without manipulation and with/without traction
closed treatment	fracture site that is not surgically opened and visualized
coccyx	caudal extremity of vertebral column
collagen	protein substance of skin
Colles' fracture	fracture at lower end of radius that displaces the bone posteriorly
colonoscopy	fiberscopic examination of the entire colon that may include part of the terminal ileum
colostomy	artificial opening between the colon and the abdominal wall
component	part
computed axial tomography	CAT or CT, procedure by which selected planes of tissue are pinpointed through computer enhancement, and images may be reconstructed by analysis of variance in absorption of the tissue
conjunctiva	the lining of the eyelids and the covering of anterior sclera
contraction	drawn together

contralateral	opposite side
cordectomy	surgical removal of the vocal cord(s)
cordocentesis	procedure to obtain a fetal blood sample; also called a percutaneous umbilical blood sampling
corneosclera	cornea and sclera of the eye
corpectomy	removal of vertebrae
corpora cavernosa	the two cavities of the penis
corpus uteri	uterus
crackles	abnormal sounds when breathing (heard on auscultation)
craniectomy	permanent, partial removal of skull
craniotomy	opening of the skull
cranium	that part of the skeleton that encloses the brain
curettage	scraping of a cavity using a spoon-shaped instrument
curette	spoon-shaped instrument used to scrape a cavity
cutdown	incision into a vessel for placement of a catheter
cyanosis	bluish discoloration
cystocele	herniation of the bladder into the vagina
cystography	radiographic recording of the urinary bladder
cystolithectomy	removal of a calculus (stone) from the urinary bladder
cystolithotomy	cystolithectomy
cystometrogram	CMG, measurement of the pressures and capacity of the urinary bladder
cystoplasty	surgical reconstruction of the bladder
cystorrhaphy	suture of the bladder
cystoscopy	use of a scope to view the bladder
cystostomy	surgical creation of an opening into the bladder
cystotomy	incision into the bladder
cystourethroplasty	surgical reconstruction of the bladder and urethra
cystourethroscopy	use of a scope to view the bladder and urethra
dacryocystography	radiographic recording of the lacrimal sac or tear duct sac
dacryostenosis	narrowing of the lacrimal duct
debridement	cleansing of or removal of dead tissue from a wound
deductible	amount the patient is liable for before the payer begins to pay for covered services
delayed flap	pedicle of skin with blood supply that is separated from origin over time
delivery	childbirth
dermabrasion	planing of the skin by means of sander, brush, or sandpaper

dermatologist	physician who treats conditions of the skin
dermatoplasty	surgical repair of skin
dialysis	filtration of blood
dilation	expansion
discectomy	removal of a vertebral disc
discography	radiographic recording of an intervertebral joint
dislocation	placement in a location other than the original location
distal	farther from the point of attachment or origin
diverticulum	protrusion in the wall of an organ
Doppler	ultrasonic measure of blood movement
dosimetry	scientific calculation of radiation emitted from various radioactive sources
drainage	free flow or withdrawal of fluids from a wound or cavity
duodenography	radiographic recording of the duodenum or first part of the small intestine
dysphagia	difficulty swallowing
dysphonia	speech impairment
dyspnea	shortness of breath, difficult breathing
dysuria	painful urination
echocardiography	radiographic recording of the heart or heart walls or surrounding tissues
echoencephalography	ultrasound of the brain
echography	ultrasound procedure in which sound waves are bounced off an internal organ and the resulting image is recorded
ectopic	pregnancy outside the uterus (i.e., in the fallopian tube)
edema	swelling due to abnormal fluid collection in the tissue spaces
elective surgery	nonemergency procedure
electrocardiogram	ECG, written record of the electrical action of the heart
electrocautery	cauterization by means of heated instrument
electrocochleography	test to measure the eighth cranial nerve (hearing test)
electrode	lead attached to a generator that carries the electrical current from the generator to the atria or ventricles
electroencephalogram	EEG, written record of the electrical action of the brain
electromyogram	EMG, written record of the electrical activity of the skeletal muscles
electronic claim submission	claims prepared and submitted via a computer
electronic signature	identification system of a computer
electro-oculogram	EOG, written record of the electrical activity of the eye

electrophysiology	study of the electrical system of the heart, including the study of arrhythmias
embolectomy	removal of blockage (embolism) from vessel
emphysema	air accumulated in organ or tissue
encephalography	radiographic recording of the subarachnoid space and ventricles of the brain
endarterectomy	incision into an artery to remove the inner lining so as to eliminate disease or blockage
endomyocardial	pertaining to the inner and middle layers of the heart
endopyelotomy	procedure involving the bladder and ureters, including the insertion of a stent into the renal pelvis
endoscopy	inspection of body organs or cavities using a lighted scope that may be inserted through an existing opening or through a small incision
enterolysis	releasing of adhesions of intestine
enucleation	removal of an organ or organs from a body cavity
epicardial	over the heart
epidermolysis	loosening of the epidermis
epidermomycosis	superficial fungal infection
epididymectomy	surgical removal of the epididymis
epididymis	tube located at the top of the testes that stores sperm
epididymography	radiographic recording of the epididymis
epididymovasostomy	creation of a new connection between the vas deferens and epididymis
epiglottidectomy	excision of the covering of the larynx
episclera	connective covering of the sclera
epistaxis	nosebleed
epithelium	surface covering of internal and external organs of the body
erythema	redness of skin
escharotomy	surgical incision into necrotic (dead) tissue
eventration	protrusion of the bowel through an opening in the abdomen
evisceration	pulling the viscera outside of the body through an incision
evocative	tests that are administered to evoke a predetermined response
exenteration	removal of an organ all in one piece
exophthalmos	protrusion of the eyeball
exostosis	bony growth
exstrophy	condition in which an organ is turned inside out
extracorporeal	occurring outside of the body
false aneurysm	sac of clotted blood that has completely destroyed the vessel and is being contained by the tissue that surrounds the vessel

fasciectomy	removal of a band of fibrous tissue
Federal Register	official publication of all "Presidential Documents," "Rules and Regulations," "Proposed Rules," and "Notices"; government-instituted national changes are published in the *Federal Register*
fee schedule	services and payment allowed for each service
femoral	pertaining to the bone from the pelvis to knee
fenestration	creation of a new opening in the inner wall of the middle ear
fissure	cleft or groove
fistula	abnormal opening from one area to another area or to the outside of the body
fluoroscopy	procedure for viewing the interior of the body using x-rays and projecting the image onto a television screen
fracture	break in a bone
free full-thickness graft	graft of epidermis and dermis that is completely removed from donor area
fulguration	use of electrical current to destroy tissue
fundoplasty	repair of the bottom of the bladder
furuncle	nodule in the skin caused by *Staphylococcus* entering through hair follicle
ganglion	knot
gastrointestinal	pertaining to the stomach and intestine
gastroplasty	operation on the stomach for repair or reconfiguration
gastrostomy	artificial opening between the stomach and the abdominal wall
gatekeeper	a physician who manages a patient's access to health care
glaucoma	eye diseases that are characterized by an increase of intraocular pressure
globe	eyeball
glottis	true vocal cords
gonioscopy	use of a scope to examine the angles of the eye
Group Practice Model	an organization of physicians who contract with a Health Maintenance Organization to provide services to the enrollees of the HMO
grouper	computer used to input the principal diagnosis and other critical information about a patient and then provide the correct DRG code
Health Maintenance Organization	HMO, a healthcare delivery system in which an enrollee is assigned a primary care physician who manages all the healthcare needs of the enrollee
hematoma	mass of blood that forms outside the vessel
hemodialysis	cleansing of the blood outside of the body
hemolysis	breakdown of red blood cells

hemoptysis	bloody sputum
hepatography	radiographic recording of the liver
hernia	organ or tissue protruding through the wall or cavity that usually contains it
histology	study of structure of tissue and cells
homograft	allograft, same species graft
hormone	chemical substance produced by the body's endocrine glands
hydrocele	sac of fluid
hyperopia	farsightedness, eyeball is too short from front to back
hypogastric	lowest middle abdominal area
hyposensitization	decreased sensitivity
hypothermia	low body temperature; sometimes induced during surgical procedures
hypoxemia	low level of oxygen in the blood
hypoxia	low level of oxygen in the tissue
hysterectomy	surgical removal of the uterus
hysterorrhaphy	suturing of the uterus
hysterosalpingography	radiographic recording of the uterine cavity and fallopian tubes
hysteroscopy	visualization of the canal and cavity of the uterus using a scope placed through the vagina
ichthyosis	skin disorder characterized by scaling
ileostomy	artificial opening between the ileum and the abdominal wall
ilium	portion of hip
imbrication	overlapping
immunotherapy	therapy to increase immunity
incarcerated	regarding hernias, a constricted, irreducible hernia that may cause obstruction of an intestine
incise	to cut into
Individual Practice Association	IPA, an organization of physicians who provide services for a set fee; Health Maintenance Organizations often contract with the IPA for services to their enrollees
inferior	away from the head or the lower part of the body; also known as caudalingual
inguinofemoral	referring to the groin and thigh
inofemoral	referring to the groin and thigh
internal/external fixation	application of pins, wires, and/or screws placed externally or internally to immobilize a body part
intracardiac	inside the heart

intramural	within the organ wall
intramuscular	into a muscle
intrauterine	inside the uterus
intravenous	into a vein
intravenous pyelography	IVP, radiographic recording of the urinary system
introitus	opening or entrance to the vagina from the uterus
intubation	insertion of a tube
intussusception	slipping of one part of the intestine into another part
invasive	entering the body, breaking skin
iontophoresis	introduction of ions into the body
ischemia	deficient blood supply due to obstruction of the circulatory system
island pedicle flap	contains a single artery and vein that remain attached to origin temporarily or permanently
isthmus	connection of two regions or structures
isthmus, thyroid	tissue connection between right and left thyroid lobes
isthmusectomy	surgical removal of the isthmus
jejunostomy	artificial opening between the jejunum and the abdominal wall
jugular nodes	lymph nodes located next to the large vein in the neck
keratomalacia	softening of the cornea associated with a deficiency of vitamin A
keratoplasty	surgical repair of the cornea
ketones	compounds that are carbon-based byproducts of fatty acid metabolism; excess ketone bodies in urine may indicate diabetes mellitus
kidney	organs that filter blood and balance the levels of water, salt, and minerals in the blood
kidney stones	formations of minerals and salt that may form in the urine
Kock pouch	surgical creation of a urinary bladder from a segment of the ileum
kyphosis	humpback
labyrinth	inner connecting cavities, such as the internal ear
labyrinthitis	inner ear inflammation
lacrimal	related to tears
lamina	flat plate
laminectomy	surgical excision of the lamina
laparoscopy	exploration of the abdomen and pelvic cavities using a scope placed through a small incision in the abdominal wall
laryngeal web	congenital abnormality of connective tissue between the vocal cords

laryngectomy	surgical removal of the larynx
laryngography	radiographic recording of the larynx
laryngoplasty	surgical repair of the larynx
laryngoscope	fiberoptic scope used to view the inside of the larynx
laryngoscopy	direct visualization and examination of the interior of larynx with a laryngoscope
laryngotomy	incision into the larynx
lateral	away from the midline of the body (to the side)
lavage	washing out
leukoderma	depigmentation of skin
leukoplakia	white patch on mucous membrane
ligament	fibrous band of tissue that connects cartilage or bone
ligation	binding or tying off, as in constricting the blood flow of a vessel or binding fallopian tubes for sterilization
lipocyte	fat cell
lipoma	fatty tumor
lithotomy	incision into an organ or a duct for the purpose of removing a stone
lithotripsy	crushing of a stone by sound waves or force
lobectomy	surgical excision of lobe of the lung
lordosis	anterior curve of the spine
lumbodynia	pain in the lumbar area
lunate	one of the wrist (carpal) bones
lymph node	station along the lymphatic system
lymphadenectomy	excision of a lymph node or nodes
lymphadenitis	inflammation of a lymph node
lymphangiography	radiographic recording of the lymphatic vessels and nodes
lymphangiotomy	incision into a lymphatic vessel
lysis	releasing
magnetic resonance imaging	MRI, procedure that uses nonionizing radiation to view the body in a cross-sectional view
Major Diagnostic Categories	MDC, the division of all principal diagnoses into 25 mutually exclusive principal diagnosis areas within the DRG system
mammography	radiographic recording of the breasts
Managed Care Organization	MCO, a group that is responsible for the health care services offered to an enrolled group of persons
manipulation	movement by hand
manipulation or reduction	alignment of a fracture or joint dislocation to its normal position

mastoidectomy	removal of the mastoid bone
Maximum Actual Allowable Charge	MAAC, limitation on the total amount that can be charged by physicians who are not participants in Medicare
meatotomy	surgical enlargement of the opening of the urinary meatus
medial	toward the midline of the body
Medical Volume Performance Standards	MVPS, government's estimate of how much growth is appropriate for nationwide physician expenditures paid by the Part B Medicare program
Medicare Economic Index	MEI, government mandated index that ties increases in the Medicare prevailing charges to economic indicators
Medicare Fee Schedule	MFS, schedule that listed the allowable charges for Medicare services; was replaced by the Medicare reasonable charge payment system
Medicare Risk HMO	a Medicare-funded alternative to the standard Medicare supplemental coverage
melanin	dark pigment of skin
melanoma	tumor of epidermis, malignant and black in color
Ménière's disease	condition that causes dizziness, ringing in the ears, and deafness
M-mode	one-dimensional display of movement of structures
modality	treatment method
Mohs surgery or Mohs micrographic surgery	removal of skin cancer in layers by a surgeon who also acts as pathologist during surgery
monofocal	eyeglasses with one vision correction
multipara	more than one pregnancy
muscle	organ of contraction for movement
muscle flap	transfer of muscle from origin to recipient site
myasthenia gravis	syndrome characterized by muscle weakness
myelography	radiographic recording of the subarachnoid space of the spine
myopia	nearsightedness, eyeball too long from front to back
myringotomy	incision into tympanic membrane
nasal button	synthetic circular disk used to cover a hole in the nasal septum
nasopharyngoscopy	use of a scope to visualize the nose and pharynx
National Provider Identifier	NPI, a 10-digit number assigned to a physician by Medicare
nephrectomy, paraperitoneal	kidney transplant
nephrocutaneous fistula	a channel from the kidney to the skin
nephrolithotomy	removal of a kidney stone through an incision made into the kidney
nephrorrhaphy	suturing of the kidney
nephrostolithotomy	creation of an artificial channel to the kidney

nephrostolithotomy, percutaneous	procedure to establish an artificial channel between the skin and the kidney
nephrostomy	creation of a channel into the renal pelvis of the kidney
nephrostomy, percutaneous	creation of a channel from the skin to the renal pelvis
nephrotomy	incision into the kidney
neurovascular flap	contains artery, vein, and nerve
noninvasive	not entering the body, not breaking skin
nuclear cardiology	diagnostic specialty that uses radiologic procedures to aid in diagnosis of cardiologic conditions
nystagmus	rapid involuntary eye movements
ocular adnexa	orbit, extraocular muscles, and eyelid
olecranon	elbow bone
Omnibus Budget Reconciliation Act of 1989	OBRA, act that established new rules for Medicare reimbursement
oophorectomy	surgical removal of the ovary(ies)
opacification	area that has become opaque (milky)
open fracture repair	surgical opening (incision) over or remote opening as access to a fracture site
open treatment	fracture site that is surgically opened and visualized
ophthalmodynamometry	test of the blood pressure of the eye
ophthalmology	body of knowledge regarding the eyes
ophthalmoscopy	examination of the interior of the eye by means of a scope, also known as fundoscopy
optokinetic	movement of the eyes to objects moving in the visual field
orchiectomy	castration; removal of the testes
orchiopexy	surgical procedure to release undescended testes and fixate them within the scrotum
order	shows subordination of one thing to another; family or class
orthopnea	difficulty in breathing, needing to be in erect position to breathe
orthoptic	corrective; in the correct place
osteoarthritis	degenerative condition of articular cartilage
osteoclast	absorbs or removes bone
osteotomy	cutting into bone
otitis media	noninfectious inflammation of the middle ear; serous otitis media produces liquid drainage (not purulent) and suppurative otitis media produces purulent (pus) matter
otoscope	instrument used to examine the internal and external ear
oviduct	fallopian tube
papilledema	swelling of the optic disc (papilla)

paraesophageal hiatal hernia	hernia that is near the esophagus
parathyroid	produces a hormone to mobilize calcium from the bones to the blood
paronychia	infection around nail
Part A	Medicare's Hospital Insurance; covers hospital/facility care
Part B	Medicare's Supplemental Medical Insurance; covers physician services and durable medical equipment that are not paid for under Part A
participating provider program	Medicare providers who have agreed in advance to accept assignment on all Medicare claims, now termed Quality Improvement Organizations (QIO)
patella	knee cap
pedicle	growth attached with a stem
Peer Review Organizations	PROs, groups established to review hospital admission and care
pelviolithotomy	pyeloplasty
penoscrotal	referring to the penis and scrotum
percussion	tapping with sharp blows as a diagnostic technique
percutaneous	through the skin
percutaneous fracture repair	repair of a fracture by means of pins and wires inserted through the fracture site
percutaneous skeletal fixation	considered neither open nor closed; the fracture is not visualized, but fixation is placed across the fracture site under x-ray imaging
pericardiocentesis	procedure in which a surgeon withdraws fluid from the pericardial space by means of a needle inserted percutaneously
pericardium	membranous sac enclosing heart and ends of great vessels
perineum	area between the vulva and anus; also known as the pelvic floor
peripheral nerves	12 pairs of cranial nerves, 31 pairs of spinal nerves, and autonomic nervous system; connects peripheral receptors to the brain and spinal cord
peritoneal	within the lining of the abdominal cavity
peritoneoscopy	visualization of the abdominal cavity using one scope placed through a small incision in the abdominal wall and another scope placed in the vagina
pharyngolaryngectomy	surgical removal of the pharynx and larynx
phlebotomy	cutting into a vein
phonocardiogram	recording of heart sounds
photochemotherapy	treatment by means of drugs that react to ultraviolet radiation or sunlight
physics	scientific study of energy
pilosebaceous	pertains to hair follicles and sebaceous glands

placenta	a structure that connects the fetus and mother during pregnancy
plethysmography	determining the changes in volume of an organ part or body
pleura	covers the lungs and lines the thoracic cavity
pleurectomy	surgical excision of the pleura
pleuritis	inflammation of the pleura
pneumonocentesis	surgical puncturing of a lung to withdraw fluid
pneumonolysis	surgical separation of the lung from the chest wall to allow the lung to collapse
pneumonostomy	surgical procedure in which the chest cavity is exposed and the lung is incised
pneumonotomy	incision of the lung
pneumoplethysmography	determining the changes in the volume of the lung
posterior (dorsal)	in back of
posterior segment	those parts of the eye behind the lens
posteroanterior	from back to front
postpartum	after childbirth
Preferred Provider Organization	PPO, a group of providers who form a network and who have agreed to provide services to enrollees at a discounted rate
priapism	painful condition in which the penis is constantly erect
primary care physician	PCP, physician who oversees a patient's care within a managed care organization
primary diagnosis	chief complaint of a patient in outpatient setting
primipara	first pregnancy
prior approval	also known as a prior authorization, the payer's approval of care
proctosigmoidoscopy	fiberscopic examination of the sigmoid colon and rectum
Professional Standards Review Organization	PSRO, voluntary physicians' organization designed to monitor the necessity of hospital admissions, treatment costs, and medical records of hospitals
prognosis	probable outcome of an illness
prostatotomy	incision into the prostate
Provider Identification Number	PIN, assigned to physicians by payers for use in claims submission
pyelography	radiographic recording of the kidneys, renal pelvis, ureters, and bladder
qualitative	measuring the presence or absence of
Quality Improvement Organizations	QIO, consists of a national network of 53 entities that work with consumers, physicians, hospitals, and caregivers to refine care delivery systems
quantitative	measuring the presence or absence of and the amount of

rad	radiation-absorbed dose, the energy deposited in patient's tissues
radiation oncology	branch of medicine concerned with the application of radiation to a tumor site for treatment (destruction) of cancerous tumors
radiograph	film on which an image is produced through exposure to x-radiation
radiologist	physician who specializes in the use of radioactive materials in the diagnosis and treatment of disease and illness
radiology	branch of medicine concerned with the use of radioactive substances for diagnosis and therapy
rales	coarse sounds on inspiration, also known as crackles (heard on auscultation)
real time	two-dimensional display of both the structures and the motion of tissues and organs, with the length of time also recorded as part of the study
reduction	replacement to normal position
Relative Value Unit	RVU, unit value that has been assigned for each service
Resource-Based Relative Value Scale	RBRVS, scale designed to decrease Medicare expenditures, redistribute physician payment, and ensure quality health care at reasonable rates
resource intensity	refers to the relative volume and type of diagnostic, therapeutic, and bed services used in the management of a particular illness
retrograde	moving backward or against the usual direction of flow
rhinoplasty	surgical repair of nose
rhinorrhea	nasal mucous discharge
salpingectomy	surgical removal of the uterine tube
salpingostomy	creation of a fistula into the uterine tube
scan	mapping of emissions of radioactive substances after they have been introduced into the body; the density can determine normal or abnormal conditions
sclera	outer covering of the eye
scoliosis	lateral curve of the spine
sebaceous gland	secretes sebum
seborrhea	excess sebum secretion
sebum	oily substance
section	slice of a frozen block
segmentectomy	surgical removal of a portion of a lung
septoplasty	surgical repair of the nasal septum
serum	blood from which the fibrinogen has been removed

severity of illness	refers to the levels of loss of function and mortality that may be experienced by patients with a particular disease
shunt	an artificial passage
sialography	radiographic recording of the salivary duct and branches
sialolithotomy	surgical removal of a stone of the salivary gland or duct
sinography	radiographic recording of the sinus or sinus tract
sinusotomy	surgical incision into a sinus
skeletal traction	application of pressure to the bone by means of pins and/or wires inserted into the bone
skin traction	application of pressure to the bone by means of tape applied to the skin
skull	entire skeletal framework of the head
somatic nerve	sensory or motor nerve
specimen	sample of tissue or fluid
spirometry	measurement of breathing capacity
splenectomy	excision of the spleen
splenography	radiographic recording of the spleen
splenoportography	radiographic procedure to allow visualization of the splenic and portal veins of the spleen
split-thickness graft	all epidermis and some of dermis
spondylitis	inflammation of vertebrae
Staff Model	a Health Maintenance Organization that directly employs the physicians who provide services to enrollees
steatoma	fat mass in sebaceous gland
stem cell	immature blood cell
stereotaxis	method of identifying a specific area or point in the brain
strabismus	extraocular muscle deviation resulting in unequal visual axes
stratified	layered
stratum (strata)	layer
subcutaneous	tissue below the dermis, primarily fat cells that insulate the body
subluxation	partial dislocation
subungual	beneath the nail
superior	toward the head or the upper part of the body; also known as cephalic
supination	supine position
supine	lying on the back
Swan-Ganz catheter	a catheter that measures pressure in the heart
sympathetic nerve	part of the peripheral nervous system that controls automatic body function and nerves activated under stress

symphysis	natural junction
synchondrosis	union between two bones (connected by cartilage)
tachypnea	quick, shallow breathing
tarsorrhaphy	suturing together of the eyelids
Tax Equity and Fiscal Responsibility Act	TEFRA, act that contains language to reward cost-conscious healthcare providers
tendon	attaches a muscle to a bone
tenodesis	suturing of a tendon to a bone
tenorrhaphy	suture repair of tendon
thermogram	written record of temperature variation
third-party payer	insurance company or entity that is liable for another's healthcare services
thoracentesis	surgical puncture of the thoracic cavity, usually using a needle, to remove fluids
thoracic duct	collection and distribution point for lymph, and the largest lymph vessel located in the chest
thoracoplasty	surgical procedure that removes rib(s) and thereby allows the collapse of a lung
thoracoscopy	use of a lighted endoscope to view the pleural spaces and thoracic cavity or to perform surgical procedures
thoracostomy	incision into the chest wall and insertion of a chest tube
thoracotomy	surgical incision into the chest wall
thromboendarterectomy	procedure to remove plaque or clot formations from a vessel by percutaneous method
thymectomy	surgical removal of the thymus
thymus	gland that produces hormones important to the immune response
thyroglossal duct	connection between the thyroid and the tongue
thyroid	part of the endocrine system that produces hormones that regulate metabolism
thyroidectomy	surgical removal of the thyroid
tinnitus	ringing in the ears
titer	measure of a laboratory analysis
tocolysis	repression of uterine contractions
tomography	procedure that allows viewing of a single plane of the body by blurring out all but that particular level
tonography	recording of changes in intraocular pressure in response to sustained pressure on the eyeball
tonometry	measurement of pressure or tension
total pneumonectomy	surgical removal of an entire lung
tracheostomy	creation of an opening into trachea

tracheotomy	incision into trachea
traction	application of pressure to maintain normal alignment
transcutaneous	entering by way of the skin
transesophageal echocardiogram	TEE, echocardiogram performed by placing a probe down the esophagus and sending out sound waves to obtain images of the heart and its movement
transmastoid	creates an opening in the mastoid for drainage antrostomy
transplantation	grafting of tissue from one source to another
transseptal	through the septum
transtracheal	across the trachea
transureteroureterostomy	surgical connection of one ureter to the other ureter
transurethral resection of prostate	TURP, procedure performed through the urethra by means of a cystoscopy to remove part or all of the prostate
transvenous	through a vein
transvesical ureterolithotomy	removal of a ureter stone (calculus) through the bladder
trephination	surgical removal of a disc of bone
trocar needle	needle with a tube on the end; used to puncture and withdraw fluid from a cavity
tubercle	lesion caused by infection of tuberculosis
tumescence	state of being swollen
tunica vaginalis	covering of the testes
tympanolysis	freeing of adhesions of the tympanic membrane
tympanometry	test of the inner ear using air pressure
tympanostomy	insertion of ventilation tube into tympanum
ultrasound	technique using sound waves to determine the density of the outline of tissue
unbundling	reporting with multiple codes that which can be reported with one code
unilateral	occurring on one side
uptake	absorption of a radioactive substance by body tissues; recorded for diagnostic purposes in conditions such as thyroid disease
ureterectomy	surgical removal of a ureter, either totally or partially
ureterocolon	pertaining to the ureter and colon
ureterocutaneous fistula	channel from the ureter to exterior skin
ureteroenterostomy	creation of a connection between the intestine and the ureter
ureterolithotomy	removal of a stone from the ureter
ureterolysis	freeing of adhesions of the ureter
ureteroneocystostomy	surgical connection of the ureter to a new site on the bladder
ureteropyelography	ureter and bladder radiography

ureterotomy	incision into the ureter
urethrocystography	radiography of the bladder and urethra
urethromeatoplasty	surgical repair of the urethra and meatus
urethropexy	fixation of the urethra by means of surgery
urethroplasty	surgical repair of the urethra
urethrorrhaphy	suturing of the urethra
urethroscopy	use of a scope to view the urethra
urography	same as pyelography; radiographic recording of the kidneys, renal pelvis, ureters, and bladder
uveal	vascular tissue of the choroid, ciliary body, and iris
varices	varicose veins
varicocele	swelling of a scrotal vein
vas deferens	tube that carries sperm from the epididymis to the urethra
vasectomy	removal of segment of vas deferens
vasogram	recording of the flow in the vas deferens
vasotomy	incision in the vas deferens
vasorrhaphy	suturing of the vas deferens
vasovasostomy	reversal of a vasectomy
vectorcardiogram	VCG, continuous recording of electrical direction and magnitude of the heart
venography	radiographic recording of the veins and tributaries
vertebrectomy	removal of vertebra
vertigo	dizziness
vesicostomy	surgical creation of a connection of the viscera of the bladder to the skin
vesicovaginal fistula	creation of a tube between the vagina and the bladder
vesiculectomy	excision of the seminal vesicle
vesiculography	radiographic recording of the seminal vesicles
vesiculotomy	incision into the seminal vesicle
viscera	an organ in one of the large cavities of the body
volvulus	twisted section of the intestine
vomer	flat bones of the nasal septum
xanthoma	tumor composed of cells containing lipid material, yellow in color
xenograft	different species graft
xeroderma	dry, discolored, scaly skin
xeroradiography	photoelectric process of radiographs

Combining Forms

abdomin/o	abdomen
acetabul/o	hip socket
acr/o	height/extremities
aden/o	in relationship to a gland
adenoid/o	adenoids
adip/o	fat
adren/o, adrenal/o	adrenal gland
albin/o	white
albumin/o	albumin
alveol/o	alveolus
ambly/o	dim
amni/o	amnion
an/o	anus
andr/o	male
andren/o	adrenal gland
andrenal/o	adrenal gland
angi/o	vessel
ankyl/o	bent, fused
aort/o	aorta
aponeur/o	tendon type
appendic/o	appendix
aque/o	water
arche/o	first
arter/o, arteri/o	artery
arthr/o	joint
atel/o	incomplete
ather/o	plaque
atri/o	atrium

audi/o	hearing
aut/o	self
axill/o	armpit
azot/o	urea
balan/o	glans penis
bi/o	life
bil/i	bile
bilirubin/o	bile pigment
blephar/o	eyelid
brachi/o	arm
bronch/o	bronchus
bronchi/o	bronchus
bronchiol/o	bronchiole
burs/o	fluid-filled sac in a joint
calc/o, calc/i	calcium
cardi/o	heart
carp/o	carpals (wrist bones)
cauter/o	burn
cec/o	cecum
celi/o	abdomen
cephal/o	head
cerebell/o	cerebellum
cerebr/o	cerebrum
cervic/o	neck/cervix
chol/e	gall/bile
cholangio/o	bile duct
cholecyst/o	gallbladder
choledoch/o	common bile duct
cholester/o	cholesterol
chondr/o	cartilage
chori/o	chorion
clavic/o, clavicul/o	clavicle (collar bone)
col/o	colon
colp/o	vagina
coni/o	dust
conjunctiv/o	conjunctiva

cor/o, core/o	pupil
corne/o	cornea
coron/o	heart
cortic/o	cortex
cost/o	rib
crani/o	cranium (skull)
crin/o	secrete
crypt/o	hidden
culd/o	cul-de-sac
cutane/o	skin
cyan/o	blue
cycl/o	ciliary body
cyst/o	bladder
dacry/o	tear
dacryocyst/o	pertaining to the lacrimal sac
dent/i	tooth
derm/o, dermat/o	skin
diaphragmat/o	diaphragm
dips/o	thirst
disc/o	intervertebral disc
diverticul/o	diverticulum
duoden/o	duodenum
dur/o	dura mater
encephal/o	brain
enter/o	small intestine
eosin/o	rosy
epididym/o	epididymis
epiglott/o	epiglottis
episi/o	vulva
erythr/o, erythem/o	red
esophag/o	esophagus
essi/o, esthesi/o	sensation
estr/o	female
femor/o	thighbone
fet/o	fetus
fibul/o	fibula

galact/o	milk
gangli/o	ganglion
ganglion/o	ganglion
gastr/o	stomach
gingiv/o	gum
glomerul/o	glomerulus
gloss/o	tongue
gluc/o	sugar
glyc/o	sugar
glycos/o	sugar
gonad/o	ovaries and testes
gyn/o	female
gynec/o	female
hepat/o	liver
herni/o	hernia
heter/o	different
hidr/o	sweat
home/o	same
hormon/o	hormone
humer/o	humerus (upper arm bone)
hydr/o	water
hymen/o	hymen
hyster/o	uterus
ichthy/o	dry/scaly
ile/o	ileus
ili/o	ilium (upper pelvic bone)
immun/o	immune
inguin/o	groin
ir/o	iris
irid/o	iris
ischi/o	ischium (posterior pelvic bone)
jaund/o	yellow
jejun/o	jejunum
kal/i	potassium
kerat/o	hard, cornea

kinesi/o	movement
kyph/o	hump
lacrim/o	tear
lact/o	milk
lamin/o	lamina
lapar/o	abdomen
laryng/o	larynx
lingu/o	tongue
lip/o	fat
lith/o	stone
lob/o	lobe
lord/o	curve
lumb/o	lower back
lute/o	yellow
lymph/o	lymph
lymphaden/o	lymph gland
mamm/o	breast
mandibul/o	mandible (lower jawbone)
mast/o	breast
maxill/o	maxilla (upper jawbone)
meat/o	meatus
melan/o	black
men/o	menstruation, month
mening/o, meningi/o	meninges
menisc/o, menisci/o	meniscus
ment/o	mind
metacarp/o	metacarpals (hand)
metatars/o	metatarsals (foot)
metr/o	uterus, measure
metr/i	uterus
mon/o	one
muc/o	mucus
my/o, muscul/o	muscle
myc/o	fungus

myel/o	bone marrow, spinal cord
myring/o	ear drum
myx/o	mucus
nas/o	nose
nat/a, nat/i	birth
natr/o	sodium
necr/o	death
nephr/o	kidney
neur/o	nerve
noct/i	night
ocul/o	eye
olecran/o	olecranon (elbow)
olig/o	scant, few
onych/o	nail
oo/o	egg
oophor/o	ovary
ophthalm/o	eye
opt/o	eye, vision
optic/o	eye
or/o	mouth
orch/i, orch/o, orchi/o, orchid/o	testicle
orth/o	straight
oste/o	bone
ot/o	ear
ov/o	egg
ovari/o	ovary
ovul/o	ovulation
ox/i, ox/o	oxygen
oxy/o	oxygen
pachy/o	thick
palat/o	palate
palpebr/o	eyelid
pancreat/o	pancreas

papill/o	optic nerve
patell/o	patella (kneecap)
pelv/i	pelvis (hip)
pericardi/o	pericardium
perine/o	perineum
peritone/o	peritoneum
petr/o	stone
phac/o	eye lens
phak/o	eye lens
phalang/o	phalanges (finger or toe)
pharyng/o	pharynx
phas/o	speech
phleb/o	vein
phren/o	mind, diaphragm
phys/o	growing
pil/o	hair
pituitar/o	pituitary gland
pleur/o	pleura
pneumat/o	lung/air
pneumon/o	lung/air
poli/o	gray matter
polyp/o	polyp
pont/o	pons
proct/o	rectum
prostat/o	prostate gland
psych/o	mind
pub/o	pubis
pulmon/o	lung
pupill/o	pupil
py/o	pus
pyel/o	renal pelvis
pylor/o	pylorus
quadr/i	four
rachi/o	spine
radi/o	radius (lower arm)
radic/o, radicul/o	nerve root
rect/o	rectum

ren/o	kidney
retin/o	retina
rhin/o	nose
rhiz/o	nerve root
rhytid/o	wrinkle
rube/o	red
sacr/o	sacrum
salping/o	uterine tube, fallopian tube
scapul/o	scapula (shoulder)
scler/o	sclera
scoli/o	bent
seb/o	sebum/oil
semin/i	semen
sept/o	septum
sial/o	saliva
sigmoid/o	sigmoid colon
sinus/o	sinus
somat/o	body
son/o	sound
sperm/o, spermat/o	sperm
sphygm/o	pulse
spir/o	breath
splen/o	spleen
spondyl/o	vertebra
staped/o	middle ear, stapes
staphyl/o	clusters
steat/o	fat
ster/o, stere/o	solid, having three dimensions
stern/o	sternum (breast bone)
steth/o	chest
stomat/o	mouth
strept/o	twisted chain
synovi/o	synovial joint membrane
tars/o	tarsal (ankle)
ten/o	tendon

tend/o, tendin/o	tendon (connective tissue)
test/o	testicle
thorac/o	thorax
thromb/o	clot
thym/o	thymus gland
thyr/o, thyroid/o	thyroid gland
tibi/o	shin bone
toc/o	childbirth
tonsill/o	tonsil
top/o	place
tox/o, toxic/o	poison
trache/o	trachea
trich/o	hair
tympan/o	eardrum
uln/o	ulna (lower arm bone)
ungu/o	nail
ur/o	urine
ureter/o	ureter
urethr/o	urethra
urin/o	urine
uter/o	uterus
uve/o	uvea
uvul/o	uvula
vagin/o	vagina
valv/o, valvul/o	valve
vas/o, vascul/o	vessel
ven/o	vein
ventricul/o	ventricle
vertebr/o	vertebra
vesic/o	bladder
vesicul/o	seminal vesicles
vitre/o	glass/glassy
vulv/o	vulva
xanth/o	yellow
xer/o	dry

Prefixes

a-	not
an-	not
ante-	before
audi-	hearing
bi-	two
brady-	slow
de-	lack of
dys-	difficult, painful
ecto-	outside
endo-	in
epi-	on/upon
eso-	inward
eu-	good/normal
exo-	outward
extra-	outside
hemi-	half
hyper-	excess, over
hypo-	under
in-	into
inter-	between
intra-	within
meta-	change, after
multi-	many
neo-	new
nulli-, nulti-	none
oxy-	sharp, oxygen
pan-	all
para-	beside

per-	through
peri-	surrounding
poly-	many
post-	after
primi-	first
pseudo-	false
quadri-	four
retro-	behind
sub-	under
supra-	above
sym-	together
syn-	together
tachy-	fast
tetra-	four
tri-	three
tropin-	act upon
uni-	one

Suffixes

-agon	assemble
-algesia	pain sensation
-algia	pain
-ar	pertaining to
-arche	beginning
-ary	pertaining to
-asthenia	weakness
-blast	embryonic
-capnia	carbon dioxide
-cele	hernia
-centesis	puncture to remove (drain)
-chezia	defecation
-clast, -clasia, -clasis	break
-coccus	spherical bacterium
-cyesis	pregnancy
-desis	fusion
-dilation	widening, expanding
-drome	run
-dynia	pain
-eal	pertaining to
-ectasis	stretching
-ectomy	removal
-edema	swelling
-emia	blood
-esthesis	feeling
-gram	record
-graph	recording instrument
-graphy	recording process

-gravida	pregnancy
-ia	condition
-iatrist	physician specialist
-iatry	medical treatment
-ical	pertaining to
-ictal	pertaining to
-in	a substance
-ine	a substance
-itis	inflammation
-listhesis	slipping
-lithiasis	condition of stones
-lysis	separation
-malacia	softening
-megaly	enlargement
-meta	change
-meter	measurement; instrument that measures
-metry	measurement of
-oid	resembling
-oma	tumor
-omia	smell
-one	hormone
-opia	vision
-opsy	view of
-orrhexis	rupture
-osis	condition
-oxia	oxygen
-para	woman who has given birth
-paresis	incomplete paralysis
-parous	to bear
-penia	deficient
-pexy	fixation
-phagia	eating
-phonia	sound
-phylaxis	protection
-physis	to grow
-plasty	repair
-plegia	paralysis

-pnea	breathing
-poiesis	production
-poly	many
-porosis	passage
-retro	behind
-rrhagia	bursting of blood
-rrhaphy	suture
-rrhea	discharge
-schisis	split
-sclerosis	hardening
-scopy	to examine
-spasm	contraction of muscle
-steat/o	fat
-stenosis	blockage, narrowing
-stomy	opening
-thorax	chest
-tocia	labor
-tom/o	to cut
-tome	an instrument that cuts
-tomy	cutting, incision
-tripsy	crush
-tropia	to turn
-tropin	act upon
-uria	urine
-version	turning

Abbreviations

ABG	arterial blood gas
ABN	Advanced Beneficiary Notice; used by CMS to notify beneficiary of payment of provider services
ACL	anterior cruciate ligament
AD	right ear
AFB	acid-fast bacillus
AFI	amniotic fluid index
AGA	appropriate for gestational age
AGCUS	atypical glandular cells of undetermined significance
AKA	above-knee amputation
ANS	autonomic nervous system
APCs	Ambulatory Payment Classifications, patient classification that provides a payment system for outpatients
ARDS	adult respiratory distress syndrome
ARF	acute renal failure
ARM	artificial rupture of membrane
AS	left ear
ASCUS	atypical squamous cells of undetermined significance
ASCVD	arteriosclerotic cardiovascular disease
ASD	atrial septal defect
ASHD	arteriosclerotic heart disease
AU	both ears
AV	atrioventricular
BCC	benign cellular changes
BiPAP	bi-level positive airway pressure
BKA	below-knee amputation
BP	blood pressure
BPD	biparietal diameter

BPH	benign prostatic hypertrophy
BPP	biophysical profile
BUN	blood urea nitrogen
BV	bacterial vaginosis
bx	biopsy
C1-C7	cervical vertebrae
ca	cancer
CABG	coronary artery bypass graft
CBC	complete blood (cell) count
CF	conversion factor, national dollar amount that is applied to all services paid on the Medicare Fee Schedule basis
CHF	congestive heart failure
CHL	crown-to-heel length
CK	creatine kinase
CMS	Centers for Medicare and Medicaid Services, formerly HCFA, Health Care Financing Administration
CNM	certified nurse midwife
CNS	central nervous system
COB	coordination of benefits, management of payment between two or more third-party payers for a service
COPD	chronic obstructive pulmonary disease
CPAP	continuous positive airway pressure
CPD	cephalopelvic disproportion
CPK	creatine phosphokinase
CPP	chronic pelvic pain
CSF	cerebrospinal fluid
CTS	carpal tunnel syndrome
CVA	cerebrovascular accident, stroke
CVI	cerebrovascular insufficiency
D&C	dilation and curettage
D&E	dilation and evacuation
derm	dermatology
DHHS	Department of Health and Human Services
DLCO	diffuse capacity of lungs for carbon monoxide
DRGs	Diagnosis Related Groups, disease classification system that relates the types of inpatients a hospital treats (case mix) to the costs incurred by the hospital
DSE	dobutamine stress echocardiography

DUB	dysfunctional uterine bleeding
ECC	endocervical curettage
EDC	estimated date of confinement
EDD	estimated date of delivery
EDI	electronic data interchange, exchange of data between multiple computer terminals
EEG	electroencephalogram
EFM	electronic fetal monitoring
EFW	estimated fetal weight
EGA	estimated gestational age
EGD	esophagogastroduodenoscopy
EGJ	esophagogastric junction
EMC	endometrial curettage
EOB	explanation of benefits, remittance advice
EPO	Exclusive Provider Organization, similar to a Health Maintenance Organization except that the providers of the services are not prepaid, but rather are paid on a fee-for-service basis
EPSDT	Early and Periodic Screening, Diagnosis, and Treatment
ERCP	endoscopic retrograde cholangiopancreatography
ERT	estrogen replacement therapy
ESRD	end-stage renal disease
FAS	fetal alcohol syndrome
FEF	forced expiratory flow
FEV_1	forced expiratory volume in 1 second
$FEV_1:FVC$	maximum amount of forced expiratory volume in 1 second
FHR	fetal heart rate
FI	fiscal intermediary, financial agent acting on behalf of a third-party payer
FRC	functional residual capacity
FSH	follicle-stimulating hormone
FVC	forced vital capacity
fx	fracture
GERD	gastroesophageal reflux disease
GI	gastrointestinal
H or E	hemorrhage or exudate
HCFA	Health Care Financing Administration, now known as Centers for Medicare and Medicaid Services (CMS)
HCVD	hypertensive cardiovascular disease
HD	hemodialysis

HDL	high-density lipoprotein
HEA	hemorrhage, exudate, aneurysm
HHN	hand-held nebulizer
HJR	hepatojugular reflux
H&P	history and physical (examination)
HPV	human papillomavirus
HSG	hysterosalpingogram
HSV	herpes simplex virus
I&D	incision and drainage
IO	intraocular
IOL	intraocular lens
IPAP	inspiratory positive airway pressure
IRDS	infant respiratory distress syndrome
IVF	in vitro fertilization
IVP	intravenous pyelogram
JBP	jugular blood pressure
KUB	kidneys, ureter, bladder
L1-L5	lumbar vertebrae
LBBB	left bundle branch block
LEEP	loop electrosurgical excision procedure
LGA	large for gestational age
LLQ	left lower quadrant
LP	lumbar puncture
LUQ	left upper quadrant
LVH	left ventricular hypertrophy
MAT	multifocal atrial tachycardia
MDI	metered dose inhaler
MI	myocardial infarction
MRI	magnetic resonance imaging
MSLT	multiple sleep latency testing
MVV	maximum voluntary ventilation
NCPAP	nasal continuous positive airway pressure
NSR	normal sinus rhythm
OA	osteoarthritis
OD	right eye
OS	left eye
OU	each eye

PAC	premature atrial contraction
PAT	paroxysmal atrial tachycardia
PAWP	pulmonary artery wedge pressure
PCWP	pulmonary capillary wedge pressure
PEAP	positive end-airway pressure
PEEP	positive end-expiratory pressure
PEG	percutaneous endoscopic gastrostomy
PERL	pupils equal and reactive to light
PERRL	pupils equal, round, and reactive to light
PERRLA	pupils equal, round, and reactive to light and accommodation
PFT	pulmonary function test
pH	symbol for acid/base level
PICC	peripherally inserted central catheter
PID	pelvic inflammatory disease
PND	paroxysmal nocturnal dyspnea
PNS	peripheral nervous system
PROM	premature rupture of membranes
PSA	prostate-specific antigen
PST	paroxysmal supraventricular tachycardia
PSVT	paroxysmal supraventricular tachycardia
PT	prothrombin time
PTCA	percutaneous transluminal coronary angioplasty
PTT	partial thromboplastin time
PVC	premature ventricular contraction
RA	remittance advice, explanation of services
RA	rheumatoid arthritis
RBBB	right bundle branch block
RDS	respiratory distress syndrome
REM	rapid eye movement
RLQ	right lower quadrant
RSR	regular sinus rhythm
RUQ	right upper quadrant
RV	respiratory volume
RVG	*Relative Value Guide*
RVH	right ventricular hypertrophy
RVS	relative value studies, list of procedures with unit values assigned to each

RV:TLC	ratio of respiratory volume to total lung capacity
SHG	sonohysterogram
sp gr	specific gravity
SROM	spontaneous rupture of membranes
subcu, subq, SC, SQ	subcutaneous
SUI	stress urinary incontinence
SVT	supraventricular tachycardia
T1-T12	thoracic vertebrae
TAH	total abdominal hysterectomy
TEE	transesophageal echocardiography
TENS	transcutaneous electrical nerve stimulation
TIA	transient ischemic attack
TLC	total lung capacity
TLV	total lung volume
TM	tympanic membrane
TMJ	temporomandibular joint
TPA	tissue plasminogen activator
TSH	thyroid-stimulating hormone
TST	treadmill stress test
TURBT	transurethral resection of bladder tumor
TURP	transurethral resection of prostate
UA	urinalysis
UCR	usual, customary, and reasonable—third-party payers' assessment of the reimbursement for health care services: usual, that which would ordinarily be charged for the service; customary, the cost of that service in that locale; and reasonable, as assessed by the payer
UPJ	ureteropelvic junction
URI	upper respiratory infection
UTI	urinary tract infection
V/Q	ventilation/perfusion scan
VBAC	vaginal birth after cesarean
WBC	white blood (cell) count

Further Text Resources

ANATOMY AND PHYSIOLOGY

Book Title	Authors	Imprint	Copyright Date	ISBN-13
The Anatomy and Physiology Learning System, 4th Edition	Applegate	Saunders	2011	978-1-4377-0393-1
Gray's Anatomy for Students, 2nd Edition	Drake, Vogl, Mitchell	Churchill Livingstone	2010	978-0-443-06952-9
Anthony's Textbook of Anatomy and Physiology, 20th Edition	Thibodeau, Patton	Mosby	2012	978-0-323-09600-3

CODING

Book Title	Authors	Imprint	Copyright Date	ISBN-13
Step-by-Step Medical Coding, 2014 Edition	Buck	Saunders	2014	978-1-4557-4635-4
2014 ICD-10-CM Draft Standard Edition	Buck	Saunders	2014	978-1-4457-2290-7
2014 ICD-10-PCS Draft Standard Edition	Buck	Saunders	2014	978-1-4457-2289-1
ICD-10-CM Online Training Modules	Buck	Saunders		978-1-4457-4384-1
ICD-10-PCS Online Training Modules	Buck	Saunders		978-1-4457-4603-3
2014 ICD-9-CM, Volumes 1 & 2 (Professional Edition)	Buck	Saunders	2014	978-0-323-18676-2
2014 ICD-9-CM, Volumes 1, 2, & 3 (Professional Edition)	Buck	Saunders	2014	978-0-323-18674-2
2014 HCPCS Level II (Professional Edition)	Buck	Saunders	2014	978-1-4557-7504-0
The Next Step, Advanced Medical Coding and Auditing, 2014 Edition	Buck	Saunders	2014	978-1-4557-5897-5
Facility Coding Exam Review 2014: The Certification Step with ICD-10-CM/PCS	Buck	Saunders	2014	978-1-4557-4574-6

Book Title	Authors	Imprint	Copyright Date	ISBN-13
Online Internship for Medical Coding, 2014 Edition	Buck	Saunders	2014	978-0-3232-3937-0
ICD-9-CM Coding: Theory and Practice with ICD-10-CM, 2013/2014 Edition	Lovaasen, Schwerdtfeger	Saunders	2013	978-1-4557-0701-0
ICD-10-CM/PCS Coding Theory and Practice, 2014 Edition	Lovaasen, Schwerdtfeger	Saunders	2014	978-1-4557-7260-5

PATHOPHYSIOLOGY

Book Title	Authors	Imprint	Copyright Date	ISBN-13
Pathology for the Health Professions, 4th Edition	Damjanov	Saunders	2012	978-1-4377-1676-4
Essentials of Human Diseases and Conditions, 5th Edition	Frazier, Drzymkowski	Saunders	2013	978-1-4377-2408-0
Pathophysiology for the Health Professions, 4th Edition	Gould	Saunders	2011	978-1-4377-0965-0
The Human Body in Health and Illness, 4th Edition	Herlihy	Saunders	2011	978-1-4160-6842-6
The Human Body in Health and Disease, 6th Edition	Thibodeau, Patton	Mosby	2014	978-0-323-10124-1

MEDICAL TERMINOLOGY

Book Title	Authors	Imprint	Copyright Date	ISBN-13
The Language of Medicine, 10th Edition	Chabner	Saunders	2014	978-1-455-2846-6
Jablonski's Dictionary of Medical Acronyms & Abbreviations, 6th Edition	Jablonski	Saunders	2008	978-1-4160-5899-1
Exploring Medical Language, 8th Edition	LaFleur, Brooks	Mosby	2012	978-0-323-07308-0
Building a Medical Vocabulary (with Spanish Translations), 8th Edition	Leonard	Saunders	2012	978-1-4377-2784-5
Quick & Easy Medical Terminology, 7th Edition	Leonard	Saunders	2014	978-1-4557-4070-3
Mastering Healthcare Terminology, 4th Edition	Shiland	Mosby	2013	978-0-323-08032-3
Dorland's Illustrated Medical Dictionary, 32nd Edition		Saunders	2011	978-1-4160-6257-8

INTRODUCTION TO COMPUTERS

Book Title	Author	Imprint	Copyright Date	ISBN-13
Computerized Medical Office Procedures: A Worktext, 3rd Edition	Larsen	Saunders	2011	978-1-4377-1608-5

BASICS OF WRITING/MEDICAL TRANSCRIPTION

Book Title	Authors	Imprint	Copyright Date	ISBN-13
Medical Transcription Guide: Do's and Don'ts, 3rd Edition	Diehl	Saunders	2005	978-0-7216-0684-2
Medical Transcription: Techniques and Procedures, 7th Edition	Diehl	Saunders	2012	978-1-4377-0439-6

COMPREHENSION BUILDING/STUDY SKILLS

Book Title	Author	Imprint	Copyright Date	ISBN-13
Career Development for Health Professionals: Success in School and on the Job, 3rd Edition	Haroun	Saunders	2010	978-1-4377-0673-4

BASIC MATH

Book Title	Authors	Imprint	Copyright Date	ISBN-13
Using Maths in Health Sciences	Gunn	Churchill Livingstone	2001	978-0-443-07074-7

MEDICAL BILLING/INSURANCE

Book Title	Authors	Imprint	Copyright Date	ISBN-13
Health Insurance Today: A Practical Approach, 4th Edition	Beik	Saunders	2013	978-1-4557-0819-2
Medical Insurance Made Easy: Understanding the Claim Cycle, 2nd Edition	Brown	Saunders	2006	978-0-7216-0556-2
Insurance Handbook for the Medical Office, 12th Edition	Fordney	Saunders	2012	978-1-4377-2256-7
Electronic Health Record "Booster" Kit for the Medical Office, 2nd Edition	Buck	Saunders	2012	978-1-4557-2301-0
Practice Kit for Medical Front Office Skills, 3rd Edition	Buck	Saunders	2011	978-1-4377-2201-7
ePractice Kit for Medical Front Office Skills with MedTrack Systems	Buck	Saunders	2012	978-1-4377-2722-7

Practice Exercises Answers and Rationales

Practice Exercise 3-1

Professional Service: 99232 (Evaluation and Management, Hospital)
ICD-9-CM: 584.9 (Failure, renal, acute), **403.90** (Hypertension, kidney, with chronic kidney disease, unspecified), **585.9** (Failure, renal, chronic), **276.50** (Depletion, volume), **443.9** (Disease, peripheral, vascular)

Rationale: The service in this an inpatient progress note is reported with 99232 because it describes an expanded problem focused history and examination. The patient has two stable chronic conditions (hypertension and peripheral vascular disease) and acute on chronic renal failure that is improving; therefore, the medical decision making is of moderate complexity.

The patient has acute renal failure (584.9) and chronic renal failure (585.9), but according to ICD-9-CM Section I.C.7.a.3. of the *Official Guidelines for Coding and Reporting,* the coder is to assign a code from the 403 category to report hypertensive kidney disease, when a hypertensive patient has a condition that is classifiable to 585. You are to assume a cause-and-effect relationship and classify the chronic renal failure with hypertension as hypertensive renal disease (403.90 and 585.9). The acute renal failure category 584 is not included in the Guideline to assume as cause-and-effect relationship. The acute renal failure would be reported because when you reference the Excludes note following 403.9, the coder is directed to assign 584.9 for acute renal failure. Note that according to ICD-9-CM Section I.B.10 of the Guidelines, when there is both an acute and chronic condition present, the acute condition is reported first.

The patient also has volume depletion (276.50), which is reported because the condition contributes to the patient's renal status. The peripheral vascular disease (443.9) is reported because it was important enough for the physician to mention it in the impression section of the report.

Practice Exercise 3-2

Professional Service: 99214 (Evaluation and Management, Office and Other Outpatient)
ICD-9-CM: 008.8 (Gastroenteritis, viral NEC)

Rationale: Code 99214 reports an office visit for an established patient. The note is titled as a follow-up clinic visit. The patient is established with this provider. The history is expanded problem focused and the examination is detailed. The medical decision making is moderate because there are possibly two new problems—gastroenteritis and possible otitis media. Prescription drugs were given—making this a moderate medical decision making. Only two components of history, exam, and medical decision making are required for an established visit.

The diagnosis is viral gastroenteritis reported with 008.8, and because the otitis media was stated as possible, that diagnosis would not be reported.

Practice Exercise 3-3
Professional Service: 99284 (Emergency Department Services)
ICD-9-CM: 787.01 (Vomiting, with nausea), **276.51** (Dehydration), **150.9** (Neoplasm, esophagus, Malignant, Primary), **198.5** (Neoplasm, bones, Malignant, Secondary), **197.8** (Neoplasm, stomach, Malignant, Secondary)

Rationale: This was a level 4 emergency department service and included a detailed history, comprehensive examination, and moderate decision making level of complexity.

The first-listed diagnosis is the primary reason the patient presented to the emergency department—vomiting and nausea, reported with 787.01. The dehydration was noted in the assessment and was treated and would be reported with 276.51. The underlying condition that is causing these symptoms is the primary malignant neoplasm of the esophagus and is reported with 150.9. She has severe pain due to the metastases being treated with morphine. Assign the codes for these conditions because they were treated. Metastases included bones (198.5) and stomach (197.8).

Practice Exercise 3-4
Professional Service: 99391 (Preventive Medicine, Established Patient)
ICD-9-CM: V20.32 (Checkup, newborn, routine, 8 to 28 days old)

Rationale: This is a routine checkup for an established infant and is considered preventive medicine. When choosing a code from this category, the age of the infant or child and whether the patient is new or established determines the code choice. Code 99391 is assigned for a newborn until 1 year of age. The diagnosis is a routine health check reported with V20.32.

Practice Exercise 3-5
Professional Service: 99469 (Critical Care Services, Neonatal, Subsequent)
ICD-9-CM: 765.17 (Preterm, infant NEC), **765.25** (Newborn, gestation, 29-30 completed weeks), **769** (Hyaline, membrane), **774.6** (Hyperbilirubinemia, neonatal), **747.0** (Patent ductus arteriosus or Botallo)

Rationale: When a critically ill newborn 30 days of age or less is either born or brought to the hospital and placed in the Neonatal Critical Care Unit, the initial care day is coded with 99468; each additional day is coded with 99469, as long as the baby is considered critically ill.

The diagnosis is preterm infant with a body weight of 1716 kg, reported with 765.17 and the fifth digit is determined by weight. (See fifth-digit subclassification preceding 764.) The code for the term weight is 765.1, with a fifth digit based on weight, in this case "7", for infants between 1750 and 1999 grams. The preterm gestation is reported with 765.25. The hyaline membrane is reported 769. Hyperbilirubinemia of the neonate is reported with code 774.6. This patient also has patent ductus arteriosus (747.0). There is mention of some type of pulmonary valve disorder which could be associated with Noonan syndrome; however, that has not been verified and we do not know what the pulmonary valve disorder is.

Practice Exercise 3-6
Professional Service: 00840-QK-P2 (Anesthesia, Abdomen, Intraperitoneal), **99100** (Anesthesia, Special Circumstances, Extreme Age)

Rationale: The surgical procedure is an abdominal procedure in which the anesthesia is reported with 00840. HCPCS modifier -QK indicates the anesthesiologist was medically directing two to four concurrent cases. 99100 is added to indicate age over 70, which is a qualifying circumstance that may impact the anesthesia service. -P2 indicates a patient with a mild systemic disease (hypertension).

Practice Exercise 3-7
Professional Service: 00400-AA-QS-P1 (Anesthesia, Integumentary System, Anterior Trunk)

Rationale: The service is an anesthesia service for a procedure to the breast reported with 00400. -AA indicates that the anesthesiologist personally performed the anesthesia service. -P1 indicates a normal healthy patient. This was a monitored anesthesia case (MAC) as noted by modifier -QS.

Practice Exercise 3-8
Professional Service: 00790-QK-P2 (Anesthesia, Abdomen, Intraperitoneal)

Rationale: The service is an abdominal anesthesia service for a procedure of the upper abdomen, reported with 00790. Modifier -QK is added to indicate the anesthesiologist was supervising more than one procedure at the same time. -P2 indicates a patient with a mild systemic disease.

Practice Exercise 3-9
Professional Service: 00902-AA-P3 (Anesthesia, Anus)

Rationale: The service is anesthesia for a procedure of the anus in which a spinal was administered and reported with 00902. -AA indicates that the anesthesiologist personally performed the anesthesia service.

Practice Exercise 3-10
Professional Service: 00211-AA-P5 (Anesthesia, Brain)

Rationale: The service was anesthesia for an intercranial hematoma reported with 00211. -AA indicates that the anesthesiologist personally performed the anesthesia service. -P5 indicates that the patient is not expected to survive without this procedure.

Practice Exercise 3-11
Professional Service: 49060-78-52 (Drainage, Abscess, Retroperitoneal), **11005-78-51** (Debridement, Skin, Subcutaneous Tissue, Infected)
ICD-9-CM: 998.59 (Infection, postoperative wound), **567.82** (Necrosis, fat, fatty [generalized], abdominal wall) or (Necrosis, peritoneum), **709.8** (Necrosis, skin or subcutaneous tissue), **569.81** (Fistula, abdominal [wall])

Rationale: The primary procedure was drainage of an abdominal abscess reported with 49060. Modifier -78 is added to indicate an unplanned return to the operating room. Modifier -52 (reduced services) is added to indicate that the abdomen was already open and it was packed and left open. This patient had debridement (11005) of an abdominal wound, which was necrotic. Modifier -51 is added to 11005 to indicate multiple procedures were performed. Modifier -78 is also added.

This is a life-threatening condition that required extensive debridement of the skin, fat, and the area behind the abdominal contents. The diagnoses codes are: 998.59 reports the postoperative wound infection, 567.82 reports fat necrosis of abdominal wall, 709.8 reports the necrosis of the skin, and 569.81 reports the fistula of the abdominal wall between the abdominal cavity and the retroperitoneal area.

Practice Exercise 3-12
Professional Service: 11404-58 (Excision, Skin, Lesion, Benign)
ICD-9-CM: 216.6 (Neoplasm, skin, arm, Benign)

Rationale: The procedure was re-excision of a benign lesion that measured 1 cm in diameter; the original procedure had 0.5-cm margins. This left a 2-cm incision that the surgeon now re-excised with a 1-cm margin. The total measurement for the re-excision is 4 cm. Modifier -58 is added to indicate that the patient was returned to the operating room during the postoperative period of the first procedure in part two of a two-part procedure.

The pathology report states fibrosis and granulation tissue, and there was no evidence of the Spitz nevus. In cases such as this, when there is excision of additional skin margins, it is acceptable to report the original diagnosis, which in this case is the Spitz nevus, a benign lesion, and reported with 216.6.

Practice Exercise 3-13
Professional Service: 93306-26 (Echocardiography, Cardiac, Transthoracic)
ICD-9-CM: 397.0 (Insufficiency, tricuspid), **427.31** (Fibrillation, atrial), **429.9** (Dysfunction, ventricular)

Rationale: This patient had an echocardiogram and the key to correctly reporting an echocardiogram is to identify whether it was performed transthoracic or transesophageal, and if it was a complete study or follow-up/limited study. The service in this case was a two-dimensional with M-mode recording complete echo—93306 for the real-time image and documentation. Code 93306 includes spectral and color flow Doppler; therefore, 93320 and 93325 are not reported separately. You would add modifier -26 because you are reporting only the physician portion of the procedure.

The patient has valvular disease, and the report indicates the specific type of valvular disease. In this case, tricuspid insufficiency (397.0), atrial fibrillation (427.31), and ventricular dysfunction (429.9).

Practice Exercise 3-14
Professional Service: 99214-24 (Evaluation and Management, Office and Other Outpatient)
ICD-9-CM: 654.63 (Abnormal, cervix, in pregnancy or childbirth), **V13.21** (History (personal) of, obstetric disorder, pre-term labor)

Rationale: This is an office visit service in which a decision was made to proceed with surgery. Modifier -57 is not assigned as the global period for 59320 (Cerclage, Cervix, Vaginal) has a 0-day global period. Use modifier -24 to indicate that this service is totally separate from the obstetric global package for a complication of the pregnancy. The examination includes a detailed history and examination, together with medical decision making complexity of a moderate level, reported with 99214.

The diagnosis is incompetent cervix, which is an abnormal cervix with a tendency to dilate prematurely in one who is pregnant, reported with 654.63. The history of pre-term labor was a factor in the decision to proceed, code V13.21 is also reported.

Practice Exercise 3-15
Professional Service: 30520 (Septoplasty), **31267-51-50** (Antrostomy, Sinus, Maxillary), **31288-51-50** (Sphenoidotomy, Excision with Nasal/Sinus Endoscopy), **31255-51-50** (Ethmoidectomy, Endoscopic), **30930-51-50** (Turbinate, Fracture, Therapeutic)
ICD-9-CM: 470 (Deviation, septum), **471.9** (Polyp, nasal), **471.8** (Polyp, sinus [accessory]), **473.8** (Pansinusitis), **478.0** (Hypertrophy, turbinate)

Rationale: The services are listed in the Procedures Performed section of the report and are supported within the body of the report as: (1) bilateral endoscopic total ethmoidectomy, 31255-51-50; (2) bilateral endoscopic maxillary antrostomy with removal of polyps from maxillary sinus, 31267-51-50; (3) bilateral endoscopic sphenoidotomy, 31288-51-50; (4) septoplasty, 30520; and (5) bilateral inferior turbinate outfracture, 30930-51-50. Note that all procedures except the primary procedure, septoplasty, have modifier -50 to indicate bilateral procedures and modifier -51 to indicate multiple procedures.

The diagnoses are listed in the Postoperative Diagnosis section of the report as: (1) septal deviation, 470; (2) bilateral sinonasal polyposis, 471.9 (nasal) and (3) 471.8 (sinus); (4) pansinusitis, 473.8, (5) bilateral inferior turbinate hypertrophy, 478.0; and nasal obstruction. The nasal obstruction is not reported because it is caused by the septal deviation.

Practice Exercise 3-16
Professional Service: 11312 (Lesion, Skin, Shaving)
ICD-9-CM: 216.3 (Neoplasm, skin, cheek [external], Benign)

Rationale: The procedure is a shave excision of a lesion on the cheek that measures 1.6 cm. When reporting lesion removal, first identify the technique used. Shaving involves transverse incision or horizontal slicing and does not involve a full-thickness (through the dermis) excision. The excision codes involve full-thickness excision and generally require suture closure. Also identify the body area on which the lesion is located, the size of the lesion, and whether the lesion is benign or malignant. Note that in the case of shavings, the nature (benign or malignant) does not influence the selection of the CPT code.

In this case, the lesion shaved was benign, as indicated by the pathology report and reported with 216.3.

Practice Exercise 3-17
Professional Service: 19120-RT (Breast, Excision, Lesion)
ICD-9-CM: 174.0 (Neoplasm, breast, nipple, Malignant, Primary)

Rationale: This patient presents for excision of a tumor of the right breast (19120-RT). The tumor is submitted for frozen section, which is an analysis performed by the pathologist during the procedure (intraoperatively). The results of the frozen section were carcinoma of the right breast nipple (174.0).

Practice Exercise 3-18
Professional Service: 15574-F7 (Pedicle Flap, Formation), **15120-51** (Split, Grafts)
ICD-9-CM: 886.0 (Amputation, finger), **E919.9** (Index to External Causes, Accident, caused by, machinery)

Rationale: While working on machinery, this patient amputated the tip of her middle finger. A flap was formed from the ulnar aspect of the hand to place over the defect of the right middle finger (15574-F7). Modifier -F7 indicates the middle finger of the right hand. The split-thickness graft is reported with 15120 with modifier -51.

The diagnosis is traumatic amputation of the finger reported with 886.0. The external cause code /E919.9 is reported to indicate the injury was sustained while working on machinery.

Practice Exercise 3-19
Professional Service: 12002-F7 (Closure)
ICD-9-CM: 883.0 (Wound, open, finger), **E920.8** (Index to External Causes, Cut, by, arrow)

Rationale: The patient presents with multiple lacerations of the finger that total 6 cm for which simple repair is performed (12002). Modifier -F7 is added to indicate the middle right finger.

Code 883.0 reports a laceration of the right finger. An external cause code (E920.8) is reported to indicate how the finger was injured (due to arrow).

Practice Exercise 3-20
Professional Service: 11005-58 (Debridement, Skin, Subcutaneous Tissue, Infected)
ICD-9-CM: 567.82 (Necrosis, fat, abdominal wall), **709.8** (Necrosis, skin or subcutaneous tissue), **998.6** (Fistula, postoperative, persistent)

Rationale: The patient returns to the operating room for additional debridement of the abdominal wound (11005). Modifier -58 indicates returning to the operating room for a related procedure by the same physician during the postoperative period.

The diagnoses are necrosis of the abdominal wall fat (567.82), necrosis of the skin/subcutaneous tissue (709.8), and postoperative fistula (998.6).

Practice Exercise 3-21
Professional Service: 29898-RT (Arthroscopy, Surgical, Ankle)
ICD-9-CM: 715.97 (Osteoarthritis), **726.91** (Exostosis, ankle), **729.90** (Disorder, soft tissue)

Rationale: The service is an arthroplasty of the right ankle by means of a scope, not an open surgical procedure as would be reported with 27700-27703. The arthroscopic procedures are located in the Endoscopy/Arthroscopy category of codes (29800-29999). When locating the service in the index of the CPT, the main term *Arthroplasty* directs the coder to the incisional procedures. The main term *Arthroscopy* directs the coder to the correct surgical and diagnostic arthroscopic procedure codes. Codes 29894-29898 are the correct range, and the code to report the services in this case is 29898, with modifier -RT to indicate right.

The first diagnosis in the Postoperative Diagnoses section of the report is osteoarthritic change of the ankle. When referencing "Osteoarthritis" the coder is directed to the Tabular of ICD-9-CM to review 715.9, with a fifth digit added to indicate the location of the condition. In this case, the location is the ankle represented by the fifth digit "7."

The second postoperative diagnosis is osteophytic spurring. When referring "Osteophyte" in the Index of the ICD-9-CM, the coder is directed to "*see* Exostosis," which is a benign bony growth that projects from the bone, commonly referred to as a spur. The "*see* Exostosis" entry directs the coder to 726.91, exostosis of unspecified site, the correct code for this condition.

The third postoperative diagnosis is impinging soft tissue, but when referencing the Index of the ICD-9-CM, the only entry under impingement is of the soft tissue between the teeth. With no more specific entry, the coder would reference a general term, such as "Disorder, soft tissue." In ICD-9-CM referencing "Disorder, soft tissue" leads to 729.90

Practice Exercise 3-22
Professional Service: 20610-LT (Injection, Joint)
ICD-9-CM: 726.19 (Bursitis, subacromial)

Rationale: This is an injection into the shoulder, which is considered a major joint. The main code 20600 states arthrocentesis, aspiration, and/or injection small joint. This was an injection, so the area is correct, but the small joints are listed in parentheses after 20600 as fingers and toes. The indented codes that follow 20600 indicate shoulder, as included in 20610.

The patient has bursitis, and this is the main heading to reference in the ICD-9 index. There is a subacromial type of bursitis listed as a subterm, and the coder is directed to 726.19. When verifying in the Tabular, the description becomes "other specified disorders" of the shoulder, rather than "bursitis."

Practice Exercise 3-23
Professional Service: 25210-LT (Carpal Bone, Excision), **25310-51-LT** (Tendon, Transfer, Wrist)
ICD-9-CM: 715.94 (Osteoarthrosis, hand)

Rationale: This is an arthroplasty of the patient's carpometacarpal joint. The trapezium, one of the carpal bones, was removed in pieces (25210). The flexor carpi radialis (FCR) tendon was transferred to the site and threaded through bone. This was harvested through two incisions at the distal wrist and in the forearm. The report states that the underlying FCR tendon was preserved and later it was cut at the floor of the thumb and transferred through the hole at the base of the first metatarsal and pinned to the second metatarsal (25310). The report is difficult to read because it appears that the "harvested" FCR is removed; however, it is just separated and the proximal end was left intact. Code 25447 involves the insertion of a prosthesis; therefore, it is not correct. Modifier -LT is appended to both procedures to indicate the procedure was performed on the left wrist. Modifier -51 indicates 25210 is a second procedure during the same session.

When referencing the index of the ICD-9-CM under the term *arthritis, degenerative,* the coder is directed to "*see* Osteoarthrosis." The term *degenerative* is included as a parenthetical word after the main term "*Osteoarthritis,*" directing the coder to 715.9. The code requires a fifth digit to indicate the location of the osteoarthritis. In this case, the location is the patient's hand, thus the correct code would be 715.94.

Practice Exercise 3-24
Professional Service: 27355-RT (Excision, Cyst, Femur)
ICD-9-CM: 213.7 (Neoplasm, bone, femur, Benign)

Rationale: This is an excision of a bone tumor of the femur. You would not use code 27328 because this code reports a procedure of the muscle of the thigh, and the tumor in this case was in the bone, reported with 27355, with -RT to indicate the right leg.

The diagnosis is a benign neoplasm (per the pathology report) of the long bone (213.7). The femur, or thigh bone, is the longest bone in the leg. It would not be correct to report 213.8 because this is for the short bones of the leg, such as the tibia or fibula.

Practice Exercise 3-25
Professional Service: 27327-LT (Excision, Tumor, Knee)
ICD-9-CM: 215.3 (Neoplasm, connective tissue, knee, Benign)

Rationale: This mass is in the subcutaneous tissue of the patient's knee, reported with 27327, with -LT added to indicate left side. You would not use code 27328 because this code is for deeper than subcutaneous.

The pathology report indicated a benign mass of the bursa, and when referencing "Neoplasm" in the Index of the ICD-9-CM, subterm *bursa,* the coder is directed to the subterm *connective tissue.* 215.3 reports a benign tumor of the connective tissue of the knee.

Practice Exercise 3-26
Professional Service: 36217-RT (Insertion, Catheter, Brachiocephalic Artery), **36216-59-LT** (Insertion, Catheter, Brachiocephalic Artery), **36215-59-LT** (Insertion, Catheter, Brachiocephalic Artery)
ICD-9-CM: 431 (Hemorrhage, intracerebral)

Rationale: You were given instructions to assign the codes for the catheterizations only. When reporting catheterizations of the carotid and peripheral arteries, carotids in this case, you need to know where the catheter tip is being placed. The arteries are listed by family and by order—the deeper the vessel, the higher the order. In this case, the third-order vessel is reported first (right internal carotid artery), the second-order vessel is reported second (left vertebral artery), and the first-order vessel (left common carotid artery) is reported last. Modifier -59 is added to 36215 and 36216 to indicate the catheterizations are in different families than 36217. Modifiers -RT and -LT indicate right or left vessels.

The procedure is being performed because the patient has an intracranial hemorrhage, reference Hemorrhage, intracerebral, 431.

Practice Exercise 3-27
Professional Service: 36580 (Vein, Catheterization, Replacement)
ICD-9-CM: V56.1 (Admission for dialysis, catheter, removal or replacement), **585.6** (Disease, renal, end stage)

Rationale: The service is a venous catheter replacement by means of a percutaneous approach reported with 36580.

In ICD-9-CM reference the Index for Admission for, dialysis, catheter, removal or replacement, extracorporeal, V56.1. The diagnosis is stated as end-stage renal failure and reported with 585.6.

Practice Exercise 3-28
Professional Service: 36558 (Insertion, Catheter, Venous), **77001-26** (Fluoroscopy, Venous Access Device), **99144, 99145** (Sedation, Moderate)
ICD-9-CM: 162.9 (Neoplasm, lung, Malignant, Primary)

Rationale: The service was the placement of a Port-a-Cath, which is a catheter that is inserted into a large central vein, such as the jugular in this case, with a pump attached to the other end of the catheter. The small pump (about the size of three silver dollars stacked) is a port or reservoir implanted under the skin.

The pump is used to infuse various substances by means of a reservoir. The substance is infused over time. In this case, the pump is being used for chemotherapy administration, and the insertion is reported with 36558. Codes 36555 and 36556 report temporary pump or port placement, 36557 and 36558 report a port or pump that is level with the skin by placing it under the skin. Codes 36560 and 36561 report ports or pumps that extend outside the skin and are not often used.

The physician fluoroscopic guidance service is reported with 77001. Modifier -26 is added to indicate that only the professional component of the service is being provided. Conscious sedation was provided as indicated in the report and was assigned code 99144 (30 minutes) and 99145 (15 minutes) because the patient was over age 5 and the sedation lasted 45 minutes.

The diagnosis is stated as primary lung cancer, reported with 162.9.

Practice Exercise 3-29
Professional Service: 36217-RT (Catheterization, Thoracic Artery), **36218-RT** (Catheterization, Thoracic Artery), **36215-51-LT** (Catheterization, Thoracic Artery)
ICD-9-CM: 433.30 (Occlusion, artery, carotid, with other precerebral artery, bilateral)

Rationale: 36200 (Insertion, Catheter, Aorta) is bundled into 36217-RT (Catheterization, Thoracic Artery), which reports the selective catheterization of the RT vertebral artery. 36218-RT (Catheterization, Thoracic Artery) reports the selective catheterization of the right common carotid artery, which is a second order; therefore, the add-on code is assigned for the additional second or third order in the same family.

36215-51-LT (Catheterization, Thoracic Artery) reports the selective catheterization of the left carotid artery. Modifier -51 is placed to indicate an additional procedure.

The Clinical Symptoms section of the report indicates carotid artery stenosis, and the Impression statement in the third item (30-40% diameter narrowing of the carotid bulb on right) and the fourth item (complete occlusion of the left internal carotid artery) supports stenosis of the carotid artery, reported with 433.30.

Practice Exercise 3-30
Professional Service: 36246-RT (Catheterization, Legs), **37211** (Transcatheter, Therapy, Infusion), **75710-59-26-RT** (Angiography, Leg Artery)
ICD-9-CM: 996.74 (Complications, due to [presence of] any device, implant or graft, arterial), **444.22** (Thrombosis, thrombotic, femoral)

Rationale: The service is a selective catheter placement of the arterial system of the second order for a diagnostic right extremity angiogram (36246-RT, 75710-59-26-RT), followed by catheter placement for infusion of tissue plasminogen activator (tPA). The catheters are placed in the common femoral through the Gore-Tex graft (36247) to below the knee. A coaxial system is one in which catheters are placed into the vessel on each side of the clot to release tPA to dissolve/lyse the clot. 36247 replaces 36246 as it is the highest order. The tPA is a thrombolytic drug used for arterial thrombotic occlusion. The infusion (37211) has a radiology component included. Modifier -59 is required on the diagnostic extremity angiogram to indicate that it was completely separate from the thrombolytic procedure. The patient returns in the morning so that the interventional radiologist can determine the extent to which the procedure was successful.

The reason for the service is a complication due to a Gore-Tex graft that is reported with 996.74. The patient has a complete occlusion of the peripheral artery of the lower extremity, reported with 444.22.

Practice Exercise 3-31
Professional Service: 43752 (Placement, Orogastric Tube)
ICD-9-CM: 536.3 (Paresis, stomach)

Rationale: The service is placement of an orogastric tube (43752), known as CORFLO placement. The tube is placed to ensure that the patient receives proper nutrition. The KUB (kidneys, ureter, bladder) would be reported separately by the radiologist.

The patient has gastroparesis (536.3).

Practice Exercise 3-32
Professional Service: 49440 (Gastrostomy Tube, Placement, Percutaneous, Nonendoscopic), **49446-51** (Gastrostomy Tube, Conversion to Gastro-jejunostomy Tube), **76942-26** (Ultrasound, Guidance, Needle or Catheter Placement)
ICD-9-CM: 263.9 (Malnutrition)

Rationale: This patient required placement of a feeding tube for nutritional support. Code 49440 is assigned to report the percutaneous placement of the feeding tube. The notes following 49440 state, "For conversion to a gastro-jejunostomy tube at the time of initial gastrostomy tube placement, use 49440 in conjunction with 49446," which is the second procedure. Modifier -51 is appended to the second procedure, 49446-51. Ultrasound guidance 76942-26 was used to locate the edge of the liver to assist with needle placement for the catheter. Modifier -26 is added to indicate that only the professional service was provided. The fluoroscopic guidance is included in codes 49440 and 49446 and is not reported separately.

This procedure was performed because the patient is malnourished, 263.9.

Practice Exercise 3-33
Professional Service: 49000-78 (Laparotomy, Exploration)
ICD-9-CM: 998.2 (Puncture, accidental, complicating surgery)

Rationale: This patient had a laparoscopy the day before this procedure. After discharge, the patient presents to the emergency department with abdominal pain and is taken to the operating room where she was found to have a large amount of urine in her peritoneal cavity. During her previous surgery the urinary bladder had been punctured. Report 49000 for the exploratory laparotomy because this is the portion of the service that Dr. Martinez performed. Add modifier -78 to indicate the return to the operating room for a related procedure during the postoperative period. The cystorrhaphy (51860) was performed by Dr. Smithson who dictated the note separately for the cystorrhaphy and intestinal adhesiolysis (44005).

The postoperative complication of the puncture of the urinary bladder is reported with 998.2.

Practice Exercise 3-34
Professional Service: 44640-22 (Repair, Intestines, Small, Fistula), **44120-51** (Excision, Intestines, Small)
ICD-9-CM: 569.81 (Fistula, intestine)

Rationale: A fistula is an abnormal communication between two epithelialized surfaces. An intestinal fistula is an abnormal anatomic connection between a part (or multiple parts) of the intestinal lumen and the lumen of another epithelialized structure or the skin. The goal of the procedure was to restore the continuity of the gastrointestinal tract and restore function to the other involved structures. There were multiple intestinal fistulas repaired and reported with 44640. The report stated that the procedure took significantly more time than would typically be required, which directs the assignment of modifier -22, increased procedural service.

The colon is the large intestine and the small bowel is the small intestine. The small intestine was resected and reported with 44120 with modifier -51 to indicate multiple procedures.

The diagnosis is 569.81 (fistula of the intestine).

Practice Exercise 3-35
Professional Service: 43117-62 (Esophagectomy, Partial), **47100** (Biopsy, Liver), **47000-59-52** (Biopsy, Liver), **44015** (Jejunostomy, Insertion, Catheter)
ICD-9-CM: 530.85 (Barrett's esophagus), **228.04** (Hemangioma, intra-abdominal structures)

Rationale: The report states that a wedge biopsy (47100) was performed on a liver mass on the right lobe of the liver. The pathology report was returned with a diagnosis of hemangioma, which is a benign neoplasm.

The report states that if the cancer has not spread to the liver, an esophagogastrectomy using the Ivor-Lewis technique (43117, partial esophagectomy) will be performed. Dr. White is a co-surgeon with Dr. Sanchez because Dr. White performed the mobilization of the stomach and the pyloroplasty for the abdominal portion of the procedure and closed the abdomen. Dr. Sanchez then performed a thoracotomy for the remainder of the procedure. Co-surgery refers to a single surgical procedure that requires the skill of two surgeons of different specialities to perform parts of the same procedure. It could be that the two surgeons perform different procedures, in which case it is not co-surgery. Co-surgery has been performed if the procedure performed is part of and would be reported using a single surgical code. Each surgeon dictates his part of the procedure and reports 43117-62. Modifier -62 is appended for co-surgeon and each surgeon will be paid 62.5 % of the procedure. Dr. White also performed the jejunostomy (44015). Code 44015 is an add-on code when the jejunostomy is performed during another procedure; therefore, modifier -51 is not reported.

Before the open biopsy, the physician attempted to perform a percutaneous biopsy of a lesion on the liver (47000), which was terminated after the start of the procedure because the patient was unable to hold his breath. Since the lesion was very close to the diaphragm, the surgeon elected to discontinue the procedure and take the patient to the operating room. An open wedge biopsy of the liver was performed and is reported with 47100, which is an add-on code when performed with another open procedure. Modifier -59 is required because 47000 is mutually exclusive of 47100. Since 47000 was performed earlier than the abdominal procedure, modifier -59 denotes that the percutaneous biopsy was performed at a different session than 47100. The surgeon elected to terminate the procedure; therefore, modifier -52 (reduced procedure) is also added to 47000-59-52. The liver biopsy was a staged procedure in that a frozen section was performed to rule out metastasis to the liver. The frozen section showed hemangioma. Had the FS showed metastasis, the procedure would have been cancelled.

Code 530.85 is reported for Barrett's syndrome, as is stated in the Postoperative Diagnosis section of the report. There is no ICD-9-CM code for severe esophageal dysplasia as it is included in Barrett's syndrome 530.85. Code 228.04 (Hemangioma, intra-abdominal structures) is reported for the liver biopsy because this is indicated in the pathology report. You would not report 150.9 (Malignant neoplasm of the esophagus) because it states possible malignancy and you cannot report possible or rule-out conditions.

Practice Exercise 3-36
Professional Service: 50280-RT (Excision, Cyst, Kidney)
ICD-9-CM: 593.2 (Cyst, kidney, acquired)

Rationale: The procedure was the excision of a cyst on the right kidney, which is reported with 50280. Modifier -RT is added to indicate that the procedure was on the right side.

The diagnosis is stated in the Postoperative Diagnosis section of the report as renal cyst, reported with 593.2.

Practice Exercise 3-37
Professional Service: 50541-RT (Kidney, Cyst, Ablation)
ICD-9-CM: 593.2 (Cyst, kidney, acquired)

Rationale: This service was a laparoscopic cyst removal reported with 50541 with modifier -RT to indicate the right side. The biopsy is included in the ablation code and is not reported separately.

The diagnosis is cyst of the kidney (593.2) and is confirmed by the pathology report.

Practice Exercise 3-38
Professional Service: 58150 (Hysterectomy, Abdominal, Total)
ICD-9-CM: 626.2 (Menorrhagia), **218.9** (Leiomyoma, uterus)

Rationale: This patient had a total abdominal hysterectomy with bilateral removal of tubes and ovaries. The report indicates this was an open abdominal approach (58150).

Code 626.2 is assigned to report menorrhagia and is listed as the first diagnosis in the Preoperative Diagnoses section of the report. The leiomyomas are listed as the second diagnosis in the Preoperative Diagnoses section and are reported with 218.9. When referencing the Index of the ICD-9-CM under "Fibroid, uterus," the coder is directed to 218.9.

Practice Exercise 3-39
Professional Service: 59515 (Cesarean Delivery, Postpartum Care)
ICD-9-CM: 641.21 (Placenta, separation), **644.21** (Pregnancy, complicated by early onset of delivery [spontaneous]), **V27.0** (Outcome of delivery, single, liveborn)

Rationale: This patient presents for an emergency cesarean section in which the OB surgeon will then follow the patient postpartum (59515).

In ICD-9-CM, the service is due to the premature separation of the placenta (641.21); the fifth digit "1" indicates delivery. The onset of preterm labor complicating pregnancy is reported with 644.21. The Outcome of delivery is reported on the mother's record with V27.0 for single liveborn.

Practice Exercise 3-40
Professional Service: 56630-RT (Vulvectomy, Radical)
ICD-9-CM: 233.32 (Neoplasm, labia, majora, Malignant, Ca in situ)

Rationale: The vulvectomy, radical/partial is the excision of a portion of the labia, reported with 56630. We are not told the size of the lesion, only that it was located at the 11 o'clock position of the right labia majora and that a 1 cm margin was taken on all sides. Even a 1 cm margin on two sides would lead to an area of 2 cm (based on size of lesion and the narrowest margin x 2). A partial radical vulvectomy involves removal of less than 80% of the vulvar area and a radical procedure involves removal of the skin and deep subcutaneous tissue. The report does indicate that "running locked suture of 2–0 Vicryl was then placed in the deeper tissues." This is correctly coded with 56630. It would not be appropriate to use the excision of malignant lesions codes (11620-11626) and the intermediate repair codes (12041-12047) because deeper tissue was involved. Modifier -RT indicates the vulvectomy was performed on the right only.

The lesion, which was sent to pathology, was returned with a diagnosis of Neoplasia III, which is carcinoma in situ of the labia majora, reported with 233.32.

Practice Exercise 3-41
Professional Service: 61313-RT (Craniotomy, Surgery)
ICD-9-CM: 431 (Hematoma, brain, nontraumatic)

Rationale: This patient had a craniotomy for evacuation of an intracerebral hematoma (supratentorial), 61313. Modifier -RT indicates the surgery was performed on the right temporal lobe. If this procedure was performed infratentorial, it would be much more extensive, and the physician service would be reported with infratentorial codes.

The diagnosis is stated as a nontraumatic intracerebral hematoma of the right temporal lobe, reported with 431. In the ICD-9-CM Index reference Hematoma, brain, nontraumatic and you are referred to – *see also* Hemorrhage, brain. 431.

Practice Exercise 3-42
Professional Service: 61154-RT (Burr Hole, Skull, Drainage, Hematoma)
ICD-9-CM: 432.1 (Hematoma, subdural, nontraumatic)

Rationale: This patient had a nontraumatic subdural hematoma drained through burr holes, which were drilled into the frontal and posterior parietal areas of the right cranium (61154). Code 61154 represents evacuation and/or drainage of either a subdural (under the dura) or extradural (on top of the dura) hematoma. This was a unilateral procedure, so the modifier -RT is appended to indicate the right side.

The diagnosis is stated as a nontraumatic subacute subdural hematoma, reported with 432.1. The ICD-9-CM Index for Hemorrhage, subdural refers to - *see* Hemorrhage, intracranial, subarachnoid.

Practice Exercise 3-43
Professional Service: 64721-LT (Carpal Tunnel Syndrome, Decompression)
ICD-9-CM: 354.0 (Carpal tunnel syndrome)

Rationale: Carpal tunnel release is performed on this patient (64721), in which the physician decompresses the median nerve by freeing the nerve inside the carpal tunnel of the wrist. Modifier -LT indicates the procedure was performed on the left wrist.

The diagnosis is stated as carpal tunnel syndrome, reported with 354.0.

Practice Exercise 3-44
Professional Service: 63709-78 (Repair, Spinal Cord, Cerebrospinal Fluid Leak)
ICD-9-CM: 997.01 (Pseudomeningocele, postprocedural)

Rationale: A pseudomeningocele is an abnormal collection of cerebrospinal fluid (CSF) without a membrane (dura) surrounding it. A leak in the dura causes the CSF to build in the extradural space or the tissues. This leak was a complication of a previous procedure. The previous incision was reopened. Repair of pseudomeningocele is performed on this patient for whom the physician repairs an opening in the dura with a fat graft which was taken from the same area; therefore, it is included in the procedure. After the repair the surgeon noticed another leak and he performed a partial hemilaminectomy of L5 on the left and closed the leak. A hemilaminectomy involves removing lamina and part of the spinal process (63709). Code 63709 describes this procedure as it states repair of pseudomeningocele, with laminectomy. Had the surgeon stopped after the repair of the first leak, you would have reported 63707 for a repair of a pseudomeningocele without laminectomy. Modifier -78 indicates that the patient has returned to the operating room for a related procedure during the postoperative period.

The diagnosis is postprocedural spinal pseudomeningocele (997.01).

Practice Exercise 3-45
Professional Service: 63047 (Laminectomy, with Facetectomy), **63048 x 2** (Laminectomy, with Facetectomy)
ICD-9-CM: 724.02 (Stenosis, spinal, lumbar, lumbosacral), **738.4** (Spondylolisthesis, acquired)

Rationale: This patient had a bilateral laminectomy with foraminotomy for spinal stenosis that was indicated on a MRI. The first segment is reported with 63047; each additional segment is reported with 63048 (this code is submitted times the number of segments involved, in this case, two). The additional segments are L4 and L5. Modifier -50 is not reported because the description in the CPT for these codes states unilateral or bilateral. Code 63048 is an add-on code; therefore, modifier -51 is not required.

The diagnosis is stated as spinal stenosis, reported with 724.02, and grade 1 spondylolisthesis of L4-5 level, reported with 738.4.

Practice Exercise 3-46
Professional Service: 70450-26 (CT Scan, without Contrast, Head)
ICD-9-CM: 780.97 (Alteration, mental status)

Rationale: This is stated as a noncontrast CT scan of the head (70450). Modifier -26 is appended to indicate the physician portion only. Code 780.97 indicates an altered mental status.

Practice Exercise 3-47
Professional Service: 76705-26 (Ultrasound, Abdomen)
ICD-9-CM: 277.4 (Findings [abnormal], bilirubin)

Rationale: This is an ultrasound of the gallbladder, which is an organ located in the right upper abdomen. The physician states that it is a limited ultrasound. Code 76705 specifies that this code is for a single organ ultrasound with modifier -26 to indicate the professional component only. You would not use code 76700 because this code describes a complete ultrasound.
The indication for the ultrasound was elevation of the patient's bilirubin (277.4).

Practice Exercise 3-48
Professional Service: 78452-26 (Stress Tests, Myocardial Perfusion Imaging)
ICD-9-CM: 786.50 (Pain, chest), **410.01** (Arteriosclerosis, coronary [artery], due to, graft, native artery), **V43.3** (Status, organ replacement, by artificial or mechanical device or prosthesis of, heart, valve)

Rationale: This report is the professional radiologic component of a Cardiolite stress test reported by the radiologist. Modifier -26 would be added to the codes indicating the radiologist's portion of the procedure. Code 78452 reports the SPECT imaging portion of the stress test with multiple studies. Although the stress study and at rest study were performed on separate days, 78452 is reported only once. Note that the code range 78451-78454 contains imaging codes that require careful reading to ensure the correct code has been assigned.

The reason for the encounter was chest pain (786.50). The report indicates that the patient has arteriosclerotic coronary artery disease (410.01) and that he has had an aortic and mitral valve replacement (V43.3). These diagnoses are reported as they may be related to the cause of the chest pain.

Practice Exercise 3-49
Professional Service: 76506-26 (Echoencephalography)
ICD-9-CM: 765.17 (Preterm infant NEC), **765.20** (Newborn, gestation, unspecified completed weeks)

Rationale: The service was an ultrasound of the head (76506) to examine the brain. The radiology technologist performs the ultrasound to detect intracranial abnormalities, determine ventricular size, and define cerebral contents. The examination (76506) includes all the various imaging methods performed, such as B-scan, A-scan, and real-time. Modifier -26 indicates the professional component.

The diagnosis is preterm newborn with body weight between 1750 and 1999 grams (765.17). Patient indicated to be preterm; however, gestational weeks not specified, code 765.20 is correctly reported.

Practice Exercise 3-50
Professional Service: 74455-26 (Urethrocystography)
ICD-9-CM: 753.29 (Hydronephrosis, congenital)

Rationale: Voiding cystourethrogram (74455) is a radiologic examination of the urethra and bladder to evaluate the voiding function. Modifier -26 indicates the professional component.

The clinical symptoms and diagnosis for this examination indicate congenital hydronephrosis (753.29).

Practice Exercise 3-51

Professional Service: 88304 (Pathology, Surgical, Gross and Micro Exam, Level III)
ICD-9-CM: 722.10 (Displacement, intervertebral disc, lumbar)

Rationale: Intervertebral disc is listed in the 88304 code description. This includes any intervertebral disc, whether lumbar, thoracic, sacral, or cervical. When reporting this code for payment of service, a word of caution is that 88304 does not mean level 4 pathology; it means level 3 pathology. There is no CPT code 88303. The pathologic findings are fragments of fibrocartilage, consistent with herniated disc L3-4.

When referencing the Index in the ICD-9-CM under the term "Hernia disc," the coder is directed to "*see* Displacement intervertebral disc." Reference "Displacement" in the Index with the subterm "*intervertebral disc, lumbar,*" directs the coder to 722.10.

Practice Exercise 3-52

Professional Service: 88307 (Pathology, Surgical, Gross and Micro Exam, Level V)
ICD-9-CM: 617.0 (Adenomyosis), **620.0** (Cyst, follicular), **218.1** (Leiomyoma, uterus, intramural)

Rationale: The specimen taken in this case was the uterus, fallopian tubes, and ovaries. Code 88305 would initially seem to be the right code because it reports the uterus, fallopian tubes and ovaries, which is the case here. However, under uterus in the description for 88305, it states "for prolapse," which was not stated in this case. Code 88307 states uterus, with or without tubes and ovaries, other than neoplastic/prolapse, which is correct.

This patient had a total hysterectomy due to menorrhagia. The pathology report indicates more definitive diagnoses of adenomyosis (617.0) and follicular cyst (620.0), so the menorrhagia would not be reported. The proliferating endometrium is included in 617.0 and not reported separately. Also reported are multiple intramural leiomyomata (218.1).

Practice Exercise 3-53

Professional Service: 88307 (Pathology, Surgical, Gross and Micro Exam, Level V)
ICD-9-CM: 658.41 (Placentitis, complicating pregnancy)

Rationale: This is a pathologic examination of a third-trimester placenta. The description for 88307 states "placenta, third trimester." Third trimester is the last 3 months of a woman's pregnancy. This woman is 31 weeks pregnant. You would not report 88305 because the code description states "placenta, other than third trimester." There was one specimen as the umbilical cord is attached to the placenta. There is only one report describing the placenta and the umbilical cord; therefore, only one unit is reported for 88307.

The findings of the pathologic examination indicate mild, early placentitis, reported with code 658.41. The fifth digit "1" indicates the fetus is delivered, with no mention of the antepartum condition.

Practice Exercise 3-54

Professional Service: 88304 (Pathology, Surgical, Gross and Micro Exam, Level III)
ICD-9-CM: 723.0 (Stenosis, spinal, cervical)

Rationale: Listed under the code description for 88304 is intervertebral disc.

Code 723.0 reports stenosis of the cervical spine.

Practice Exercise 3-55
Professional Service: 88304 (Pathology, Surgical, Gross and Micro Exam, Level III)
ICD-9-CM: 431 (Hematoma, brain, nontraumatic)

Rationale: Listed in the code description for 88304 is hematoma; this is the only code that lists hematoma. Nowhere in the description of the code does it state cerebral hematoma. Even though this hematoma was located in the patient's brain, you would still report 88304 because the specimen was the hematoma, not brain tissue.

In the ICD-9-CM Index, reference the main term "Hematoma" with subterm "cerebral," which directs the coder to "*see* Hematoma, brain." Reporting 853.0 would be incorrect, as it refers to a traumatic injury. Instead, you index "Hematoma, brain, nontraumatic," reported with 431. The Tabular supports selection of 431, Intracerebral hemorrhage.

Practice Exercise 3-56
Professional Service: 93458-26 (Catheterization, Cardiac, Left Heart, with Ventriculography)
ICD-9-CM: 411.1 (Angina, unstable), **414.01** (Arteriosclerosis, coronary [artery], due to, graft, native artery)

Rationale: This patient is having a left heart catheterization (LHC) and coronary artery angiography. The placement of the catheter into the left side of the heart and the injection of contrast and the selective catheterization of the coronary arteries followed by the injection of contrast is reported with 93458. All components of the cardiac catheterization (placement, injection, imaging) are reported with 93458. Modifier -26 is added to indicate only the physician portion of this procedure is being reported.

Report the diagnosis of unstable angina (411.1) and coronary artery atherosclerosis (414.01).

Practice Exercise 3-57
Professional Service: 93971-26-LT (Duplex Scan, Venous Studies, Extremity)
ICD-9-CM: V72.81 (Examination, preprocedural, cardiovascular), **414.01** (Arteriosclerosis, coronary, due to, graft, native artery), **786.50** (Pain, chest)

Rationale: This patient is in need of a bypass procedure on his heart. Before this can be performed, the lower extremity veins need to be mapped to see whether they can be used as bypass grafts. You would not code 93970 because this is for a complete bilateral study and the service was a unilateral service. It states specifically in the note that only the left side was assessed, so you would use code 93971, which is for just one side. You would then add -26 to indicate that only the professional component was provided and -LT to indicate the left side.

The patient has atherosclerotic heart disease of the native coronary arteries (414.01) and chest pain (786.50). V72.81 (Examination, preoperative, cardiovascular) indicates that this is a preoperative examination to assess the veins in the lower extremities before the patient's bypass procedure.

Practice Exercise 3-58
Professional Service: 93971-26 (Duplex Scan, Venous Studies, Extremity)
ICD-9-CM: 729.5 (Pain, leg), **729.81** (Swelling, leg)

Rationale: This is an ultrasound on the veins of the leg that is performed as a diagnostic test to rule out deep vein thrombosis. The procedure in this report was performed bilaterally and is reported with 93970; however, the ultrasound was a limited study, so rather than 93970, you would report 93971 because that code description indicates a unilateral or limited study. Modifier -26 is assigned to indicate that only the professional component is being reported.

Outpatient coders do not report rule out diagnoses, rather, you report the presenting symptoms, which in this case are leg pain (729.5) and leg swelling (729.81).

Practice Exercise 3-59
Professional Service: 93970-26 (Duplex Scan, Venous Studies, Extremity), **76700-26** (Ultrasound, Abdomen)
ICD-9-CM: 729.81 (Swelling, leg), **786.09** (Breathing, labored), **789.59** (Ascites)

Rationale: Code 93970 reports the ultrasound of both legs that was performed to diagnose deep vein thrombosis (DVT). Modifier -26 is added to indicate that only the professional component of the service is being reported. An ultrasound of the abdomen was performed (76700) and modifier -26 is added to indicate the professional component of the service. The ultrasound included the liver, spleen, bile ducts, gallbladder, pancreas, kidneys, and abdominal aorta, which is a complete examination reported with 76700.

The diagnosis is 729.81 (swelling of the legs to rule out DVT) and 786.09 (difficulty breathing). The ascites was diagnosed and is reported with 789.59.

Practice Exercise 3-60
Professional Service: 90966 (Dialysis, End Stage Renal Disease)
ICD-9-CM: 585.6 (Disease, renal, end-stage), **285.21** (Anemia, in, end-stage renal disease)

Rationale: This patient is on home peritoneal dialysis and presents for a monthly checkup. Usually peritoneal dialysis is performed by the patient at his/her home. The patient is over 20 years of age. The code for the office evaluation is 90966 (Dialysis, End Stage Renal Disease). Although 90945 reports a physician evaluation of a patient one time during dialysis, this would not be the correct code to report because the patient is not receiving dialysis at the time of this visit.

The patient is receiving dialysis for end-stage renal disease (585.6). Code 285.21 is also reported for the anemia in end-stage renal disease because the physician is managing this condition.

Index

Pancreas, 163f, 164, 212, 433
  disorders, 186–187
Pancreatitis, 186–187
Panels, organ or disease oriented, 456–457
Papilledema, 259
Papule, 9, 10f
Papulosquamous disorders, 15–16
Paraesophageal hernia, 168
Paranasal sinuses, 55
Paraphimosis, 133–134
Parathyroid, 198, 212
  disorders, 223–224
Parietal bone, 30, 31f, 32f
Parietal pericardium, 76
Paring or cutting, 354
Parkinson's disease, 238–239
Passive immunization, 467
Past, family and social history (PFSH), 305–306,
    307f
Patella, 34
Patent ductus arteriosus, 93
Pathology and laboratory section, 456–466
  anatomic pathology, 459
  consultations, 457–458
  cytogenetic studies, 460
  cytopathology, 460
  drug testing, 457
  evaluation of specimens to determine disease
      pathology, 460
  evocative/suppression testing, 457
  facility indicators, 456
  hematology and coagulation, 459
  immunology, 459
  microbiology, 459
  organ or disease oriented panels, 456–457
  practice exercises, 462–466
  therapeutic drug assays, 457
  tissue typing, 459
  transfusion medicine, 459
  types of pathologic examination, 460–461
  urinalysis, 458
Pathophysiology
  cardiovascular system, 85–96
  digestive system, 171–190
  endocrine system, 219–228
  female genital system and pregnancy,
      107–121
  hemic and lymphatic system, 201–210
  integumentary system, 9–28
  male genital system, 129–140
  musculoskeletal system, 47–54
  nervous system, 237–252, 251–252
  respiratory system, 65–72
  senses, 263–270
  urinary system, 149–160

Patient-controlled analgesia (PCA), 328
Patient self-management, 477
PCA (patient-controlled anesthesia), 328
Pectoralis major, 40
Pedicle, 6
Pelvic girdle, 34, 35f
Pelvic inflammatory disease (PID), 109
Pelvis, 34, 35f
Penis, 123–124, 133–135
  male genital system subsection, 417
Penoscrotal, 125
Peptic ulcers, 175–176
Percussion, 61
Percutaneous, 44
Percutaneous fracture repair, 44, 369
Percutaneous skeletal fixation, 44
Pericardial cavity, 76
Pericardial effusion, 93
Pericardiocentesis, 81
Pericarditis, 91, 92–93
Pericardium, 76, 81
  cardiovascular in surgery section, 386–387
Perinatal period, 509
Perineum, 98, 103
  female genital system subsection, 418
Periosteum, 29
Peripheral arterial disease, 89
  rehabilitation, 395
Peripheral nerves, 233
Peripheral nervous system (PNS), 231
Peritoneal dialysis, 470
Peritoneum, 164–165, 164f
Peritonitis, 178–179
Pernicious anemia, 201–202
Peroneus group, 40
Perpendicular plate, 32f
Pertussis, 61
Peyronie's disease, 134
PFSH (past, family, and social history),
    305–306, 307f
Phalanges, 34, 35f, 36
Pharyngolaryngectomy, 61
Pharynx, 55, 163
Phimosis, 133–134
Phlebitis, 88
Photochemotherapy, 476
Photodynamic therapy, 476
Physical medicine and rehabilitation, 476–477
Physical status modifiers, 329
Physician status, types of, 314
PID (pelvic inflammatory disease), 109
Pilonidal cyst, 356
Pilosebaceous, 6
Pineal gland, 213, 433
  tumors, 249

Make the most of your physician coding exam review!

1. Assess!
Take the Pre-Exam

Use the Pre-Exam located on the companion Evolve site to gauge your strengths and weaknesses, develop a plan for focused study, and gain a better understanding of the testing process.

2. Study!

Use the quizzes in this book to sharpen your skills and build competency.

3. Apply!
Take the Post-Exam

After studying, apply your knowledge to the Post-Exam located on the companion Evolve site. When finished, you'll receive scores for both the Pre- and Post-Exams and a breakdown of incorrect answers to help you identify areas where you need more detailed study and review.

4. Test!
Take the Final Exam

Gauge your readiness for the actual physician coding exam with the Final Exam, located in Unit 4, and boost your test-taking confidence and ensure certification success.

2014

PHYSICIAN CODING EXAM REVIEW

THE CERTIFICATION STEP
with ICD-9-CM

Carol J. Buck
MS, CPC, CPC-H, CCS-P

ELSEVIER

http://evolve.elsevier.com

ISBN: 978-1-4557-2287-7

Perfect your understanding and prepare for certification— start your review now!